Study Guide for the

Core Curriculum for Oncology Nursing

Updated Fifth Edition

Editor, Updated 5th Edition

Suzanne M. Mahon RN DNSc AOCN® AGN-BC
Professor
Division of Hematology/Oncology
Department of Internal Medicine
Professor
Adult Nursing, School of Nursing
Saint Louis University
St. Louis, Missouri

Contributors, Updated 5th Edition

Erin Dickman, MS, RN, OCN®
Nurse Manager
The Ohio State University Wexner Medical
Center – James Cancer Hospital
Columbus, Ohio

Mallory Dye, MS, RN, OCN®
Nurse Manager, Oncology Emergency Department
The Ohio State University Wexner Medical
Center – James Cancer Hospital and Richard J.
Solove Research Institute
Columbus, Ohio

Editors, 5th Edition

June Eilers, PhD, APRN-CNS, BC
Research Associate Professor
University of Nebraska College of Nursing
Omaha, Nebraska

Martha E. Langhorne, MSN, RN, FNP, AOCN®
Nurse Practitioner
Binghamton Gastroenterology
Binghamton, New York;
Oncology Unit
United Health Services
Johnson City, New York

Regina M. Fink, RN, PhD, AOCN®, FAAN
Research Nurse Scientist
University of Colorado Hospital;
Associate Professor
University of Colorado, College of Nursing
Aurora, Colorado

ELSEVIER

ELSEVIER

3251 Riverport Lane
St. Louis, Missouri 63043

Notices

Previous editions copyrighted 2016, 2005, 1998, 1992, 1987

Executive Content Strategist: Lee Henderson
Content Development Specialist: Marybeth Thiel
Publishing Services Manager: Deepthi Unni
Project Manager: Radhika Sivalingam
Cover Designer: Gopalakrishnan Venkatraman

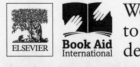
Printed in United States of America

Last digit is the print number: 9 8 7 6 5 4 3 2 1

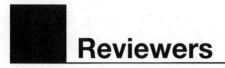

Reviewers

Karen J. Abbas, MS, RN, AOCN®
Oncology Clinical Nurse Specialist
University of Rochester Medical Center
Rochester, New York

Paula J. Anastasia, RN, MN, AOCN®
Gyn-Oncology Clinical Nurse Specialist
Cedars-Sinai Medical Center
Los Angeles, California

Ashley Leak Bryant, PhD, RN-BC, OCN®
Assistant Professor
School of Nursing
The University of North Carolina at Chapel Hill
Chapel Hill, North Carolina

Susan DeCristofaro, RN, MSN, OCN®
Professional Advancement Coordinator
Boston Medical Center;
Dana Farber Cancer Institute;
Mass College of Pharmacy School of Nursing;
Boston, Massachusetts

Seth Eisenberg, RN, ASN, OCN®, BMTCN
Professional Practice Coordinator
Infusion Services
Seattle Cancer Care Alliance
Seattle, Washington

Michele E. Gaguski, MSN, RN, AOCN®, CHPN, APN-C
Clinical Director
Medical Oncology/Infusion Services
Atlanticare Cancer Care Institute
Egg Harbor Township, New Jersey

Marcelle Kaplan, MS, RN, AOCN®, CBCN®
Advanced Practice Oncology Nurse Consultant
Merrick, New York

Valerie Kogut, MA, RD, LDN, CTTS
Nutrition Instructor
University of Pittsburgh School of Nursing
Pittsburgh, Pennsylvania

Denise Scott Korn, MSN, RN, OCN®
Education Specialist
High Point Regional Health UNC Health Care
High Point, North Carolina

Sandra A. Mitchell, PhD, CRNP, AOCN®
Research Scientist
National Cancer Institute
Bethesda, Maryland

Kimberly A. Rumsey, RN, MSN, OCN®
Professor
Lone Star College—Tomball
Tomball, Texas;
Houston Methodist Willowbrook Hospital
Houston, Texas

Carol S. Viele, RN, MS, OCN®
Clinical Nurse Specialist
Associate Clinical Professor
Department of Physiological Nursing
UCSF School of Nursing
San Francisco, California

Michele A. B. Voss, RN, BSN, OCN®
Blood Marrow and Transplant Coordinator
Saint Louis University Hospital
St. Louis, Missouri

Renee Yanke, ARNP, MN, AOCN®
Cancer Program Manager & Oncology Advanced
Practice Nurse
Whidbey General Hospital
Medical Ambulatory Care & Oncology
Coupeville, Washington

Preface

The content in this Study Guide is a companion text to the *Core Curriculum for Oncology Nursing*, Fifth Edition. Each chapter in this new edition has a corresponding chapter in that text, reflecting content updates in the practice of oncology nursing since the previous edition. Among the changes, you will notice totally new chapters with content that is critical to our work. Both texts have used the OCN® Test Blueprint established in 2013 for versions of the examination through 2017 to organize the framework and material provided.

This is the only study guide that accompanies the *Core Curriculum for Oncology Nursing,* Fifth Edition, and is created in conjunction with the Oncology Nursing Society. This user-friendly guide will serve nurses who are preparing to make that professional commitment and take the OCN® Examination.

In addition, the use of this Study Guide and corresponding text can guide the development of an educational plan to enhance the knowledge and understanding of nurses as individuals and groups providing care for people with cancer and their family members. This process addresses the recommendation in the 2013 Institute of Medicine report, *Delivering High-Quality Cancer Care: Charting a New Course for a System in Crisis,* that all individuals caring for cancer patients should have appropriate core competencies. An emphasis on QSEN competencies is designed to reduce errors in oncology nursing practice with a focus on safety and evidence-based practice. Safety-related content has been highlighted through new *Safety Alert* icons. ⚠

Contents

1 Epidemiology, Prevention, and Health Promotion

1. Which of the following statements are true about cancer mortality in the United States?
   A. Cancer is the leading cause of death.
   B. Among women, the five leading causes of cancer-related death are lung, breast, colorectal, pancreas, and ovary.
   C. One in every three deaths is caused by cancer.
   D. Among men, the five leading causes of cancer-related death are lung, prostate, colorectal, head or neck, and bladder.

2. Breast cancer lifestyle-related risk factors include which of the following?
   A. Long-term use of hormone replacement therapy
   B. Use of selective estrogen receptor modulators (↓ Breast CA)
   C. Certain fertility drugs (e.g., Pergonal) (↑ risk for ovarian ca)
   D. African American ethnicity
      (white women are more likely)

3. The five most common cancer diagnoses worldwide are
   A. lung, breast, stomach, liver, and prostate.
   B. lung, breast, colorectal, stomach, and prostate.
   C. lung, colorectal, pancreatic, breast, prostate.
   D. lung, colorectal, breast, prostate, and cervix.

4. When comparing the United States and worldwide trends in cancer incidence, which of the following is true?
   A. The cancer incidence rate in the United States decreased from 1998 to 2008; the worldwide cancer incidence increased.
   B. The cancer incidence rates in both the United States and worldwide increased.
   C. The cancer incidence rates in both the United States and worldwide decreased.
   D. The cancer incidence rate in the United States increased from 1998 to 2008; the worldwide cancer incidence decreased.

5. After taking a patient's health history, the nurse discovers that the patient, a 58-year-old postmenopausal woman, has never had a mammogram or colonoscopy; drinks at least 2 glasses of wine a day; has a history of hepatitis B infection; and follows a diet that is high in fat and low in whole grains, vegetables, and fruits. Of these risk factors, which has been specifically linked with one particular type of cancer?
   A. Lack of adherence to screening guidelines (e.g., mammography and colonoscopy)
   B. Alcohol consumption
   C. Infection with hepatitis B
   D. A diet high in fat and low in fiber, fruits, and vegetables

6. Your employer has asked the nurse to develop a survivorship program for cancer patients. After conducting an evidence-based literature review, the nurse finds some interesting facts about cancer survivorship that must be considered in program planning. Which of the following statements is true?
   A. More men than women survive cancer.
   B. Approximately one third of cancer survivors are living more than 5 years later.
   C. The most common cancer site in the survivor population is colorectal cancer.
   D. The majority of cancer survivors in the United States are elderly (65 years or older).

7. A smoking cessation program developed at the nurse's hospital is offered to employees, patients, family members, and the public. The purpose is to significantly reduce the number of cancer-related diagnoses and deaths caused by tobacco use. A focus on which of the following would potentially have the greatest impact?
   A. Using the U.S. Public Health Service 5A model (Ask, Assess, Alert, Assist, Advise)
   B. Showing the patient pictures of diseased lungs from smoking
   C. Offering relevant and culturally appropriate cessation materials and tobacco dependence medications (over-the-counter, prescription, or both)
   D. Recommending the use of battery-operated electronic cigarettes to dispel craving behaviors

8. Cancer health disparities exist in certain population groups. Which of these statements is accurate?
   A. African American women have the highest incidence rate of breast cancer.
   B. African American men have the lowest incidence and mortality rates than other ethnic groups in the United States.
   C. Hispanic women have the lowest incidence rate of cervical cancer.
   D. Asian and Pacific Islanders have the highest incidence and mortality rate for liver and stomach cancer.

9. Risk factors associated with oral cancer include
   A. cigarette smoking, consumption of processed and red meats, and history of diabetes mellitus.
   B. obesity, history of human immunodeficiency virus (HIV) infection, and exposure to asbestos.
   C. human papillomavirus (HPV) infection, tobacco use, and alcohol consumption.
   D. tobacco use, history of exposure to ultraviolet radiation, and Epstein-Barr virus.

10. Which of the following measures should be instituted to try to prevent skin cancer? ⚠
    A. Minimize indoor tanning booth use. Only use it for 1 week before going on a beach vacation.
    B. Cover exposed skin using a sunscreen lotion with sun protection factor (SPF) of 30 or higher.
    C. Avoid direct exposure to the sun between 9 AM and 1 PM, when ultraviolet rays are the most intense.
    D. Only use sun lamps, as prescribed by dermatologists, to reduce acne.

11. One of the nurse's patients is concerned that her children are properly vaccinated to prevent viral infections that may predispose them to certain cancers. What are the correct recommendations for vaccinating young children? ⚠
    A. Routine vaccination for boys and girls ages 11 to 12 years (may start at 9 years of age) with three doses of Gardasil or Cervarix to prevent HPV
    B. Hepatitis B vaccination for babies at 2 months
    C. Three doses of hepatitis B vaccine for children starting at age 3
    D. Children should receive their first hepatitis A vaccine at 3 years of age.

12. The local news station is having its yearly health fair, and the nurse is a volunteer. What are some key dietary strategies the nurse can teach the public to prevent cancer?
    A. Minimize consumption of processed and red meats; choose fish, poultry, or beans as alternatives to red meat.
    B. Eat at least 1½ cups of vegetables and fruits daily.
    C. Limit alcohol to three drinks a day for men and two drinks a day for women.
    D. Limit whole-grain products; use refined-grain foods.

13. A nurse in a public health setting is asked to perform a comprehensive cancer risk assessment on each new patient seen. The biggest benefit to the patient undergoing this assessment is to
    A. document lifestyle risk factors.
    B. record the personal or family history of cancer.
    C. choose appropriate cancer prevention strategies.
    D. verify occupational exposures.

14. Obesity is considered a major risk factor for cancer. Which of the following should be included in an educational session on obesity and its association with cancer?
    A. A person is considered obese when his or her body mass index (BMI) is 28 or greater.
    B. Obesity is responsible for 50% of all cancers in the United States, breast cancer particularly.
    C. More women are obese than men.
    D. African American men and women have higher rates of obesity than non-Hispanic white and Hispanic men and women.

15. The nurse works at a safety net hospital where there is a predominance of poor clients with a low socioeconomic status (SES); few have health insurance. Which of the following is true about the association of low SES, cancer risk, and cancer incidence?
    A. There is decreased tobacco use among poor populations.
    B. High SES is associated with an increased risk of lung and cervical cancers.
    C. More advanced disease at diagnosis is found among poor populations.
    D. Low SES is associated with an increased risk of breast and prostate cancers.

16. The American Cancer Society (ACS) has outlined specific physical activity guidelines to promote a healthy lifestyle. These include which of the following?
    A. Children should have at least 30 minutes of moderate or vigorous intensity activity each day; vigorous activities should occur on at least one day per week.
    B. Adults should have at least 150 minutes of moderate intensity activity per week or 75 minutes of vigorous intensity activity per week.
    C. Sedentary behavior (e.g., sitting, lying down, watching television) should be encouraged, especially while patients are taking chemotherapy and radiation therapy.
    D. Cancer survivors should return to normal activity as soon as possible after diagnosis, exercise at least 300 minutes per week, and participate in strength training at least 3 days per week.

17. Tobacco use is the single largest preventable cause of cancer, accounting for 30% of all cancer deaths. Which statements about smoking are true of United States populations?
    A. The highest percentage of cigarette smokers is found in the American Indian and Alaskan Native population.
    B. Cigar use is highest among Asians.
    C. Adults with college degrees are five times more likely to smoke than those in high school.
    D. A greater percentage of women smoke than men.

18. Occupational exposure increases the risk of certain cancers. Which of these statements about occupational exposure are accurate?
    A. Increased rates of gastric cancer are seen in chemical workers.
    B. Rubber workers have increased rates of prostate cancer.
    C. Miners have increased rates of bladder cancer.
    D. Steel workers have increased rates of esophageal cancer.

19. The nurse is in an influential role to determine a person's motivation to engage in cancer prevention behaviors. Which of the following questions might be most appropriate to use to gauge a person's interest in changing his or her lifestyle and decreasing cancer risk?
    A. Cancer is a serious problem, don't you think?
    B. Do you think you are at risk of developing cancer?
    C. Do you know any family or friends who had a cancer diagnosis? How did they do with treatment?
    D. Do you believe your risk of developing cancer will decrease by not smoking or engaging in other risky behavior? Why or why not?

20. The worldwide cancer rate is projected to increase by 75% in 2030 because of which of the following factors?
    A. Aging population
    B. Decreased tobacco use
    C. Increased screening
    D. Fluoridated water

2 Screening and Early Detection

1. Cancer incidence is defined as
   A. the number of new and existing cancer cases identified in a specified population during a defined period of time.
   B. the percentage of all individuals with cancer at a given point in time in a specified population.
   C. the number of new cancer cases identified in a specified population during a defined period of time.
   D. the number of cancer deaths in a population.

2. The nurse suggests to a woman at high risk for developing breast cancer that she begin annual mammography at age 30 years. This is an example of
   A. primary prevention.
   B. secondary prevention.
   C. tertiary prevention.
   D. quaternary prevention

3. Which of the following is true about a screening test's sensitivity?
   A. Sensitivity is a measure of the test's ability to correctly identify persons with the disease among the population screened.
   B. Sensitivity is a measure of the test's ability to correctly identify persons who do not have the disease among the population screened.
   C. Sensitivity is not reliant on the competency of the person interpreting the study.
   D. A screening test that has 100% sensitivity has no false positives.

4. Which screening test has the strongest evidence (randomized clinical trial) to decrease mortality in a defined population?
   A. Mammography for breast cancer
   B. Prostate-specific antigen (PSA) for prostate cancer
   C. Pap test for cervical cancer
   D. Colonoscopy for colorectal cancer

5. Which statement best describes lead-time bias?
   A. Bias that occurs in an elderly individual who has undergone screening and has been diagnosed with a slow growing cancer that may have not otherwise been detected, and treatment may not be necessary
   B. Bias that occurs when a cancer is diagnosed early before any symptom development, giving the appearance of improved survival when actually there is no decrease in mortality attributed to early diagnosis
   C. Bias that occurs when screening is more likely to pick up slower growing, less aggressive cancers that have an extended asymptomatic period and can exist in the body longer than fast-growing cancers before symptoms develop
   D. Bias that occurs when a cancer is diagnosed in an individual who has better access to screening than the general population

6. Which of the following lung cancer screening guidelines does the National Comprehensive Cancer Network (NCCN) recommend?
   A. Individuals with moderate risk (age older than 50 years old with 20 or more pack-year history of smoking or secondhand smoke exposure) should be screened every 5 years using chest radiography.
   B. Individuals with moderate risk should be screened with yearly sputum cytology and chest radiography, which is more beneficial than chest radiography alone in diagnosing lung cancer earlier.
   C. Individuals with low risk (age younger than 50 years or less than 20 pack-year history of smoking) should be screened every 5 years with chest radiography.
   D. Individuals between 55 and 74 years of age with at least a 30-pack-year smoking history who either continue to smoke or have quit less than 15 years ago should consider screening using low-dose computed tomography.

7. Which of the following is true about genetic testing for *BRCA1* and *BRCA2* mutations?
   A. These mutations are responsible for approximately 50% of hereditary breast cancers.
   B. This testing is recommended for the general population.
   C. These mutations are responsible for approximately 5% to 10% of all breast cancers in women.
   D. These mutations are responsible for 50% of breast cancer in men.

8. *BRCA1* and *BRCA2* mutation testing should be offered to family members of persons with features indicating an increased likelihood of a *BRCA* mutation. Which individuals should be considered for testing?
   A. A woman with multiple cases of early breast cancer in her family
   B. An individual with a strong family history of lung cancer
   C. An individual with Eastern European heritage
   D. A man diagnosed with testicular cancer

9. According to the American Cancer Society, which of the following are breast cancer screening recommendations using mammography?
   A. High-risk women (those with a greater than 15% to 20% lifetime risk or family history) should begin annual mammography at age 30 years.
   B. Patients with lobular cancer in situ should begin mammography at age 40 years.
   C. All women age 50 years and older should have an annual mammogram.
   D. Men with a genetic predisposition to breast cancer should receive an annual mammogram starting at age 25 years.

10. What statement is true about guaiac-based fecal occult blood test (gFOBT) for colorectal (CRC) screening?
    A. Two consecutive stool samples are optimal.
    B. It is procured by rectal examination.
    C. The gFOBT is not affected by diet, any medications, or both.
    D. The gFOBT is the only proven CRC screening method that is consistently effective in RCTs.

11. According to the NCCN, how often is a screening colonoscopy recommended for colorectal cancer prevention in individuals 50 years of age and older?
    A. Every 3 years
    B. Every 5 years
    C. Every 7 years
    D. Every 10 years

12. Which is true about CT colonography (also known as virtual colonoscopy)?
    A. This CT does not require a bowel preparation.
    B. This test is not a good alternative for elderly or frail patients.
    C. If a lesion is detected, further testing is required.
    D. This CT may be used as a solitary screening tool.

13. Which of the following factors may affect the sensitivity and specificity of PSA levels?
    A. Nonsteroidal antiinflammatory drugs (NSAIDs)
    B. Inflammation
    C. Recent ejaculation (within 72 hours)
    D. Ethnicity

14. A 64-year-old African American patient was recently diagnosed with prostate cancer. He asks if his 45-year-old son should be screened for prostate cancer. What should the nurse tell him?
    A. "Your son should receive a digital rectal examination and PSA at age 50 years."
    B. Your son is at an increased risk of developing prostate cancer because he is African American and has a family history, but there are potential risks versus benefits associated with screening. It's a personal preference."
    C. "I think you should ask your doctor what the screening guidelines are. They are very confusing and controversial."
    D. "Your son has a few risk factors for developing prostate cancer. He is African American, he has a family history of prostate cancer, and you were diagnosed before age 65 years. He should receive a PSA and digital rectal examination now. The frequency of continued testing will depend on his PSA level. I would have him consult with his physician to gather more information."

15. Which of the following screening tests for cervical cancer is recommended in women between the ages of 30 and 65 years?
    A. Pap test yearly for 3 years. If the result is normal, then Pap tests should be done every 10 years.
    B. Pap test every 5 years with human papillomavirus (HPV) testing or Pap test every 3 years without HPV testing
    C. Pap test every 3 years with HPV testing
    D. Pap test yearly with HPV testing

16. The American Cancer Society, the National Comprehensive Cancer Network (NCCN), and the American College of Obstetrics and Gynecologists support the discontinuation of cervical cancer screening in which situation?
    A. Postmenopausal women who had three consecutive normal Pap test results and no abnormal Pap test results within the past 10 years
    B. Women older than age 65 years who have undergone regular cervical cancer testing with normal results
    C. Women who have had a hysterectomy to remove cervical cancer or precancerous lesion
    D. Women who are not sexually active

17. Mr. S is an 83-year-old retired chemist who went to his primary care doctor for an annual examination. He had a slightly elevated PSA and positive digital rectal examination, and upon ultrasound-guided prostatic biopsy, he was diagnosed with an early stage prostate cancer. This is an example of
    A. lead-time bias.
    B. length-time bias.
    C. selection bias.
    D. overdiagnosis.

5

18. The ideal screening examination for cancer will have the following characteristics? ⚠
    A. The screening should be annual.
    B. Patients should be informed that the risks associated with screening may outweigh the benefits.
    C. It will be cost effective.
    D. It will occur within the hospital setting.

19. Which of the following is the only biomarker used for cancer screening?
    A. PSA
    B. CA 19-9
    C. CA-125
    D. HPV

20. Which of the following is true about breast cancer screening recommendations?
    A. Mammography remains the primary screening modality.
    B. Breast ultrasonography should be used regularly in conjunction with mammography in moderate-risk populations.
    C. Breast self-examination is routinely endorsed and recognized as a reliable screening tool.
    D. Preliminary results suggest that digital mammography is more effective than traditional mammography for breast cancer screening.

21. Mrs. B is 58 years old and has been diagnosed with stage III colorectal cancer (CRC). Her mother had a history of polyps, and her father was diagnosed with prostate cancer. She asks the nurse if she should undergo genetic testing. The nurse tells Mrs. B that according to the National Cancer Institute, genetic testing is recommended for individuals with one or more of the following.
    A. The general population
    B. Having a personal history of ulcerative colitis or diverticulitis
    C. Having a strong family history of CRC, polyps, or other cancers consistent with an inherited risk of CRC
    D. Age at CRC diagnosis 60 years of age or older

22. A nurse volunteers at a community health fair, providing education about cancer screening to the public. An individual asks why the general population is not screened annually for all cancer types because many cancers can be detected earlier with proper screening techniques. Which of the following rationales for cancer screening might the nurse provide?
    A. Annual pap tests are recommended because cervical cancer is a fast-growing cancer.
    B. The costs associated with routine lung cancer screenings (radiographs, CT scans, or both) are very high. False positives have occurred, which result in patients enduring unnecessary tests. Screenings have achieved only a small number of prevented deaths. Therefore, annual lung cancer screening is not used.
    C. It is a well-known fact that annual colonoscopies decrease cancer-related deaths.
    D. There is strong evidence to support breast cancer screening using annual mammography in women indefinitely.

23. According to the NCCN guidelines, besides smoking history, what additional factors are associated with a high risk of developing lung cancer?
    A. Family history of chronic obstructive pulmonary disease (COPD)
    B. Personal history of leukemia or hepatoma
    C. Occupational exposure (e.g., arsenic, asbestos, coal smoke)
    D. Living in the southwest region of the United States

24. The nurse completes an assessment of a patient's history for each new patient who comes to the cancer clinic. Which of the following elements should be included?
    A. Chief complaint
    B. Physical examination
    C. Allergies
    D. Complete breast examination

25. The percentage of persons who screen positive for a particular cancer and actually have that disease is the
    A. positive predictive value.
    B. negative predictive value.
    C. specificity.
    D. sensitivity.

26. The nurse examines Ms. Y. in the clinic and identifies which of the following that may be indicative of cancer?
    A. Enlargement and darkening of a mole
    B. History of skin cancer
    C. Dry, flaky skin
    D. Increased tanning booth usage

27. Mrs. G, is 52 years old and has never had a screening baseline mammogram or colonoscopy. The nurse encourages her to schedule an appointment with her primary care physician (PCP) for a history and physical examination, but she refuses. What should the nurse do?
    A. Schedule an appointment for Mrs. G and offer to pick her up.
    B. Leave a copy of the American Cancer Society Cancer Facts and Figures and screening recommendations in her mailbox.
    C. Assess barriers to participation in screening programs (e.g., transportation, child care, and costs) and work with her to overcome them.
    D. Call Mrs. G's primary care office and ask them to reach out to her to schedule an appointment.

28. The nurse is writing a grant proposal to the state's Department of Health to provide cancer screening to uninsured individuals. Which of the following is a short-term variable or outcome important to measure to determine the program's success?
    A. Cost per cancer detected
    B. Stage of detected cancer
    C. Cancer site-specific mortality rate of the target population
    D. Impact of early detection on symptom management and quality of life

29. When conducting a clinical examination, which of the following findings would be considered suspicious for a brain tumor or brain metastasis?
    A. Visual disturbances, cognitive deficits, headache
    B. Decreased performance status, fatigue, malaise
    C. Loss of appetite, weight loss, mouth lesions
    D. Dyspnea, edema, cough

30. A nurse in a public health setting is asked to perform a comprehensive cancer risk assessment on each new patient seen. A key component of the client history to be obtained during the cancer-oriented screening examination is
    A. socioeconomic and insurance status.
    B. marital status.
    C. current medications.
    D. personal and family history of cancer.

31. A cancer-oriented physical examination should include which of the following?
    A. Assessment of cranial nerves
    B. Assessment of physical activity
    C. Hearing assessment
    D. Visual examination

3 Carcinogenesis

1. Which of the following chronic inflammatory conditions are associated with tumor development?
   A. Bronchitis and lung cancer
   B. Hashimoto thyroiditis and acute myelogenous leukemia
   C. Lichen sclerosus and primary liver cancer
   D. Reflex sympathetic dystrophy and primary brain tumor

2. What is the process of initiating and promoting cancer through the action of biological, chemical, or physical agents?
   A. Mutagenesis
   B. Teratogenesis
   C. Carcinogenesis
   D. Immune surveillance

3. Which of the following is true about genetic changes in cells?
   A. When mutated in cancer cells, tumor suppressor genes stop cell division and proliferation.
   B. Epigenetic changes modify the activity of a gene and DNA sequencing.
   C. DNA repair genes are caretaker genes and are necessary to correct mistakes made during replication that may have been caused by carcinogens.
   D. Cancers are not associated with hypomethylation of regulatory genes.

4. What is the term used to describe an abnormal number of chromosomes?
   A. Polymorphism
   B. Pleomorphism
   C. Aneuploidy
   D. Amplification

5. Nowell's theory of clonal evolution explains how and why cancer occurs. Which of the following statements support the evidence?
   A. Clonal cells cannot be traced to a single origin.
   B. Clonal cells have mutations that can give their cell lineage a survival advantage.
   C. Clonal cells with differing characteristics cannot arise from the same tumor.
   D. Clones do not change over time.

6. Which of the following are true about the clinical usefulness of tumor antigens?
   A. Are not used as an indicator or marker of tumor presence
   B. Are not found in benign conditions
   C. Are mostly used as screening tools
   D. Monitor response to therapy

7. Cancer can arise because of the combination of which three pathophysiologic factors?
   A. Apoptosis, inflammation, and genomic instability
   B. Genomic instability, contact inhibition, and inflammation
   C. Inflammation, genomic instability, and multiple mutations in regulatory cells
   D. Apoptosis, genomic instability, and multiple mutations in regulatory cells

8. Mr. C is a 25-year-old man diagnosed with a non-seminomatous (germ cell) testicular cancer. The nurse should assess which tumor markers to monitor his response to treatment?
   A. Carcinoembryonic antigen (CEA)
   B. β-Human chorionic gonadotropin (β-HCG)
   C. Cancer antigen 19-9 (CA 19-9)
   D. Adrenocorticotropic hormone (ACTH)

9. Which viruses are associated with nasopharyngeal cancer?
   A. Epstein Barr virus (EBV)
   B. Hepatitis B virus (HBV)
   C. Hepatitis C virus (HCV)
   D. Human T-cell lymphotropic virus-1 (HTLV-1)

10. Which primary site tumors commonly metastasize to the brain?
    A. Breast
    B. Pancreatic
    C. Endometrial
    D. Multiple myeloma

11. Which of the following viruses are associated with particular cancer types?
    A. EBV and gastric cancer
    B. Adenovirus and lung cancer
    C. HTLV-1 and primary liver cancer
    D. BK virus and nonmelanoma skin cancer

12. *Ras* is an example of a
    A. mutated tumor suppressor gene.
    B. mutated oncoprotein gene.
    C. mutated DNA repair gene.
    D. chromosome translocation.

13. A 68-year-old man presents at the clinic with a diagnosis of stage IV non–small-cell lung cancer (NSCLC). In taking his history, the nurse learns that he has worked in a coal mine for 45 years and was a Marine in the Vietnam War where he was overseas for 2 years. He drinks socially on weekends and has an occasional drink with his friends after work. He smoked one-half pack of cigarettes a day for 10 years from age 15 to 25 years but has not smoked since. What is this client's most influential risk factor for lung cancer?
    A. Smoking history
    B. Alcohol consumption
    C. Occupational exposure to coal
    D. Vietnam war experience

14. A cancer arising from mesenchymal origin and connective tissue may be called a(n)
    A. adenocarcinoma.
    B. squamous cell carcinoma.
    C. mesothelioma.
    D. fibrosarcoma.

15. Which of the following tumor markers are used to monitor disease progression or recurrence in specific cancer types?
    A. Homovanillic acid/vanillylmandelic acid (HVA/VMA) and hepatoma
    B. Carcinoembryonic antigen (CEA) and pancreatic cancer
    C. Bence Jones protein in the urine and bladder cancer
    D. Carcinoma antigen 125 (CA-125) and endometrial cancer

16. A 1-cm-diameter mass is equal to how many doublings?
    A. 20 tumor doublings
    B. 30 tumor doublings
    C. 40 tumor doublings
    D. 50 tumor doublings

17. Which of the following statements is true about the tumor, node, metastasis (TNM) system for staging solid tumors?
    A. N denotes the absence or presence of regional lymph node metastasis.
    B. M denotes the absence or presence of regional lymph node metastasis.
    C. N denotes the absence of regional lymph node metastasis.
    D. N denotes the presence of regional lymph node metastasis.

18. The oncogene hypothesis explains that
    A. all cells in a tumor can be traced to a single origin. Mutations occur in the genetic material in these cells that give their lineage a disadvantage.
    B. cells of the immune system patrol the body looking to destroy cancer cells and precancerous cells.
    C. cancer can be caused by factors that don't change the DNA but change the way it is translated and expressed in proteins.
    D. all cells have genes that are involved in cell growth signaling and proliferation. Mutations of these genes can result in cancer.

19. What is NOT a characteristic of a cancer cell?
    A. Cancer cells have mutations that disable gatekeeper proteins controlling mitoses.
    B. Cancer cells contain a high level of telomerase, allowing continued cell replication and contributing to immortalization.
    C. Cancer cells regulate proliferation with growth, signaling the beginning and end of mitosis.
    D. Cancer cells induce the creation of new blood vessels to support the continued growth of tumors.

20. Which of the following is true about cell differentiation?
    A. Well-differentiated tumor cells grow and spread at a slower rate than undifferentiated tumor cells.
    B. The greater the degree of a cell's differentiation, the less likely it will have some part of the functional capabilities of its normal counterpart.
    C. Tumor differentiation or grade is more important than cancer stage to define a treatment plan and determine a patient's prognosis.
    D. Grade III tumors are moderately differentiated.

21. A patient with newly diagnosed ovarian cancer tells the nurse she exercises, has healthy eating habits, and does not smoke or drink. She is surprised she has been diagnosed with cancer and asks, "how long has my cancer been around and how fast did it grow?" What explanation should the nurse provide about average tumor growth using the Gompertzian growth theory?
    A. Tumor growth constantly triples over time; this is called tripling time.
    B. Tumor growth increases very quickly and exponentially at first but then slows because of the decreased availability of nutrients and growth factors.
    C. Tumor growth increases because of faulty cell-to-cell communication.
    D. Tumor growth is hastened because of hypoxia.

22. What tumor growth patterns are associated with noncancerous or precancerous changes?
    A. Metamorphism
    B. Anaplasia
    C. Metaplasia
    D. Pleomorphism

23. Which of the following is a characteristic of a normal cell?
    A. Normal cells do not experience apoptosis.
    B. Normal cells use autophagy to survive in nutrient deprived conditions.
    C. Normal cells secrete vascular endothelial growth factor (VEGF) to decrease angiogenesis.
    D. Normal cells have limited number of growth and division cycles because of senescence.

24. Which of the following statements is true about radiation exposure? ⚠
    A. Age influences the likelihood of developing cancer after ionizing radiation exposure, with elderly people being more susceptible.
    B. Ionizing radiation causes cancer by damaging DNA.
    C. Diagnostic radiographs and CT scans are not associated with radiation exposure.
    D. Breast, lung, and salivary gland tumors are the most common cancers associated with radiation exposure.

25. Which of the following statements are true about metastasis?
    A. Approximately 20% of circulating tumor cells eventually succeed in forming secondary growth factors.
    B. "Skip" metastasis occurs when cells bypass the first node and spread to more distant sites.
    C. Tumors spread through the arterial rather than the venous system.
    D. Breast and brain are the most frequent sites of metastasis.

26. A graduate nurse on the oncology unit has questions about cancer staging. The preceptor nurse explains that the tumor, node, metastasis (TNM) staging system is intended to
    A. predict the growth fraction of a tumor.
    B. be a staging system used in all cancer types.
    C. determine a plan for cancer treatment.
    D. determine the degree of differentiation of the tumor cells.

27. The oncology nurse should understand that biomarkers are
    A. not valuable in establishing a diagnosis.
    B. routinely used in all solid tumors.
    C. beneficial in directing treatment options.
    D. not useful in prognostication.

4 Immunology

1. Which of the following are natural barriers to prevent damage by environmental substances and thwart infections by pathogens?
   A. Histochemical
   B. Physical
   C. Nonmechanical
   D. Skeletal

2. Which of the following result in the rapid activation of several plasma protein symptoms, mast cell degranulation, vascular changes, and the influx of leucocytes?
   A. Human stress response
   B. Krebs citric acid cycle
   C. Hepatolenticular degeneration
   D. Inflammatory response

3. A 77-year-old patient was diagnosed with prostate cancer 14 years ago. He had a partial suprapubic prostatectomy and did not require chemotherapy or radiation. He has taken two separate hormonal therapies since that time. He recently had a change in urinary and bowel habits with increased urinary frequency, smaller caliber stools, soft to diarrhea stools, and he has noticed intermittent blood in his urine. A colonoscopy did not show any abnormalities. An advance in his prostate cancer is suspected because of the presence of
   A. tumor protective antigens.
   B. mononuclear phagocytes.
   C. tumor-associated antigens (TAAs).
   D. immature dendritic cells.

4. The regulation, production, and development of blood cells is
   A. self-regulation.
   B. hematopoiesis.
   C. homeostasis.
   D. immune surveillance.

5. A 67-year-old male patient recently tested positive for hepatitis C. He denies any IV drug use, tattoos, or piercings. He was wounded during the Vietnam War and remembers receiving several blood transfusions. He does not have a viral load for hepatitis C and does not need treatment. Which immune system modulators most likely allowed him to "clear his virus?"
   A. Mast cells
   B. Phagocytes
   C. Interferons
   D. Platelets

6. The process of hematopoiesis begins with
   A. polymorphonuclear neutrophils (PMNs).
   B. noncommitted stem cells.
   C. a pluripotent stem cell.
   D. B lymphocytes.

7. The formation of antibodies resulting from active infection is an example of
   A. acquired or specific immunity.
   B. innate immunity.
   C. passive immunity.
   D. T helper cell–modulated immunity.

8. Which of the following best describes the monocyte/macrophage? These cells
   A. are distributed throughout tissue and are capable of ingesting foreign cells or particles.
   B. produce antibodies specific to an antigen and are involved in the humoral response.
   C. release histamine and chemotactic factors.
   D. release a substance that triggers cellular lysis.

9. An immune system that is impaired or unhealthy will prevent the body from adequately responding to all of the following except
   A. allergens.
   B. antibodies.
   C. antigens.
   D. infectious microbes.
   E. tumor cells.

10. When mature, these cells migrate through lymphatic organs to adjacent lymphoid tissue to present antigen proteins.
    A. Dendritic cells
    B. Lymphoid tissue
    C. Null cells
    D. T helper cells

11. Which of the following describes an organ of the immune system rather than a barrier to bacterial invasion?
    A. Mucous membranes
    B. Lymphoid tissues
    C. Saliva
    D. Gastric secretions

12. A patient with breast cancer is taking a trip to South Africa. She has received immunization against small pox, diphtheria, and malaria. These vaccinations provide what type of immunity?
    A. Latent immunity
    B. Acquired immunity
    C. Inherited immunity
    D. Innate immunity

13. An inflammatory response would be considered an
    A. innate immune process.
    B. infectious process.
    C. flare reaction.
    D. photosensitivity reaction.

14. Primary lymphoid organs
    A. are the sites where foreign antigens encounter lymphocyte immune responses.
    B. are the main area for generating circulating blood cells in adults.
    C. allow for the maturation of lymphocytes, including antigen receptors.
    D. include bone marrow, the spleen, and Waldeyer's ring.

15. In acquired immunity, a unique antigen is phagocytized (engulfed and destroyed) by a macrophage and presented to B or T lymphocytes and T helper cells. For this to take place, what two antigen characteristics must be present?
    A. Low molecular weight and made of recurring molecules called epitopes
    B. High molecular weight and composed of tumor associated antigens
    C. Low molecular weight and contain tumor associated antigens
    D. High molecular weight and consist of recurring molecules called epitopes

16. Which of the following function as antigen-producing cells for naïve T cells?
    A. Null cells
    B. Auxiliary cells
    C. Dendritic cells
    D. NK cells

5 | Genetic Risk Factors

1. Which statement is true about chromosomes in the human body?
   - A. The human body is made up of 40 chromosomes composed of 20 pairs.
   - B. Each parent contributes half of each pair to the offspring, including a sex chromosome.
   - C. Hereditary cancers are the primary reason for a patient to try to understand genetics.
   - D. Three growth codons are associated with the growth of amino acid chains in cancer.

2. Which is the true statement about DNA?
   - A. DNA contains two types of bases, adenine (A) and thymine (T).
   - B. The base pairs are complementary on the double strand.
   - C. Messenger DNA contains the information about the order of amino acids in a protein.
   - D. There are two nucleotide chains running in the same direction, held together by hydrogen bonds.

3. Which statement is true about ribonucleic acid (RNA)?
   - A. RNA is a double chain that represents a complimentary copy of a strand of DNA.
   - B. Transcription refers to the process of making proteins from RNA.
   - C. Translation refers to the process of making RNA from DNA.
   - D. The sequences of the amino acid chains determine the function of the proteins.

4. Messenger RNA (mRNA)
   - A. is created through a process called translation.
   - B. is a template created by transcription.
   - C. contains information about the order of the proteins in amino acids.
   - D. strands with nucleotide changes frequently cause amino acid changes.

5. Messenger ribonucleic acid (mRNA) codons
   - A. are sets of four nucleotides that act as a template for protein synthesis, providing structure for genetic material.
   - B. consist of four common bases that correspond with matching bases on a tRNA anticodon attached to a specific amino acid.
   - C. may function as "stop" codons. Examples include transfer RNA (tRNA), ribosomal RNA (rRNA), and several small silencing RNAs.
   - D. are each coded for a specific amino acid in the transcription process for DNA to RNA.

6. Which statement accurately defines a gene?
   - A. A threadlike structure that contains genetic information on exons and introns
   - B. An individual unit of hereditary information that codes for a specific protein
   - C. A specific sequence of amino acids that have a predetermined function
   - D. Two nucleotide chains coiled around one another to form a double helix

7. Understanding the role of the basic mechanisms of carcinogenesis, mutations, and heredity in cancer builds on knowing that
   - A. somatic mutations are usually considered acquired in body cells after a relatively brief period of carcinogenesis.
   - B. inherited mutations play a stronger role in cancer development than genetic mutations and instability.
   - C. acquired genetic mutations are associated with exogenous and indigenous factors.
   - D. germline reproductive cells are often involved in someone who develops cancer without a predisposition to cancer.

8. Which type of mutation results in the absence of RNA transcribed from a gene copy?
   - A. Frameshift mutations
   - B. Splicing mutations
   - C. Nonsense mutations
   - D. RNA-negative mutations

9. In someone with a genetic predisposition to cancer, a mutation
   - A. was inherited in the germline, reproductive cells.
   - B. occurred sometime during the life of the individual.
   - C. resulted from a nonsense change in an amino acid signal.
   - D. occurred through polymorphisms involving DNA sequence of a gene.

10. Chromosomal abnormalities include which of the following?
    - A. Translocation, which is the loss of a segment of both copies of a chromosome
    - B. Loss of heterozygosity in which segments of one chromosome break off
    - C. Microsatellite instability segments, repetitive pieces of DNA scattered throughout the genome in noncoding regions
    - D. Polymorphisms leading to segments of one chromosome breaking off and attaching to other chromosomes

11. What is true between proto-oncogenes and tumor suppressor genes?
   A. Proto-oncogenes function as regulators of cell growth.
   B. Proto-oncogenes have a role in DNA repair.
   C. Proto-oncogenes are normal genes essential for normal cell growth.
   D. Tumor suppressor genes convert to oncogene activation and can cause uncontrolled growth.
   E. Tumor suppressor genes are a type of repair genes associated with microsatellite instability in some syndromes.

12. What is a change in a gene's DNA pattern called?
   A. Tumor suppressor gene
   B. Proto-oncogene
   C. Mismatch repair gene
   D. Mutation

13. If a parent has a hereditary cancer that is autosomal dominant inheritance, what is the percent chance of transmitting that gene mutation to a child?
   A. 75%
   B. 50%
   C. 25%
   D. 10%

14. In genetic testing for inherited cancer risk, informed consent is very important. One critical component of informed consent is
   A. confirmation of the family history for cancer.
   B. overview of the risks, benefits, and limitations of predisposition genetic testing.
   C. recommending an individualized cancer risk management plan before testing.
   D. completion of a full history and physical examination to rule out any suspicion of cancer.

15. The primary role of the nurse in predisposition genetic testing includes
   A. establishing a cancer risk management plan.
   B. determining which members of a family should be tested for a genetic alteration.
   C. facilitating informed decision making without being directive.
   D. selecting the laboratory to perform the test.

16. What role does apoptosis play in cancer?
   A. It is the activation of a program causing abnormal mutations in genes.
   B. As cells age, apoptosis is repressed and gradually lost at the cell level.
   C. In cancer, apoptosis is reactivated, triggering cell death.
   D. Malfunctions result in uncontrolled cell proliferation of malignant cells.

17. What role does telomerase play in cancer?
   A. It is reactivated in cancer, which keeps telomeres intact, facilitating cell immortalization.
   B. It plays a role in cellular aging through the telomeres, which are at the ends of the chromosomes.
   C. Malfunction in telomerase leads to uncontrolled cell proliferation of malignant or damaged cells.
   D. It determines the sensitivity of the malignant cells to the chemotherapy and radiation therapy.

18. Which statement best describes penetrance of a gene?
   A. It is the record of an individual's ancestral history, showing inheritance patterns for a given trait.
   B. It is the proportion of individuals with a given genotype that express the corresponding phenotype.
   C. It includes the characteristics (appearance and activity) of an organism that result from the interaction between that organism's genotype and the environment.
   D. It is the degree to which a single individual with a specific genotype will exhibit a specific trait.

19. Which of the following items represents one application of pharmacogenetics in clinical practice?
   A. Drugs intended to treat a genetic change or altered protein product in a tumor
   B. Introduction of a functioning gene into cells to replace missing function
   C. Introduction of a functioning gene into the egg or sperm to prevent transmission of a gene mutation
   D. Measurement of the structure, composition, and function of proteins that are made from genes

20. Key technical characteristics of predisposition genetic testing and tumor profiling include
   A. direct sequencing that detects one single specific mutation that involves a short sequence of DNA.
   B. genome-wide association studies that detect small mutations to determine association with disease.
   C. single-strand confirmation polymorphism analysis designed to offer faster and cheaper ways to obtain genetic data.
   D. microarray techniques that detect large rearrangements, deletions, and duplications.

21. Considerations for recommending a clinical laboratory for genetic testing include all of the following except
   A. Clinical Laboratory Improvement Act (CLIA)–approved laboratory.
   B. DNA Laboratory Proficiency Certification by genetic testing review association.
   C. laboratory director certified by the American Board of Medical Genetics.
   D. evidence of meeting NIH Guidelines for Research Involving Recombinant DNA Molecules.

22. The use of genetic markers for diagnosis of cancer includes
    A. cytogenetics, which uses a personalized approach to diagnose cancer and suggest the best treatment regimen for a person's cancer.
    B. cytogenetics, which focuses on the structure, function, and abnormalities of the chromosomes to diagnose both solid and hematologic malignancies.
    C. karyotyping, which focuses on techniques such as DNA microarray or serial analysis of gene expression.
    D. gene expression profiling to identify the genetic basis for differences in the metabolism of cancer cells.

23. Mutations in which gene have been correlated with an increased risk for both breast and ovarian cancer?
    A. p53
    B. PTEN
    C. *BRCA1*
    D. APC

24. Which of the following is a clinical feature of hereditary cancer?
    A. Older age of cancer onset
    B. Telomerase
    C. Multiple primary cancers in a single individual
    D. The presence of metastasis at the time of diagnosis

25. What type of mutation adds or deletes one or more bases from the normal gene sequence?
    A. Frameshift
    B. Missense
    C. Splicing
    D. Translocation

26. An individual who has known colon cancer susceptibility in his family has tested negative. His colon cancer risk
    A. cannot be established.
    B. is at least equivalent to the general population.
    C. is nil.
    D. is still elevated.

27. Mutations in *MSH2* have been associated with an increased risk for which form of cancer?
    A. Sarcoma
    B. Ovary
    C. Lung
    D. Thyroid

28. Pharmacogenomics identifies genetic differences that influence cancer treatment, including
    A. how the body absorbs, distributes, metabolizes, and excretes the drug, called pharmacodynamics.
    B. the biochemical and physiological effects of drugs on the body, referred to as pharmacokinetics.
    C. genetic variations such as the role of decision peptide driver (DPD) protein in the inactivation of active 5 FU for decreased toxicity.
    D. genetic testing to identify the extent of disease to assist with determining the cancer diagnosis.

29. Pharmacogenomic testing is required for some cancer therapies, including
    A. Irinotecan and Nilotinib for colorectal cancer.
    B. Tyrosine kinase inhibitors for gastrointestinal stromal tumors.
    C. Busulfan in chronic myelogenous leukemia (CML).
    D. Arsenic trioxide for promyelocytic leukemia (PML).

30. The son of a patient with a known *MSH2* mutation is happy to see the results of his genetic testing were negative. What is important for him to understand about his level of risk?
    A. A negative test result in the presence of a known genetic mutation indicates that the client is within the general population risk of cancer associated with that branch of the family.
    B. Because the results of the test are negative, his risk for cancer is minimal.
    C. You do not need to know the type of cancer his parent has; you can give accurate information about his risk level regardless.
    D. It is still important for him to have the surgery for removal of tissue at risk for the cancer.

31. What role does medical management play for individuals with a mutation in a cancer susceptibility gene?
    A. Surveillance is not necessary.
    B. Prophylactic surgery to remove as much of the tissue at risk as possible to reduce the risk of developing a specific cancer.
    C. Discourage the individual from having children, who might develop the inherited cancer.
    D. There is nothing that can be done to mitigate risk.

32. Nurses can advocate for individuals with known cancer risk mutations by
    A. referring them to the NCI Physician Data Query Summaries on Genetics.
    B. supporting Health Insurance Portability and Accountability Act (HIPAA) guidelines for the use of genetic information.
    C. discouraging them from sharing their information with others.
    D. encouraging them to have their test repeated in 6 months to see if the results are consistent.

6 Research Protocols and Clinical Trials

1. What information is correct regarding research protocols and clinical trials (CTs)?
   A. Quality of life and supportive care studies are observational research, not clinical trials.
   B. Consent is not always required for research in human subjects.
   C. Clinical research may be interventional or observational and epidemiologic in nature.
   D. Clinical trials usually involve treatment aimed at improving cancer outcomes.

2. The nurse is interested in assessing biomedical and health outcomes in groups of humans. An institutional review board (IRB) proposal will need to be written to conduct what type of research?
   A. A phase IV clinical trial
   B. An interventional study
   C. An observational study
   D. A behavioral intervention study

3. A colleague indicates she would like to conduct a research study, but she does not want to do all of the work of an IRB application. What should be the priority message for the nurse's response? ⚠
   A. The research must involve no risk to the subjects, or it must be submitted for IRB review and approval.
   B. The purpose of the IRB review is to protect and safeguard the rights and welfare of human subjects.
   C. If it is not an interventional study, IRB review and approval will not be required; it's okay to start data collection.
   D. With electronic medical records, it is very easy to just extract the data on the clients the nurse is already seeing.

4. What is the purpose of a Data Safety and Monitoring Board (DSMB)? ⚠
   A. To provide assistance with analyzing research data before the publication of the findings in a professional journal
   B. To assess the effectiveness of interventions in clinical trials involving medications during the post-marketing period
   C. To assist with development of a research plan to evaluate the safety of early phase drugs for human research
   D. To provide oversight and monitoring to confirm the safety of subjects and the validity and integrity of data in a research study

5. Which of the following are applicable regarding adverse events (AEs) in a clinical trial?
   A. They include any unfavorable or unintended sign, symptom, or disease temporarily linked with the intervention being evaluated that is likely related to the study.
   B. The primary investigator (PI) has the sole responsibility for adverse event identification, documentation, grading, and assignment of attrition to the intervention.
   C. The assessment of adverse events is conducted according to each individual institution
   D. Dose modifications for adverse events, described in National Cancer Institute (NCI) CTCAE terms, must be stated for each study agent in the clinical trial.

6. J.B. indicates that Dr. M discussed participation in a research study. He asks the nurse what she thinks because he thinks the physician believes it is really important. What should be the priority to communicate as the nurse working with Dr. M's clients?
   A. That as his personal physician, Dr. M would never recommend anything he thought was too risky for his clients
   B. That the most important thing is for J.B. to feel personally informed and comfortable with his decision
   C. That research is especially important so that we can continue to improve the outcomes of cancer care
   D. That Dr. M would be willing to return and re-explain anything that JB did not understand

7. Which of the following are regarded as vulnerable populations in terms of informed consent for research studies? ⚠
   A. Children
   B. Women
   C. Individuals who do not speak English
   D. Elderly individuals

8. Which of the following is true about Comparative Effectiveness Research (CER)?
   A. CER is dependent on the findings of established research, not generating information regarding the benefits and harms of interventions.
   B. CER uses typical patients to identify the most efficacious, safe, and cost-effective care for an individual.
   C. The goal of CER is to evaluate a new medication or device against one that has been previously established as effective.
   D. The purpose of CER is to evaluate two new medications or devices against each other for their effectiveness in a new population.

9. The role of the oncology nurse in clinical trials includes which of the following? ⚠
   A. Advocate for client safety through the promotion of ethical care per state standards of professional nursing practice.
   B. Promote the success of the clinical trial by identifying potential subjects and encouraging them to participate in the study to advance cancer care.
   C. It is not necessary to consult with the clinical trials nurse before administering any new medications to a client enrolled in a clinical trial.
   D. Encourage family members of potential subjects in a clinical trial to inform the client what their decision would be if it were them.

10. How would the nurse respond to a comment by family members that a phase IV clinical trial is really making a "guinea pig" out of their loved one?
   A. Encourage them to talk about the study in more detail with the study coordinator to address any concerns.
   B. Ask them about their experience with involvement in research studies in the past.
   C. Reassure them that research in cancer treatment over the past years has led to many advances.
   D. Explain that this trial involves agents that have been already tested and approved by the FDA for use in a clinical setting.

11. The U.S. Food and Drug Administration (FDA) approval for expanded access involves which of the following?
   A. Access of research medications for subjects who do not have insurance coverage for expensive agents
   B. Compassionate use of study agents in individual patients who are too ill to participate in a clinical trial, who have disease for which no effective treatment agent is available, or who have a therapeutic response at the end of a clinical trial
   C. A process for allowing a principal investigator to expand eligibility for participation in the study based on research expertise
   D. Use of a study agent in an individual who has recently experienced progression of disease on another study agent

12. Based on prior involvement with DF, who has limited cognitive ability, the nurse knows that she tends to be very agreeable even if she does not understand the details of what she is being asked. What would be the priority as a nurse regarding research studies?
   A. Sit down with her and re-explain the study to her so she can sign the consent form to participate.
   B. Determine who her legal representative is and make certain he or she is involved in the consent process.
   C. Make sure the study involves minimal risks to subjects and then support her involvement in the research.
   D. Be certain the study involves a data safety and monitoring board.

7 Breast Cancer

1. Breast milk is produced by
   A. terminal duct lobular units (TDLUs).
   B. adipose tissue.
   C. glandular tissue.
   D. sebaceous tissue.

2. Breast cancer is
   A. the second most common cancer in women worldwide and the leading cause of cancer-related deaths in women in the United States.
   B. the leading cause of cancer in women worldwide and the third leading cause of cancer-related deaths in women in the United States.
   C. experiencing an increase in incidence due to a reduction in the use of hormone replacement therapy.
   D. the second leading cause of cancer related deaths in U.S. women, with approximately 65,000 newly diagnosed cases in 2013.

3. J.S. is a 45-year-old woman who is being seen for a new diagnosis of breast cancer. Her twin sister was diagnosed with breast cancer 2 years ago. J.S. has the *BRCA1* gene mutation. Which of the following tests would be most pertinent for her to complete?
   A. Bence Jones urine
   B. Complete metabolic profile including lipase and amylase
   C. Philadelphia chromosome and a complete blood cell count
   D. Pelvic examination and CA-125

4. C.W. is a 47-year-old woman who has been diagnosed with lobular carcinoma in situ after having had a chest radiograph because of a lingering cough. The chest radiography was followed by chest computed tomography (CT), which revealed a nodule, found later to be a lesion in the breast. She will likely receive
   A. trastuzumab (Herceptin) to improve her clinical outcome.
   B. surgical excision.
   C. fine needle aspiration.
   D. adjuvant endocrine therapy.

5. J.K. is a 39-year-old man with breast cancer who is *BRCA1* positive. He is at increased risk for
   A. prostate cancer.
   B. thyroid cancer.
   C. renal cell cancer.
   D. melanoma.

6. A 39-year-old woman who has been treated for *BRCA2*-positive breast cancer is planning a vacation to Florida. The nurse is most concerned with her increased risk of
   A. malignant melanoma.
   B. ovarian cancer.
   C. fallopian tube cancer.
   D. pancreatic cancer.

7. S.F. is a 24-year-old African American woman, the mother of two children (ages 9 and 4 years). Her mother and aunt had breast cancer. She has smoked since age 14 years and is taking Synthroid for an underactive thyroid gland. The nurse should counsel her about her increased risk for breast cancer based on which factors?
   A. Hyperthyroidism, second-degree relative with breast cancer, early pregnancies
   B. Hypothyroidism, smoking, her two pregnancies, mother and aunt with breast cancer
   C. African American, first-degree relative with breast cancer, smoking at an early age
   D. First- and second-degree relative with breast cancer, early smoking history, African American, early pregnancies

8. G.C. is a 47-year-old woman survivor of Hodgkin lymphoma who presents to the hospital's breast care center. She has abnormal mammography findings and is scheduled to have a repeat mammogram in 3 months. She is in the process of moving households and will likely put it off for a full 6 months. The most appropriate response by the nurse is to tell her that
   A. her primary care provider will receive a copy of these results and can better advise her.
   B. she can attend an educational session to learn the technique of self-breast examination, which should suffice for the next year.
   C. she should keep the 3-month mammography appointment because of her increased risk for breast cancer because of radiation treatments for Hodgkin disease.
   D. she should decrease her weight by reducing her intake of saturated fats for the next 6 months and then have the mammography repeated.

9. R.M. is a 77-year-old woman who was diagnosed and treated for HER-2 positive breast cancer 2 years ago. She appears at her appointment complaining of feeling worn out, not able to do her usual light housework because her back hurts, and she appears short of breath while at rest. R.M. had received trastuzumab within the past year but has not been seen in recent months because of the death of her spouse. Considering her symptoms, the nurse should be most concerned about the possibility of ⚠
   A. axillary involvement, liver metastasis, and cardiac failure.
   B. brain metastasis, bone metastasis, and lung metastasis.
   C. axillary and supraclavicular lymph node involvement and colon metastasis.
   D. cardiac failure, lung metastasis, and spinal cord involvement.

10. Given the description of symptoms for R.M. above, the nurse would expect which of the following tests to be ordered to evaluate her present condition? ⚠
   A. Electrocardiography, complete blood count (CBC), chest radiography, abdominal ultrasonography
   B. Echocardiogram, chemistry profile (COMP), computed tomography of the chest, bone scan
   C. Computed tomography of the abdomen and pelvis, sentinel lymph node biopsy
   D. Mamma print, magnetic resonance imaging (MRI), pulmonary function test

11. Which of the following racial and ethnic groups have the highest breast cancer mortality rates?
   A. African Americans
   B. Native Americans
   C. Asian and Pacific Islanders
   D. Hispanics

12. Which of the following factors affect the prognosis and treatment of breast cancer?
   A. History of gouty arthritis
   B. Alcohol intake
   C. History of other cancer treatment
   D. Tumor histology

13. J.P. is a 54-year-old woman with a new diagnosis of early stage, node-negative, estrogen receptor positive (ER+1) invasive breast cancer. Her family history includes her mother and a maternal aunt with breast cancer and three sisters with no history of breast cancer. J.P. has had an "Oncotype" test to predict her risk of breast cancer recurrence and asked the nurse what a score of 32 indicates. The most appropriate response by the nurse is that J.P. has
   A. no risk of recurrence after her initial surgery is complete.
   B. a low risk of recurrence.
   C. an intermediate risk of recurrence.
   D. a high risk of recurrence.

14. A female patient has been diagnosed with stage III A breast cancer. Her tumor measures 45 mm, with one small axillary lymph node involved. Her anatomic stage of IIIA means she has
   A. T2, N2A, M0.
   B. T1c, N 2, M1.
   C. T3, N1, M0.
   D. T1a, N3, M1.

15. Basal-like breast cancer cells are *(Select all that apply.)*
   A. found in triple-negative breast cancer.
   B. responsive to hormonal therapy.
   C. often diagnosed in men.
   D. known to respond to Herceptin.

16. Histologic characteristics of breast cancer are often determined by the Bloom-Richardson system and are categorized as grade 1, 2, or 3. Which statement correctly reflects this histologic classification?
   A. Grade 1: low grade or poorly differentiated
   B. Grade 1: well differentiated or low grade
   C. Grade 1: high grade or poorly differentiated
   D. Grade 1: poorly differentiated or low grade

17. E.P. is a 70-year-old woman with *HER2*-positive breast cancer. She has been treated with anthracycline, a taxane, and trastuzumab, but her cancer progressed while on therapy. She was switched to capecitabine plus lapatinib 3 weeks ago. E.P. presents to the breast center with shortness of breath, mild jaundice, and reports she is ambulating more slowly than usual. The nurse should monitor her for the most frequently occurring side effects of lapatinib. Which of the following is not a side effect of lapatinib?
   A. Anemia and neutropenia
   B. Diarrhea, nausea, and vomiting
   C. Interstitial lung disease and pneumonitis
   D. Fatigue

18. K.L. is a 56-year-old woman diagnosed with breast cancer, Stage IIA. She is scheduled to have a total mastectomy with axillary staging. She may also undergo radiation and chemotherapy. In providing pre-operative instructions, the nurse finds she is crying and distressed. Her aunt had breast cancer many years ago. She remembers that her aunt lost the entire function of her arm after having a mastectomy. The most appropriate statement by the nurse is that
    A. there is no way to guarantee the outcome of the surgery, and it is possible that she could also have no use of her arm after surgery.
    B. surgical techniques have improved a great deal over the past 40 years, and the risk of losing arm function has greatly decreased.
    C. the surgeon who performed her aunt's surgery must have removed too much tissue during the procedure and the patient should consider herself fortunate that he is no longer practicing.
    D. the hospital where her surgery is being performed has a new patient relation's department, which can help her if she has any ill effects from the surgery.

19. K.L. (from the previous question) is being seen for her first postoperative visit after her mastectomy 10 days ago. Which of the following patient educational tips is most relevant in preventing lymphedema?
    A. Teaching the patient to measure the affected arm and notify her physician if the diameter increases
    B. Teaching the patient to take precautions to prevent trauma and infection in the affected arm
    C. Teaching the patient to monitor her temperature and the color and warmth of the extremity
    D. Teaching the patient to reduce her sodium intake as a preventative measure against lymphedema

20. Postoperatively after mastectomy, some patients experience altered arm and breast sensations such as numbness and tingling of the arm and a lack of chest wall sensation. These sensations may persist indefinitely after surgery and are called
    A. pain funnel.
    B. pleuritic chest pain.
    C. phantom breast sensation.
    D. postoperative neuropathic pain syndrome.

21. Breast cancers have long been divided into three categories depending on the presence or absence of hormone receptors—estrogen receptor, progesterone receptor, and HER2 receptors. Recently, five additional subgroups have been developed that carry distinct clinical outcomes and biological features. If a patient in the clinic has a "luminal A" tumor, how best would it be to describe the biological features?
    A. Gene expression profile similar to normal breast tissue epithelium
    B. Decreased expression of ER and PR, increase of VEGF, poor prognosis
    C. Tumors tend to be high grade and may benefit from targeted HER2 therapy and chemotherapy
    D. High levels of ER expression, PR-positive and HER2-negative, low grade, favorable prognosis

22. L.K. a 59-year-old woman, recently had a lumpectomy, and is meeting with the nurse for patient education prior to starting treatment with the aromatase inhibitor (Arimidex). The nurse should explain to L.K. that patients who are prescribed aromatase inhibitors
    A. are hormone receptor negative.
    B. take the drug Arimidex to reduce the risk of recurrence.
    C. may take the medication indefinitely.
    D. will experience an increase in bone density.

23. After taking the medication for approximately 3 months, L.K. (from the question above) returns for a follow-up appointment and tells the nurse that she has joint aches and back pain. The nurse would expect the physician to order a
    A. bone scan.
    B. calcium supplement.
    C. complete blood count.
    D. Bence Jones urine.

8 | Lung Cancer

1. G.W., who is retired from the local paint factory, appears at the oncology clinic. He insists he is fine, but then he admits to some recent weight loss, lethargy, occasional recent cough, and shortness of breath on exertion. His only work up thus far has been chest radiography with some suspicious findings. He states that he has not smoked in over 10 years; however, the nurse notices some tobacco stains on his fingers. She suspects he may have lung cancer because
   A. of the patient's double risk of working in a chemically toxic environment and an admitted history of smoking.
   B. after completing his history and physical examination, there is no evidence of substantial comorbidities that explain his symptoms.
   C. his major symptoms seem to be related to the respiratory tract.
   D. the patient has both respiratory and constitutional symptoms, exposure to carcinogens, and some suspicious findings on chest radiography.

2. A recent development in lung cancer diagnosis comes from the area of cellular biology and mutations. Advances in this area include targeted therapies, which attack cell growth. In describing these advances, the term *multi-hit theory* refers to
   A. the necessity of providing multiple rounds of chemotherapy, with several different agents over time to combat the lung cancer.
   B. carcinogen exposure resulting in deoxyribonucleic acid (DNA) damage and mutation.
   C. the multiple changes that occur in tumor repressor cells resulting in carcinogenesis.
   D. the downward spiral that is often seen in the care of oncology patients, which includes diagnosis, treatment, remission, retreatment, palliative care, and end-of-life care.

3. A 55-year-old single woman is seen today in her primary provider's medical practice. She has worked most of her adult life in a commercial advertising agency and has had daily exposure to paints, acrylics, spray finishes, shellac, polyurethane, and numerous other chemicals for more than 30 years. She denies a personal history of smoking but grew up in a household where her dad smoked "like a chimney." She has been troubled for several months with a persistent, nonproductive cough, and a recent constant tingling sensation in her right upper arm. The patient is awaiting results from a chest radiography. She appears tired, pale, haggard, and older than her years. On chest auscultation, crackles are heard in her lungs. The nurse suspects a lung cancer diagnosis due to
   A. pallor, fatigue, and lung crackles.
   B. appearance of being older than her stated age.
   C. family history of father's smoking.
   D. long chemical exposure, cough, and arm tingling.

4. Which of the following facts are accurate regarding lung cancer in the United States?
   A. Lung cancers account for 25% of all cancer cases diagnosed annually.
   B. Lung cancer accounted for 27% of cancer deaths projected for 2013.
   C. Overall survival rate at 5 years for localized disease is 20%.
   D. Hispanics have poorer outcomes than other ethnic groups.

5. The overall patient survival rates for lung cancer are based on stage of disease at diagnosis—localized versus regional or advanced disease. Patients with small cell lung cancer have a poorer survival rate. Positive prognostic factors include
   A. female gender, less than 5% weight loss, and good performance status.
   B. either gender, less than 10% weight loss, and early stage of disease.
   C. male gender, less than 15% weight loss, and localized or regional disease.
   D. female gender, less than 10% weight loss, and good performance status.

6. The diagnostic workup for lung cancer would include
   A. tumor markers, chest radiography, complete blood count (CBC), and complete metabolic profile (COMP).
   B. chest and abdominal computed tomography (CT) scans and α-feta protein.
   C. chest CT, positron emission tomography (PET) scan, and magnetic resonance imaging (MRI) of the brain.
   D. pulmonary function testing.

7. Lung cancer is the leading cause of cancer-related deaths worldwide. The main factor that causes this high mortality rate is
   A. that the cancer is diagnosed at advanced stages and survival rates are poor.
   B. the worldwide long-term exposure to toxins, specifically cigarette smoking.
   C. decreased access to diagnostic services in underdeveloped countries.
   D. a lack of information on specific process by which cigarette smoking causes cancer.

8. Which of the following tools can aid in determining lung cancer as a primary site?
   A. PET scan
   B. Thyroid transcription factor-1 (TTF-1) and cytokeratin (CK) stains
   C. Sputum for cytology
   D. Full-body bone scan

9. The nurse has attended a lunch and learn in-service provided by one of the hospital pathologists. He explained small cell lung cancer (SCLC) from the pathology standpoint using a case study model. The nurse is caring for J.W., a 66-year-old man who has been diagnosed with limited stage SCLC. The nurse is aware that the patient's disease is
   A. located in more than one lung and in one distant organ.
   B. located in more than one lung and lymph nodes on the same side of the mediastinum.
   C. scattered throughout the lungs and in the mediastinal lymph nodes.
   D. limited to one site in one lobe on the right side and one lobe on the left side.

10. Smoking is the greatest risk factor for developing lung cancer, followed by exposure to secondhand smoke in nonsmokers. The risk increases cumulatively over the years. The smoking pack-year history is used to quantify tobacco exposure. The formula for determining one's smoking pack history is
    A. number of cigarettes smoked in a day multiplied by the number of days per month the patient has smoked, multiplied by total years smoking.
    B. number of packs of cigarettes smoked in a day multiplied by the number of years the person has smoked.
    C. number of packs of cigarettes smoked in a week multiplied by the number of months smoking in the current year and then divided by the patient's age.
    D. number of total cigarettes the patient smokes in a month divided by the total years the patient has smoked.

11. If an individual is a candidate, surgery is the treatment of choice for lung cancer because
    A. lung cancer is often a localized disease.
    B. chemotherapy is ineffective for lung cancer.
    C. surgery offers the best potential for cure.
    D. surgery has few complications and few side effects.

12. J.J. is a 59-year-old man who worked in the coal mines for more than 25 years. He was a smoker but quit about 2½ years ago because the cigarettes just got "too pricey." He asks the nurse about his quitting smoking and his own risk for getting lung cancer. It is impossible to determine his exact risk for lung cancer related to his occupational exposure. Regarding his smoking, the nurse tells him that
    A. quitting smoking shows an immediate reduction in the risk of lung cancer regardless of the length of time or the amount one has smoked.
    B. at the 10-year mark after quitting smoking, an individual's risk for lung cancer is the same as someone who has never smoked.
    C. the cessation of symptoms related to smoking, such as cough and production of sputum, are not usually noticeable until for an interval of 6 to 9 months after the person has stopped smoking.
    D. 5 or more years must elapse before an appreciable decrease in risk occurs.

13. The National Cancer Institute conducted a clinical trial regarding detection of lung cancer using low-dose CT scans, called the National Lung Screening Trial (NLST). It showed that screening with low-dose CT scans could detect many tumors in the early stages and could possibly lead to a reduction in lung cancer mortality rates. From this data, the American Lung Association recommends screening for current or former smokers. Which is the correct guideline for these screenings?
    A. Former smokers who have not smoked within the past 3 years should have chest radiography every 2 years and low-dose chest CT on alternate years for at least 5 years after smoking cessation.
    B. Current smokers ages 55 to 74 years should have chest CT every 2 years.
    C. Current or former smokers (>30 pack or <15 years since quitting) who are apparently healthy and between the ages of 55 and 74 years should have an annual screening with low-dose CT.
    D. Former smokers, regardless of the time since quitting, should have annual chest radiography and sputum for cytology screenings.

14. A.C. is 72 years old with an extensive history of heart disease. He has smoked a pipe for more than 30 years but quit when he turned 65 years. He also worked as a foreman at the fertilizer plant for almost 50 years. He and his son were pruning some trees in his yard when he got "bumped in the chest." A biopsy revealed stage II non–small cell lung cancer (NSCLC). He will start radiation treatments next week. He explains to the nurse that he is healthy and feels well. He states it is a small spot in the center of his chest. He does not understand why he needs anything done because he has no symptoms. Radiation treatments are indicated for him because of which factors?
    A. Comorbidities and stage of disease
    B. Location, stage of disease, and size of tumor
    C. Stage of disease, age, and performance status
    D. Possible bruising from accident with tree limb, performance status, and stage of disease

15. Limited stage disease in SCLC means the disease is located in
    A. in one lung, and the mediastinal and supraclavicular lymph nodes on the same side.
    B. two of the three lobes of the lung.
    C. above the diaphragm with no distant metastasis.
    D. one lung and lymph nodes on the same side of the mediastinum.

16. A common metastatic site for SCLC patients is the brain. What type of radiation therapy would most likely be ordered to reduce that risk?
    A. Stereotactic ablative radiation therapy (SRT)
    B. Radiofrequency ablation radiation therapy
    C. Prophylactic cranial irradiation (PCI)
    D. Radioactive seed implant therapy (brachy therapy)

17. H.W. presented to the emergency department (ED) with shortness of breath and was diagnosed with a pleural effusion. She was admitted, and after an intensive workup, she now has a diagnosis of NSCLC. She is coming to the outpatient chemotherapy clinic for her first visit and is going to receive combination chemotherapy with cisplatin and docetaxel, which is often referred to as a doublet. What side effects are most likely to occur with cisplatin?
    A. Neurotoxicity, nausea, and vomiting
    B. Nausea and vomiting, neurotoxicity, and immunosuppression
    C. Immunosuppression, neurotoxicity, and thrombocytopenia
    D. Thrombocytopenia and pruritus

18. A patient asks the nurse what targeted therapy means. The nurse explains that
    A. targeted therapy consists of biologic agents designed to target pathways or mutations that allow lung cancer cells to grow.
    B. targeted therapy means that her chemotherapy drugs are given on a very strict schedule, designed to target the cancer cells.
    C. targeted therapy refers to the administration of additional drugs aimed at targeting distant metastases.
    D. the term *targeted therapy* was coined because of the potential for target-like bruises as a side effect.

19. A patient with a new diagnosis of advanced lung cancer who is ALK positive will likely receive which of the following agents? ⚠
    A. Bevacizumab
    B. Crizotinib
    C. Erlotinib
    D. Gefitinib

20. B.C., a 72-year-old woman, was diagnosed with NSCLC and started chemotherapy about 8 weeks ago. She had a PET scan last week and was told that her disease is not responding well to the chemotherapy. The doctor says he would like to switch her to another medicine. She asks how long she will need to receive the new medicine. She wants this to be done so she can go to Florida with her family. The nurse responds by
    A. telling her, for the time being, we have to look at short-term goals, and the emphasis right now should be on attending to her treatments, nothing else.
    B. asking to sit down to talk with her and her family about her disease.
    C. saying that Florida is absolutely out of the question and it is likely she will not be going there again.
    D. explaining that even though she may feel well now, this is not likely to last. Her cancer is advancing, and she has hard times in store ahead.

21. C.G. is a 78-year-old woman who has small cell lung cancer. She has a history of peripheral vascular disease, diabetes, obesity, and a heart arrhythmia. The nurse is working in tandem with the oncologist as the patient comes into the clinic to review all of the results of her tests. The oncologist begins to sort through her laboratory test results and starts to talk about treatment options. The patient raises her hand and explains that she does not want any treatment at all. The oncologist says that is definitely her decision, but he requests that the patient spend some more time with the nurse before she leaves. The nurse then responds by
    A. encouraging the patient to reconsider treatment.
    B. acknowledging her decision and asking the social worker to join her.
    C. asking that she consider a clinical trial so others may benefit.
    D. contacting the psychiatric intervention team to assess her mental status.

22. According to the American Cancer Society (2013), what is the average 5-year survival rate for lung cancer?
    A. 5%
    B. 16%
    C. 22%
    D. 27%

23. The histopathologic diagnosis of small cell lung cancer (SCLC) as distinct from non–small cell lung cancer (NSCLC) is important because
    A. only patients with SCLC are at risk for metabolic emergencies.
    B. patients with SCLC are not at risk for metabolic emergencies.
    C. patients with SCLC tend to have a more aggressive disease course than patients with NSCLC.
    D. patients with SCLC tend to have a less aggressive course than patients with NSCLC.

24. A clinical trial should always be considered as a treatment option for an individual with lung cancer because
    A. clinical trials are available for all individuals.
    B. phase I clinical trials have a goal to cure.
    C. standard treatment options are not available.
    D. current treatment options have a low cure rate.

9 | Cancers of the Gastrointestinal Tract

1. *H. pylori* infection is a risk factor for which gastrointestinal cancer?
   A. Pancreatic
   B. Liver
   C. Colorectal
   D. Gastric

2. L.P. is a 70-year-old retired plumber and a former alcoholic who has been diagnosed with gastric cancer. He is scheduled to have subtotal gastrectomy. He says he has been told that this Oxaliplatin medication is supposed to make things easier for his surgery, but he does not understand why. The nurse reviews the chart and explains that Oxaliplatin is
   A. being used to prevent nausea before and after his surgery.
   B. used to eradicate any possible *H. pylori* organisms in his stomach.
   C. being used to treat and reduce the tumor size of his gastric cancer before surgery.
   D. used to control gastric acid secretions and thereby reduce pain.

3. The most common type of gastric cancer is
   A. adenocarcinoma.
   B. gastrointestinal stromal tumors (GISTs).
   C. neuroendocrine tumors (NETS).
   D. lymphoma.

4. L.P. tells the nurse he was really shocked by his diagnosis of gastric cancer because he felt so well. The nurse replies that is not unusual because
   A. people who have cancer for the first time are usually in denial that a problem exists.
   B. gastric cancer usually exhibits nonspecific symptoms that lead to a late diagnosis.
   C. he would have less of a tendency to have gastric pain or discomfort because of his history of alcohol abuse.
   D. his exposure to solvents and chemicals in the plumbing industry has decreased the gastric nerve receptor and any symptoms.

5. Hepatocellular cancer in the United States is projected to number 33,190 new cases and 23,000 deaths in 2014. It is the third leading cause of cancer-related deaths worldwide with over 500,000 cases. The main factor causing an increase in the incidence of hepatocellular cancer is an increase in
   A. tobacco use in underdeveloped countries.
   B. use of "statin" drugs for cholesterol.
   C. incidence of hepatitis C.
   D. exposure to chemical carcinogens such as nitrates, hydrocarbons, pesticides, and solvents.

6. G.J. is 67 years old and has had cirrhosis for more than 3 years. He has recently been diagnosed with hepatocellular carcinoma. He is coming to the outpatient GI facility for a core needle biopsy of the liver. His magnetic resonance imaging (MRI) report shows multiple tumors, with at least one larger than 5 cm. The nurse is aware that this means he
   A. is at stage T0.
   B. has no need of the core needle biopsy of the liver.
   C. is at stage T3a.
   D. should have α-fetoprotein drawn every 6 weeks.

7. I.G., an 81-year-old woman, presents in the emergency room with lightheadedness and is found to be anemic. After detection of heme-positive stools, she was diagnosed with rectal cancer. She cares for her disabled husband, has been very active, and is concerned about "wearing a bag." She asks the nurse what is meant by a colon resection. The nurse replies that the patient will
   A. definitely not have a colostomy.
   B. have a low anterior resection.
   C. have a right-sided hemicolectomy.
   D. have an extended right hemicolectomy.

8. P.R. is 55 years old and had colon cancer with previous surgery and radiation approximately 3 years ago. He is having a bowel movement daily but in smaller amounts and with misshapen stool. He has some blood mixed in with his stools and a change in the amount of stool he passes. According to these symptoms, the nurse suspects he has a recurrence of his cancer in the
   A. transverse colon.
   B. descending colon.
   C. rectum.
   D. ascending colon.

9. The nurse educator is preparing slides to teaching a nursing class regarding screening and detection for colon cancer. As a tool, the nurse compares the recommendations between the American Cancer Society (ACS) and the National Comprehensive Cancer Network (NCCN) and sees that
   A. the ACS recommends a colonoscopy every 10 years and a flexible sigmoidoscope every 3 years.
   B. the NCCN recommends a double-contrast barium enema every 10 years and a colonoscopy every 5 years.
   C. the ACS recommends a fecal occult blood test (FOBT) every 3 years and a double-contrast barium enema every 3 years.
   D. the NCCN recommends a colonoscopy every 10 years and a flexible sigmoidoscope every 5 years.

10. Persons working in the dry cleaning industry have an occupational risk factor for which type of gastrointestinal malignancy?
    A. Colon cancer
    B. Gastric cancer
    C. Esophageal cancer
    D. Pancreatic cancer

11. The nurse works in the GI outpatient laboratory and assisted the gastroenterologist who was doing an upper endoscopy on a 25-year-old patient with achalasia. His history form states that he is also a smoker. The nurse is aware that he is at increased risk for
    A. pancreatic cancer.
    B. gastric cancer.
    C. esophageal cancer.
    D. liver cancer.

12. A 78-year-old woman who is a long-time smoker is going to have an upper endoscopy because of swallowing difficulties, indigestion, and loss of appetite. Her symptoms have gradually worsened over the past 6 to 8 months. Her daughter reveals to the nurse that she has not kept up with her usual activities and her diet currently consists of soups, milkshakes and smoothies. The patient has recently lost 11 lbs. Upon review of her intake history form, the nurse sees that the patient had a previous partial gastrectomy for a gastric ulcer, and she receives shots every month for vitamin B_{12} anemia. The patient has several risk factors for gastric cancer which include
    A. previous gastric surgery, pernicious anemia, and history of gastric ulcers.
    B. inadequate intake of fruits and vegetables, age older than 50 years, and physical inactivity.
    C. history of previous gastric polyps, smoking, and alcohol.
    D. gastroesophageal reflux disease and smoking.

13. Gastric cancer has the potential to spread via
    A. direct extension to adjacent organs such as the liver or pancreas.
    B. direct penetration into the perineum.
    C. hematologic spread to the liver and the lung.
    D. distant metastasis through lymphatics and bloodstream.
    E. All of the above.

14. A patient with gastric cancer has now been found to have metastatic disease in the lymph nodes of her peritoneal cavity. She will have chemotherapy and biotherapy to reduce the risk of further metastatic spread and to offer palliative symptom management. Possible treatment combinations include
    A. Herceptin and docetaxel.
    B. interleukin and epirubicin.
    C. Rituxan and etoposide.
    D. leucovoran and 5 FU.

15. M.L. is a 57-year-old woman with a history of pancreatic cancer. She had a Whipple procedure about 2 years ago. She is seen in the clinic after having returned from India 10 days ago. She is concerned that the foods she ate abroad affected her—she has lost 11 lbs over the past month, has pains in her upper epigastric area, and appears jaundiced. The nurse believes her symptoms are caused by
    A. a recurrence in the pancreas.
    B. food poisoning, which has impacted the liver.
    C. a recurrence of her cancer with metastatic disease in the liver.
    D. a reaction to her statin medications which she has taken for years.

16. Risk factors for colorectal cancer include
    A. chemical exposure to agricultural products, a high-protein diet, and a history of IV drug use.
    B. high content of fruits and vegetables in diet, previous gastric bypass surgery, and a previous history of vitamin B_{12} deficiency anemia.
    C. smoking, use of statin drug for hyperlipidemia, and a personal history of irritable bowel syndrome.
    D. high-fat, red meat diets; physical inactivity; alcohol use; and smoking.

17. H.C. is 78 years old, has alcoholism, and has smoked his entire adult life. He has a history of GERD. He has been diagnosed with esophageal cancer and likely has
    A. adenocarcinoma of the upper two thirds of the esophagus.
    B. squamous cell carcinoma of the upper two thirds of the esophagus.
    C. squamous cell carcinoma of the lower third of the esophagus.
    D. adenocarcinoma carcinoma of the lower third of the esophagus.

18. G.H. has hepatocellular (liver) cancer that is very advanced. He is not a candidate for surgery, liver transplant, or any type of ablation therapy. The nurse has collaborated with his oncologist and wants to discuss the possibility of palliative and hospice care. His wife wants to know why he cannot have chemotherapy like his cousin who had colon cancer. Why is chemotherapy not appropriate for G.H.?
    A. Chemotherapy for liver cancer could compromise his kidney function and likely place him on dialysis.
    B. Chemotherapy would be an option if G.H.'s cancer was not as advanced.
    C. Chemotherapy in liver cancer is contraindicated because it can become trapped in his abdomen in the form of ascites.
    D. Chemotherapy is not effective in liver cancer; research has not demonstrated improved response rates or survival benefit.

19. In a patient with colorectal cancer who is having a colon resection, the appropriate number of lymph nodes examined to complete an adequate lymph node dissection would be ⚠
    A. controversy remains regarding the correct number of lymph nodes.
    B. six.
    C. eight.
    D. twelve.

20. In patients who have advanced colorectal cancer and have had previous chemotherapy, biotherapy may be an option. Of the agents listed, which drug is used as a single agent?
    A. Avastin (Bevacizumab)
    B. Erbitux (Cetuximab)
    C. Stivarga (Regorafenib)
    D. Vectibix (Panitumumab)

21. J.S. was diagnosed with locally advanced and nonresectable pancreatic cancer 5 months ago. He has had treatment with radiation and chemotherapy, and has lost 30 lbs since his diagnosis, mostly owing to loss of appetite. The nurse has spoken to the oncologist, who agrees that a PEG tube would be appropriate if the patient and family are agreeable. The most important points the nurse needs to teach the patient and his wife are those regarding
    A. complications of constipation, such as nausea and bowel obstruction.
    B. the need for a swallowing evaluation.
    C. the care of the PEG tube and the administration of tube feeding.
    D. proper diet choices related to disease process.

22. Which tumor marker is commonly used as an indicator of tumor burden and for the monitoring of recurrence in colorectal cancer?
    A. CA 19-9
    B. CA 27-29
    C. Carcinoembryonic antigen (CEA)
    D. α-Fetoprotein (AFP)

23. Which of the following is considered a late symptom of colorectal cancer?
    A. Flatulence
    B. Change in bowel habits
    C. Blood in the stool
    D. Weight loss

10 Cancers of the Reproductive System

1. D.E. is a 70-year-old widow who was treated for cervical cancer for 5 years. Her treatment at the time was radiation and a partial hysterectomy. She has been treated for rheumatoid arthritis for at least 20 years with steroid therapy. She wants to know how many more years she will have to have a Pap smear. The best response is
   A. because she is older than the age 65 years, it is no longer necessary for her to have any additional Pap smears.
   B. because she is a widow and no longer sexually active, she does not need to continue Pap smears.
   C. her previous history of cervical cancer requires her to have Pap smears every 3 years for 20 years beyond diagnosis.
   D. because she has had cervical cancer, she should have a Pap smear and human papillomavirus (HPV) testing each year for 5 years after diagnosis.

2. M.F. is a 68-year-old female smoker who has a previous history of CIN3 cancer of the cervix. She had radiation and surgery 3 years ago. She has a new onset of edema in her left leg, difficulty ambulating, back pain, and reports she feels very bloated. The nurse believes she has
   A. signs of recurrent disease.
   B. developed ascites from metastatic disease to the liver.
   C. a new diagnosis of back pain caused by arthritis, which has impaired her walking ability.
   D. developed deep vein thrombosis.

3. What is a risk factor for cervical cancer?
   A. Tobacco use
   B. No full-term births at age 35
   C. No history of sexual intercourse
   D. Intermittent use of oral contraceptives for less than 1 year

4. Which of the following statements regarding cervical cancer is correct?
   A. Cervical cancer is a hereditary disease.
   B. Oral contraceptives are protective against cervical cancer.
   C. Cervical cancer is caused by the Epstein Barr virus.
   D. Certain HPV subtypes are known to be oncogenic.

5. Which statements regarding risk for cervical cancer are accurate?
   A. The risk of cervical cancer increases with the number of sexual partners.
   B. Screening for cervical cancer to determine premalignant changes is not recommended.
   C. Vaccination for HPV can alter the screening recommendations.
   D. Heterosexual women are less likely to follow routine screening guidelines.

6. A patient is referred for a colposcopy after having an abnormal Pap test result. Preprocedure education should include
   A. avoiding vaginal intercourse for 1 month before the colposcopy.
   B. expecting copious vaginal drainage after the colposcopy.
   C. expecting a swabbing of the cervix with acetic acid solution during the procedure.
   D. douching with Betadine solution every night for 1 week before the procedure.

7. What are the risk factors for endometrial cancer?
   A. History of an abnormal Pap smear
   B. Obesity
   C. Long-term use of oral contraceptive
   D. History of cervical cancer

8. A patient recently diagnosed with endometrial cancer says she does not understand how she can now have cancer when her Pap test result was negative 8 months ago. Which of the following is the most appropriate response?
   A. Many Pap tests are not interpreted correctly.
   B. Endometrial cancer can develop in a short time.
   C. The Pap test may have been obtained incorrectly.
   D. Pap tests do not commonly detect endometrial cancer.

9. Patients with cervical cancer who are treated with radical hysterectomy may have difficulty voiding or fail to sense the need to void after surgery because of changes in the autonomic innervations of the bladder. This can leave the patient with long-term functional complications of the lower urinary tract. A suprapubic catheter is often placed postoperatively. Educational pointers that the nurse would present to the patient and caregiver include:
   A. Initiate bladder training by clamping the catheter for 4 to 5 hours.
   B. Encourage the patient to limit her fluid intake.
   C. Catheter removal after less than 150 mL of residual urine remains after voiding as ordered
   D. Teach intermittent self- catheterization.

10. Ovarian cancer most commonly metastasizes in all of the following ways except
    A. local extension into an adjacent organ.
    B. exfoliation of the ovarian capsule.
    C. serosal seeding throughout the peritoneal cavity, including the omentum.
    D. hematologic spread.
    E. lymphatic spread.

11. All of the statements regarding reproductive cancers are true except
    A. Vulvar cancer comprises 8.5% of all cancers in women, and survival rates are 80% to 90% for stage I and II disease.
    B. Ovarian cancer is the leading cause of death from gynecologic cancers in the United States.
    C. Cervical cancer is the fourth most frequent cause of cancer-related deaths in women worldwide.
    D. Endometrial cancer is the most common gynecologic malignancy among women in the United States.
    E. Testicular cancer is the most commonly occurring cancer among men ages 15 to 35 years.

12. After surgery, patients who have undergone radical hysterectomy must be assessed for possible bowel obstruction. The side effect of severe constipation can contribute to increased postoperative pain, nausea and vomiting, and prolonged hospitalization. This is primarily caused by ⚠
    A. poor preoperative bowel cleansing before surgery.
    B. postoperative use of narcotic analgesia.
    C. manipulation of the bowel that takes place during surgery.
    D. the patient's preoperative NPO status and decreased oral intake postoperatively.

13. Which of the following tumor markers are usually elevated in 80% of patients with advanced epithelial ovarian cancer?
    A. CA-125
    B. CEA
    C. CA 19-9
    D. CA 27-29

14. P.W. was recently diagnosed with ovarian cancer. She knows she needs surgery but wonders why she is being asked to travel to a large medical center several hours away. Her daughter had an appendectomy locally, and she does not understand why she cannot see that surgeon. The nurse explains that
    A. her upcoming surgery is intricate and can best be performed by a gynecologic oncologist who has experience in optimal tumor debulking.
    B. the insurance coverage the patient currently has will allow her to attend the larger medical center.
    C. her access to possible clinical trials will only be available at the larger medical center.
    D. the surgical schedule at the hospital requires several weeks' delay in her surgery.

15. Vaginal cancer
    A. is a very common cancer in postmenopausal women.
    B. usually presents as a squamous carcinoma.
    C. is commonly a metastatic disease from cervical cancer.
    D. is not associated with diethylstilbestrol use.

16. P.G. is a 51-year-old woman who was diagnosed with ovarian cancer 4 years ago. She has had extensive surgeries and several different chemotherapy regimens. Approximately 8 months ago, she again had surgical debulking followed by intraperitoneal chemotherapy, including cisplatinum 100 mg/m^2 and docetaxel 60 mg/m^2 every 3 weeks for 6 cycles. She felt well during this time and was even able to travel. Today she appears at the clinic complaining of feeling fatigued and very bloated in her abdomen, and she appears pale. The patient feels very constipated and is eating very little. The nurse suspects the patient has
    A. developed abdominal carcinomatosis.
    B. acute cholecystitis.
    C. Crohn's disease.
    D. developed metastatic disease to her colon.

17. Intraperitoneal chemotherapy for patients who have abdominal malignancies such as ovarian cancer offers what advantages?
    A. Can eliminate the need for other chemotherapy
    B. An increased concentration of the drug to the surface of the tumor
    C. Less frequent treatments
    D. Can be done at home

18. The nurse educator is preparing a set of slides to teach baccalaureate nursing students a primer on ovarian cancer. The slide for risk factors should include
    A. history of two or three live births.
    B. personal history of breast, endometrial, or colon cancer.
    C. peak incidence is age 65 to 70 years.
    D. maternal history of elevated CA-125.

19. Gestational trophoblastic neoplasia (GTN) is a group of rare diseases that arise from the abnormal growth of cells in a woman's uterus. These cells would normally develop into the placenta during pregnancy. M.K. is a 43-year-old woman who is pregnant for the first time and has been diagnosed with a hydatidiform mole. She and her spouse are very surprised by both the fact that she is pregnant and by the diagnosis. Prior to treatment, the nurse will want to discuss and clarify
   A. the importance of the patient's staying on treatment until completion.
   B. factors regarding sexual activity treatment leading up to diagnosis.
   C. that first pregnancy is the greatest risk factor for recurrence.
   D. hydatidiform mole is a risk factor for ovarian cancer.

20. S.M. is 42 years old and has gestational trophoblastic neoplasia (GTN). She married recently and was very excited about her pregnancy. She is being seen in the clinic for her first chemotherapy treatment after having had a suction evacuation of the uterus 1 week ago. She weeps as she tells the nurse this has been devastating and that she and her husband are never going to recover. The nurse responds saying:
   A. You and your husband should plan a vacation as soon as possible, just for a change of scenery to forget about this.
   B. It is really quite surprising that you became pregnant at the age of 42 anyway; did you really think you would be able to have a baby?
   C. You should know that every pregnancy carries risk factors, especially in women older than 40 years of age; perhaps you should have been preventing pregnancy.
   D. You and your spouse need time to think and come to terms with this unexpected outcome. It will be a challenge but is one you will surely meet.

21. A.D. is a healthy 30-year-old woman who presents for a routine health maintenance exam. A screening Pap smear showed low-grade squamous epithelial lesion (cervical intraepithelial neoplasia [CIN 1]). Which of the following is most likely related to Pap smear finding?
   A. Intake of oral contraceptives
   B. History of multiple sexual partners
   C. Treated basal cell carcinoma
   D. Diethylstilbestrol (DES) exposure

22. Risk factors and incidence data for testicular cancer include which of the following?
   A. Most common cancer for men age 20 to 35 years
   B. Achondroplasia
   C. History of Lynch syndrome
   D. 75% are seminomas with rapid lymphatic spread

23. Fertility issues may be of concern to male patients diagnosed with testicular cancer. In speaking to a young married couple, the nurse realizes that they wish to have a family eventually. If the couple is interested in sperm banking, when is the best time to make a sperm bank deposit?
   A. Before initiating chemotherapy treatments
   B. During chemotherapy treatments
   C. At completion of chemotherapy treatments
   D. When tumor markers return to normal range

11 Cancers of the Urinary System

1. MRI is used as a diagnostic tool in renal cell cancer
   A. in cases with compromised renal function, contrast allergy, or suspected vena cava involvement.
   B. if a renal artery embolization is planned.
   C. if KUB results are nondiagnostic.
   D. in patients presenting with hematuria and low hemoglobin and hematocrit.

2. For many years, the standard surgical treatment for renal cell carcinoma was a radical nephrectomy. This has come under question during the past decade because
   A. 25% of patients have metastatic disease at diagnosis.
   B. cytoreductive nephrectomy is also an option for a wide range of patients.
   C. the oncologic efficacy is similar to that of partial nephrectomy for small renal tumors.
   D. the option of "active surveillance" is preferred in patients younger than the age of 60 years.

3. Young African American men with sickle cell disease are most susceptible to which type of renal cell cancer?
   A. Papillary renal cell carcinoma
   B. Clear cell carcinoma
   C. Chromophobe renal cell carcinoma
   D. Renal medullary carcinoma

4. A 66-year-old woman, active and in good health until recently, has been diagnosed with renal cell cancer. Tumor activity was identified in both of her kidneys, and she is now scheduled for a partial nephrectomy. In providing patient education, the nurse explains that
   A. cytoreductive nephrectomy is also an option for a wide range of patients.
   B. partial nephrectomy is the treatment of choice in those with bilateral renal tumors.
   C. partial nephrectomy is associated with less morbidity, increased blood loss, and longer recovery times.
   D. radiation therapy will be planned after she recovers from her partial nephrectomy.

5. Which is the preferred method for surgically managing patients with renal cell cancer?
   A. Radical nephrectomy
   B. Cryosurgery or radiofrequency ablation (RFA)
   C. Partial nephrectomy
   D. Radiosurgery

6. When teaching nursing students regarding renal cell cancer, the nurse educator emphasizes the fact that
   A. renal cell cancer is relatively rare in the United States, comprising 6% of all cancers.
   B. there is decreased incidence of RCC caused by high-resolution imaging.
   C. there is decreased incidence of RCC due to OSHA safety standards in the electrical and chemical industry.
   D. incidence and mortality have increased in the past 20 years.

7. A 77-year-old man has a new diagnosis of renal cell cancer, a small lesion on one kidney. His daughter tells the nurse that he is a new widower who lives alone. He has a cardiac arrhythmia and takes Clopidogrel (Plavix). He also uses insulin daily. The patient ambulates with a cane. His weight is 340 lb, and he is 6 feet tall. On physical assessment, there is chest congestion and ankle edema. The treatment option most beneficial for him would likely be
   A. active surveillance.
   B. radical nephrectomy.
   C. partial nephrectomy.
   D. cryosurgery or radiofrequency ablation.

8. A 70-year-old man presents at the clinic with a diagnosis of stage 1 bladder cancer. For 37 years he worked in a tannery. He consumed a "beer or two on Fridays" and drinks 2 cups of coffee per day. He quit smoking 2 years ago but has a 30 pack year history and his wife smokes 2 packs per day. He also reports using acetaminophen "about once a month" for arthritic knee pain. This client's most important risk factor for bladder cancer is
   A. occupational exposure to chemical carcinogens.
   B. smoking and exposure to secondhand smoke.
   C. coffee consumption of more than 5 cups per day.
   D. long-term use of acetaminophen.

9. Transurethral resection of bladder cancer (TURBT) is the treatment of choice for urothelial cancer of the bladder. Which of these is most likely to occur after TURBT?
   A. Bleeding and infection
   B. Urinary incontinence
   C. Urethral discharge
   D. Cloudy urine containing sediment

10. When considering the current practice trends in the management of patients with non–muscle invasive bladder cancer (NMIBC), the decision to use intravesical therapy is based on which factors?
    A. Patient comorbid conditions such as diabetes, hypertension, and renal failure
    B. The probability of recurrence and progression to muscle invasive disease
    C. The patient's age and any previous treatment for bladder cancer
    D. Recent findings of digital rectal examination (DRE) and the patient's recent PSA levels

11. A male patient has a new diagnosis of bladder cancer with muscle wall involvement. The patient is retired but leads a very active life style. He is extremely reluctant to undergo bladder surgery and does not want to "wear a bag." One surgical option for this patient may be a(n)
    A. ileal conduit.
    B. double-barrel colostomy.
    C. continent ileal reservoir.
    D. radical cystectomy.

12. J.G. had a transurethral resection of the bladder (TURBT) 18 months ago. He appears well, but his wife mentions the patient noticed a painless swollen area in his groin about 3 months ago. Because it did not hurt and he seemed to have no problems voiding, they decided not to call or come in. The nurse notifies the oncologist and
    A. calls laboratory personnel to draw stat blood cultures.
    B. suggests he contact his urologist for a repeat cystoscopy.
    C. seeks insurance authorization for a CT scan of the abdomen and pelvis
    D. sends the patient home with supplies to collect urine for cytology.

13. The U.S. Preventative Service Task Force (USPSTF), along with the American Urologic Association published new guidelines in 2013 regarding Prostate Cancer Screening. These new recommendations include which of the following?
    A. The need for PSA starting at age 40 years in men who have one or more second-degree relatives with prostate cancer
    B. Digital rectal examination (DRE) as a screening tool in all men starting at age 40 years and if there are any abnormal findings, proceed with PSA
    C. Screenings are not recommended for men younger than the age of 40 years regardless of family history.
    D. Men who have started PSA screening at the age of 40 years do not need to continue this after age 54 years.

14. A patient with a new diagnosis of prostate cancer will undergo a radical prostatectomy. The most common postoperative side effects include
    A. incontinence.
    B. myelosuppression.
    C. urethral stricture.
    D. hot flashes.

15. A 71-year-old patient recently noticed some blood in his urine. He has been told he may have bladder cancer, and he is scheduled for a cystoscopy. In his preoperative teaching, the nurse explains that the cystoscopy has been planned to
    A. determine his risk for urinary incontinence.
    B. decipher the presence, location, and size of tumor.
    C. collect specimens of any purulent urethral discharge.
    D. attempt to obtain urine containing sediment.

16. A 66-year-old man is having a physical examination after not seeing a health care provider for many years. Patient education included the importance of screenings for prostate cancer, particularly a DRE and PSA. He is concerned about the cost of having too many laboratory tests and wants to know why the DRE alone will not suffice. The nurse explains that
    A. he is correct; the DRE will be sufficient to determine whether he has prostate cancer.
    B. the DRE is only required in patients who are having painful urination, burning urination, lower abdominal pain, or back pain.
    C. there is no benefit to DRE in men older than the age of 50 years because of physiologic changes in the prostate gland.
    D. the DRE assesses symmetry, size, texture, and lesions of the prostate, but only the posterior and lateral areas are palpable. A PSA is also necessary.

17. D.C. is an 80-year-old patient with COPD and rheumatoid arthritis. He has also had prostate cancer for several years. His oncologist has managed his disease by watching for new symptoms, monitoring his PSA levels, and observing his overall performance status. Two months ago, his PSA level rose sharply; his disease was advancing. He received a leuprolide (Lupron) injection 1 week ago. Today, his wife drove him to the clinic during a snowstorm. She reports that her husband cannot walk well. D.C. appears to be in severe discomfort, is not able to stand, and reports having back pain and decreased urination. The nurse suspects that the patient is ⚠
    A. experiencing an exacerbation of his rheumatoid arthritis because of the change in barometric pressure related to the unexpected snowfall.
    B. simply exhausted because of his long-term COPD status and does not have the energy to walk and move around as usual.
    C. having back pain and difficulty walking because of a recent fall.
    D. experiencing a flare reaction from the leuprolide (Lupron) injection, causing his back pain, immobility, and urinary retention.

18. Upon reviewing D.C.'s chart, suspicion for a flare reaction increases when the nurse sees he did not receive which of the following? ⚠
    A. Flutamide
    B. Dexamethasone
    C. Leucovorin
    D. Finasteride

19. Which of the following is the most frequent first-line treatment for advanced prostate cancer?
    A. Strontium
    B. Medical castration with leuprolide (Lupron) or goserelin (Zoladex).
    C. Surgery
    D. Total-body irradiation

20. Which of the following statements apply to prostate cancer?
    A. 35% of all cancers in men, usually beginning in the peripheral zone. Early bone metastasis is common.
    B. 50% of all cancers in men. A total of 50% of prostate cancers are adenocarcinomas. Survival rates have decreased steadily since 1974.
    C. 30% of all cancers in men. A total of 95% of prostate cancers are adenocarcinomas. Malignant growth initially spreads to the bladder and peritoneum.
    D. 40% of all cancers in men. A total of 55% of prostate cancers are sarcomas, mucinous, or signet ring tumors. Prostate cancer has early spread via hematologic and lymphatic pathways to the lung.

21. B.K., who is 81 years old, had brachytherapy for prostate cancer 2½ years ago. After a winter in Florida, he recently drove back north. He tells the nurse that he is starting to notice his age and reports that driving back in his mobile home caused some leg and back pain, which he never noticed before. He also noticed shoulder pain when he was turning the wheel on the trailer. He is tired from the long trip but also wonders if he has the flu. He denies stomachache and feeling feverish. His most recent PSA, drawn a few days ago, shows his PSA is 21. The nurse is aware that the patient will likely be scheduled to have
    A. transrectal ultrasonography (TRUS).
    B. repeat PSA.
    C. pelvic MRI.
    D. bone scan.

22. Which of the statements below are accurate regarding prostate cancer?
    A. About 50% of prostate cancers are diagnosed in men after the age of 50 years. The disease causes higher mortality rates in populations from Asia, South America, and the Middle East. There is no known genetic link in men related to prostate cancer.
    B. Eating a high-fat diet has been known to decrease the progression of prostate cancer. About 30% of prostate cancers are diagnosed in men after the age of 65 years. There is no benefit in using PSAs after a diagnosis of prostate cancer has been made.
    C. The mortality rate for prostate cancer is higher in developed than in developing countries. The highest incidence and mortality rates in the world are among African Americans. More than 75% of prostate cancers are diagnosed in men after the age of 65 years.
    D. Diets high in vitamins E and D, as well as selenium, may increase a risk for prostate cancer in men older than 50 years of age. There are higher mortality rates for prostate cancer in developing countries because of poorer health care access.

23. E.W., a 73-year-old patient, has been admitted from the emergency department (ED) following a fall in which he fractured his right hip. During workup in the ED, bone lesions were found on his spine and on his opposite hip. His family history shows that his father and paternal uncle had prostate cancer. Laboratory tests are pending, but he has been told he may have prostate cancer. EW is angry and shocked. He was planning a trip to Europe soon. Which are important initial nursing interventions for this patient?

A. Encourage him to verbalize his feelings, give him literature regarding screening tools for prostate cancer, and ask when he was last screened.

B. Arrange with his permission for the oncology social worker to speak to him. Provide answers to questions he may ask, encourage him to report symptoms, and provide pharmacologic and non-pharmacologic pain management.

C. Ask the patient if he ever heard of the term hospice and ask if he has a will prepared.

D. Arrange for a consult by the orthopedic surgeon. Notify discharge planning to prepare for his discharge.

24. P.C., a 66-year-old male patient, is a bachelor and lives alone. He is retired from the printing business. He has had a recent prostate biopsy 1 week ago and is attending a urology appointment this afternoon. He is overwhelmed. He is asking the nurse what his Gleason score of 8 means. The nurse responds that a Gleason score

A. of 8 means that the prostate cancer is not likely to spread and can be easily contained.

B. is used to indicate the ability of a prostate cancer to respond to radiation therapy.

C. is used to indicate how well the prostate cancer will respond to hormonal therapy.

D. of 8 is high and indicates that the prostate cancer is aggressive with a poorer prognosis.

12 Skin Cancer

1. When does melanoma require sentinel lymph node biopsy in the diagnostic workup?
   A. When melanoma lesions are smaller than 3 mm in thickness
   B. Melanoma lesions larger than 1 mm in thickness
   C. Melanoma lesions that are spread on a surface area larger than ½ inch (12.5 mm)
   D. When melanoma lesions present in a patient with any type of previous cancer

2. Which are correct statements about skin cancer?
   A. Basal cell carcinoma arises from the dermis and is caused by cumulative ultraviolet (UV) exposure over one's lifetime.
   B. Squamous cell carcinoma starts in the dermis layer of the skin. Incidence rates in women younger than 40 years of age are increasing.
   C. Melanoma starts in the dermis layer and is the most common form of skin cancer.
   D. Basal cell cancer is common in older persons, but the average age at diagnosis is decreasing.

3. There are four types of basal cell cancers. Which statements correctly differentiate these types?
   A. Superficial basal cell cancers are commonly found on the trunk; lesions progress slowly and appear as a bright red to pink patch.
   B. Micronodular basal cell cancer is nonaggressive and appears yellowish-white when stretched.
   C. Nodular basal cell cancer occurs on the back and chest areas and comprises 30% of all basal cell cancers
   D. Pigmented basal cell cancers are more common in lighter pigmented individuals.

4. A fair skinned 17-year-old high school student who swims and frequents tanning booths presents in the clinic for evaluation of a potential melanoma in a lesion she noticed on her inner left thigh. She feels healthy and is being uncooperative regarding her appointments and diagnostic workup. The nurse realizes that a biopsy of the lesion is very important to determine the ⚠
   A. presence of distant lymph node metastasis.
   B. Breslow depth.
   C. presence of telangiectasias.
   D. irregularity of lesion borders.

5. In melanoma, the choice of biopsy technique depends on which of these factors?
   A. Location, size, and shape of the lesion
   B. Pigment or color of the lesion
   C. Closeness to other skin pigmentations such as freckles, other moles, or keloids
   D. Preference of the dermatologist

6. Sentinel lymph node biopsy is an integral part of the staging process for melanoma. It has replaced elective lymph node dissection. If a positive sentinel lymph node is found, the next step is usually
   A. a complete node dissection of the involved lymph node basin.
   B. a lymph node dissection of up to 12 lymph nodes in the region.
   C. evaluation and initiation of regional radiation therapy.
   D. surgical excision of the melanoma lesion with minimum of 5-mm margins.

7. What is the most important factor in making treatment decisions for a patient with basal cell lesions?
   A. Size, location, and primary versus recurrent lesion
   B. Perineural invasion
   C. Physician decision
   D. Patient's diabetic status

8. Of the following persons, who would be at the highest risk of having nonmelanoma skin cancers (NMSCs)?
   A. A 35-year-old white ski instructor
   B. A 60-year-old white grain farmer in the midwestern United States
   C. A 40-year-old Mexican American ranch hand in the southwestern United States
   D. A 62-year-old African American cotton farmer in the southern United States

9. Which of the following lesions is the most common type of skin cancer?
   A. Basal cell carcinoma
   B. Squamous cell carcinoma
   C. Nodular melanoma
   D. Superficial spreading melanoma

10. What major factors should the nurse emphasize in teaching self-skin examination at a community forum?
    A. Self-skin examination should be done every 2 weeks.
    B. Skin cancers present with pain.
    C. Self-skin examination should start with the head and end with the feet.
    D. The most common skin cancers are psoriasis, malignant melanoma, and squamous cell.

11. The nurse should understand that the ABCDEs of Melanoma recognition include which of the following characteristics?
    A. Alignment
    B. Border
    C. Contrast
    D. Dimpling
    E. Exudate

12. A 70-year-old man who had malignant melanoma treated in his early 60s is attending a health fair. What is the most appropriate instruction for the nurse to provide to him?
    A. Do weekly systematic self-examination of the skin for suspicious lesions.
    B. Limiting daily sun exposure to 2 hours during the summer months
    C. Evaluation at regular intervals by a physician or nurse
    D. Use of sunscreens and sunblocks when outside during the summer months

13. A fair-skinned woman comes to the dermatology clinic because of a brown lesion on her left shoulder. She says it started out as a mole that she has had for years but that it has changed shape and color intensity over the past 3 months. The nurse understands this could be a superficial spreading melanoma (SSM) because
    A. the majority of SSMs arise in preexisting lesions.
    B. SSM comprises 60% to 70% of all melanomas.
    C. lesion borders are usually symmetrical.
    D. SSMs begin as a pearly pink lesion.

14. A 54-year-old patient with HIV is being seen for routine health screening in the internal medicine clinic. In providing patient teaching guidance, the nurse should include information regarding which type of skin cancer?
    A. Squamous cell
    B. Malignant melanoma
    C. Basal cell carcinoma
    D. Actinic keratosis

15. In presenting information on the risks associated with the development of malignant melanoma, nurses should particularly target which group?
    A. Senior citizens
    B. Mothers of adolescents
    C. Construction workers
    D. Mothers of infants and young children

16. Treatment options for patients with malignant melanoma who are candidates for metastasectomy have
    A. multiple metastases.
    B. brain metastases.
    C. solitary metastases to lung, distant lymph nodes, or gastrointestinal tract.
    D. short disease-free intervals.

17. In the initial treatment of skin cancer, which of the standard therapies is most effective?
    A. Biotherapy
    B. Chemotherapy
    C. Radiotherapy
    D. Surgical excision

18. In teaching a group of nursing students about the prevention of skin cancer, the nurse should make sure to include which of these points?
    A. Length of exposure to sunlight, use of sunscreen SPF (sun protective factor) of 15 or more, use of protective clothing, and use of sunglasses
    B. Weather conditions during sun exposure and recreational activities
    C. Skin type, genetic history, family pedigree about skin cancer, and use of tanning parlors
    D. Skin assessment, effects of altitude during sun exposure, time of year during sun exposure, and time of day during sun exposure

19. Acral lentiginous melanoma (ALM) appears as an enlarging hyperpigmented macule or plaque on the palms, soles, nail unit, and mucous membranes. Lesions can also present under the nails as longitudinal melanonychia, a brown or black pigmentation of the nail plate, or hyperpigmentation extending beyond the proximal nail. This is a rare and uncommon form of melanoma and is often mistaken for a benign lesion. This condition is seen in
    A. Whites.
    B. Africans.
    C. predominately the Americas.
    D. Ashkenazi Jews.

20. Which of the following is not a risk factor for malignant melanoma?
    A. Personal history of melanoma and family history
    B. Fair skin, red hair, and freckling
    C. Women at greater risk than men
    D. Immunosuppression
    E. Risk decreases with age after 30 years

21. Which statements are correct about malignant melanoma?
    A. The risk of death from cutaneous melanoma is primarily determined by the color and border of the lesion.
    B. Micrometastases of melanoma from the primary tumor migrates through the vasculature to distant organs.
    C. Malignant melanoma is restricted to areas exposed to sunlight.
    D. Melanoma accounts for 5% of skin cancers diagnosed in the United States.

22. Nurses can play a key role in prevention of skin cancer by educating patients on proper skin care and prevention techniques. Which of the following is a correct statement?
    A. Maximize exposure to sunlight between the hours of 10 a.m. and 4 p.m.
    B. Use sunscreen with an SPF of 15+ and reapply every 1.5 to 2 hours.
    C. A base tan helps reduce the risk of developing skin cancer.
    D. Regularly wear a baseball cap to protect the face and neck.

23. A sunscreen's SPF is a measurement of
    A. the amount of emollient cream compared to sun screen contained in the preparation.
    B. the duration of time the sunscreen can offer protection (in minutes) before it needs to be reapplied.
    C. the duration of time the screen needs to be making contact with the skin before it offers protection.
    D. the measurement of how long unprotected skin can be exposed to ultraviolet rays before burning compared with how long it takes to burn without protection.

13 Head and Neck Cancers

1. J.M. is a 74-year-old man who is retired from a lumber mill. He had previous head and neck cancer about 5 years ago, which was treated with radiation therapy. He presents to the clinic after returning home from visiting family in Florida. The patient reports he must have "gotten into" some allergies because he has had a sore throat since he left 3 months ago. The nurse suspects
   A. that his sore throat is caused by environmental allergies and that he was exposed to several allergens while he was away and on the way home.
   B. his sore throat is a late-term effects of the previous radiation therapy that he received more than 5 years ago.
   C. the patient may have developed a new primary cancer somewhere in the region of the head and neck.
   D. that he was exposed to a strep throat infection from his grandchildren in Florida.

2. Which of the following are risk factors for head and neck cancer?
   A. *Helicobacter pylori* infection and history of herpes zoster
   B. Human papillomavirus (HPV) infection, alcohol use, and all forms of tobacco use
   C. Petroleum cleaning solvents, asphalt paving, and painting supplies
   D. Gluten allergies and dairy allergies

3. Tobacco and excessive alcohol use increase the risk of head and neck cancers and oral or pharyngeal cancers, respectively. To what extent do these substances increase the risk for head and neck cancers?
   A. Tobacco use corresponds with a 30-fold increased risk; excessive alcohol users have a 40-fold increased risk.
   B. Tobacco use corresponds with a 25-fold increased risk; excessive alcohol users have a 30-fold increased risk.
   C. Tobacco use corresponds with a 70-fold increased risk; excessive alcohol users have a 50-fold increased risk.
   D. Tobacco use corresponds with a 25-fold increase risk; excessive alcohol users have a 9-fold increased risk.

4. J.N. is a 63-year-old female bank teller who has been recently diagnosed with laryngeal cancer. She was raised around heavy smokers. She is scheduled to have a hemilaryngectomy. Her job at the bank is the center of her life. She is very concerned about losing her position. In the preoperative teaching the nurse explains that after her recovery period, she
   A. should be able to speak, perhaps in a hoarse voice, and have minimal or no swallowing problems.
   B. will not have her voice, and she should consider retirement.
   C. should have her normal, preoperative voice.
   D. will have a permanent tracheostomy, which can be unsightly.

5. Chemotherapy as a single-treatment modality is not effective to cure head and neck cancers, but it has been used in combination with radiation therapy (RT). One advantage of this approach is that the chemotherapy
   A. is sequestered in the lymph nodes directly encasing the head and neck area.
   B. is given as a follow-up after the last RT treatment is complete.
   C. acts to sensitize the cancer cells to the RT, making the RT more effective.
   D. is not used in patients who have recurrent or metastatic disease.

6. J.H. is a 54-year-old man with alcoholism who has been diagnosed with cancer of the larynx. He is also a heavy smoker and has been told that he will be having a total laryngectomy. One year ago he had surgery on a cancerous posterior tongue lesion. His wife appears with him today and tells the nurse that he had some problems communicating at work after the surgery and eventually left his position. She believes he is depressed and that he is very worried about the laryngectomy. He has continued to drink alcohol. She requests a private room at the end of the hall so he can get his rest and not be concerned with visitors and ancillary workers seeing him after surgery. The nurse explains ⚠
   A. he will return to the floor wearing a tracheostomy collar with humidified air for 24 hours.
   B. he should not experience any postoperative effects and could likely go home the day of the surgery.
   C. he should be near the nurse's station postoperatively because of the altered airway with a tracheostomy, and he could also experience delirium tremens (DTs).
   D. the nurse can honor his request and provide a private room at the end of the hall where he will get the rest he needs and have his privacy.

7. Which of these statements is accurate regarding tracheostomy care?
   A. Suction the patient every hour for the first 2 days postoperatively.
   B. Observe the patient and request that he cough and raise and expectorate any secretions through his mouth.
   C. Insert the suction catheter carefully without disturbing any crusty secretions, which are involved in wound healing.
   D. Suctioning is based on the need for airway clearance. Accumulation of mucous and crusted secretions causes infection.

8. R.C. is 59 years old and is being transferred back to the nursing unit from the intensive care unit (ICU) after having had radical neck dissection with flap and a temporary tracheostomy. In organizing his nursing care, the nurse is aware that the important aspects of wound care involve
   A. suctioning, airway maintenance, and humidification.
   B. assessment of the surgical wound, surgical flap, and integrity of and cleaning of suture lines.
   C. administration of prescribed antibiotics and replacing soiled tracheostomy ties.
   D. removing, cleaning, and replacing the inner cannula and clearing mucus secretions.

9. Patients who are having surgery for any type of head and neck cancer need to be assessed at diagnosis and before therapy for their nutritional status. What percentage of these patients will present with malnutrition?
   A. 60%
   B. 40%
   C. 30%
   D. 25%

10. The nurse educator is teaching nursing students who will be working on a surgical ENT (ear, nose, and throat) unit. They have had some practice with tracheostomy care and suctioning on mannequin patients. In answering their questions regarding dysphagia and aspiration, the nurse educator explains that during swallowing food
    A. the vocal cords open, and the larynx moves down and forward.
    B. the vocal cords open, and the larynx moves upward and back.
    C. the vocal cords close, the larynx moves upward and back.
    D. the vocal cords close, the larynx moves upward and forward.

11. J.Y. is a 76-year-old man who has had previous surgery for cancer of the oral cavity 6 years ago. He had had a long-standing issue with alcohol abuse and smoking and worked in the petroleum business for approximately 50 years. He is now being seen for head and neck cancer. He has received 11 radiation treatments and is seen in clinic for a routine oncology appointment. The patient reports that his mouth is sore; he can eat, but everything seems to burn his tongue and the inside of his mouth. He has been using some glycerin-type oral lozenges. When the nurse inspects his oral cavity, the nurse expects to see
    A. indentation.
    B. a fungal infection.
    C. inflammation. → mucositis
    D. an allergic reaction.

12. C.R. is a 72-year-old retired chicken farmer. He appears at this intake appointment with his wife. He is scheduled to have a radical neck dissection. Mrs. R reports they do not understand why he needs to have his neck operated on when he only had the lump under his tongue. He has had many tests, which have "only found a few spots on his bones." The nurse is aware that
    A. his disease has likely spread to the lymphatics and the bone.
    B. the surgery on his neck will allow placement for a tracheostomy tube.
    C. the neck surgery is needed for placement of a PEG feeding tube.
    D. the disease has spread to the lymph nodes; the surgery will stop this spread.

13. A nurse educator from the American Cancer Society is planning to conduct free community outreach education classes on head and neck cancer. In preparing materials, which statement should be included regarding long-term survival?
    A. Oral pharyngeal cancers have a 1-year survival rate of 50%.
    B. All stages of laryngeal cancer have a 5-year survival rate of 40% to 50% if localized when detected.
    C. The overall 5-year survival rate for thyroid cancer is 75%.
    D. There is a decrease of 2% to 3% per year in new cases of laryngeal cancer.

14. Which statement about screening and detection for head and neck cancers is correct?
    A. There are no definitive screening practices for early detection of head and neck cancer.
    B. Early detection of head and neck cancer can be accomplished with yearly panoramic radiography.
    C. An oral examination by a dentist performed every 2 years in adults is the current screening recommendation.
    D. A thorough patient history regarding the digestive tract and dietary practices constitutes current head and neck screening recommendations.

15. A patient had a recent external-beam radiation to the head and neck for cancer of the tongue. This is a new primary treatment for him, although he previously had cancer of the lip about 9 years ago. He comes in today and asks if it is normal for him to have trouble swallowing. The nurse explains that this could be due to
    A. xerostomia.
    B. hypoxemia.
    C. phonation.
    D. dysphonia.

16. Those who are diagnosed with head and neck cancer are at an increased risk of developing other primary tumors because of
    A. the immunosuppressive side effects of treatment for head and neck cancer.
    B. the prolonged exposure of the mucosal surface to carcinogens.
    C. human papillomavirus 16.
    D. repeated exposure to petroleum products.

17. Head and neck cancers represent several different types of cancer, all of which have different incidence and prevalence rates, diagnostic techniques, and treatment options. Initial treatment options for naso-pharyngeal cancers include
    A. surgical resection to eliminate the tumor and ensure clean margins.
    B. chemotherapy as a single treatment modality.
    C. seed implantation with brachytherapy.
    D. radiation therapy.

18. A 32-year-old patient has a new diagnosis of a can-cer at the base of the tongue. He is being seen for an initial visit before starting targeted therapy. He re-ports that he has a coworker who had cancer on his tongue, and he remembers the patient having many treatments, but he is only scheduled for a few. He is concerned that something is wrong or someone has made an error. The nurse reviews his chart and finds that he is HPV positive and therefore
    A. he will receive a targeted therapy, but he cannot receive radiation.
    B. he needs stronger, more intense treatment.
    C. he has a better prognosis and requires less in-tense treatment.
    D. he has a poorer prognosis and may not receive any treatment.

19. A 73-year-old widow has cancer of the larynx. The patient has been transferred to nurse's floor postopera-tively from the ICU. She has had a temporary trache-ostomy for 3 days, and she has a cuffed tube. The chart was just reviewed by her doctor who mentions that we will start weaning off the tracheostomy by the end of the week. The nurse should anticipate all of the following, except
    A. the nurse will be expected to change this initial tracheostomy tube from a cuffed to a noncuffed tube sometime tomorrow.
    B. the tube will likely be downsized to a number 4 or 5 fenestrated tube.
    C. the tube will be plugged and if tolerated for 24 hours without incident, the cannula can be removed.
    D. humidification continues to be a concern for this patient.

20. Patients with head and neck cancers are at risk for being nutritionally compromised and may require oral, enteral, or parenteral nutritional supplements. One parameter used to determine nutritional status is
    A. greater than 10% body weight loss during any treatment phase.
    B. more than 10% below ideal body weight.
    C. greater than 5% body weight loss during any treatment phase.
    D. more than 15% below ideal body weight.

21. A patient in the ENT unit has had a partial laryngec-tomy and is frustrated with her inability to communi-cate. She has been reluctant to see a speech therapist but agrees to try. The nurse explains that she will need to
    A. practice throat exercises that have been demon-strated to her.
    B. become familiar with and learn esophageal speech.
    C. learn how to use a tracheoesophageal prosthesis.
    D. use an artificial larynx, which will be ordered for her.

22. Which of the following are signs and symptoms of cancer of the oral cavity?
    A. White or red patch on the gums, tongue, or lining of the mouth
    B. Swelling under the chin or around the jawbone
    C. Sinuses that are blocked and do not clear
    D. Chronic sinus infections that do not respond to antibiotics

23. R.W. has had a supraglottic laryngectomy. The postop-erative effects most likely to observe include
    A. aspiration.
    B. a decreased sense of smell.
    C. hoarseness.
    D. shoulder droop.

14 Cancers of the Neurologic System

1. The cerebrum is one of the main structures of the brain. It is
   A. located at the base of the brain.
   B. located at the top of the spinal cord.
   C. the large outer part of the brain.
   D. located in the posterior fossa at the back of the brain.

2. Which of the following viruses is considered a known situational risk factor for central nervous system (CNS) tumors?
   A. Anopheles B virus
   B. Epstein Barr virus
   C. Macropodid herpesvirus 1
   D. Human papillomavirus

3. Which of the following diagnostic measures also carry an increased risk for CNS tumors?
   A. Chest radiography in children younger than the age of 7 years
   B. Mammography in female patients over the age of 50 years
   C. Computed tomography (CT) of the abdomen and pelvis without contrast
   D. Panorex radiographs before the age of 10 years

4. What part of the brain connects the anterior and posterior arteries to provide alternative routes if blood flow to a single vessel is blocked?
   A. Dural sinuses
   B. Circle of Willis
   C. Ependymal cells
   D. Broca area

5. The nurse is assigned to care for M.S., who is a 44-year-old female patient diagnosed with a meningioma. Symptoms the nurse would expect her to display include all of the following except
   A. being irrational and having mood swings.
   B. headache and seizure activity.
   C. arm and leg weakness.
   D. vision loss.

6. The portion of the brain that regulates the sleep–wake cycle is the
   A. hypothalamus.
   B. cerebellum.
   C. temporal lobe.
   D. parietal lobe.

7. Which groups have known intrinsic risk factors for CNS tumors?
   A. Middle-aged adults
   B. Hispanic or Asian heritage
   C. Children and elderly adults
   D. Males for meningioma, females for glioma

8. Tumors of the neurologic system are not staged by the TNM system because
   A. neurologic tumors are usually in the advanced stage at diagnosis.
   B. the Hooper Crane staging criteria are implemented.
   C. there are not usually extra cranial metastases and there are no nodes.
   D. the Ann Arbor Staging system is used.

9. The most important prognostic indicators for primary brain tumors include
   A. astrocytoma versus primitive neuroectodermal cell tumor.
   B. degree of confusion and personality changes.
   C. size of the lesion (single vs. multifocal), location, and degree of malignancy.
   D. the length of time exposed to toxic substances.

10. Which statements are true about lung cancer and brain metastases?
    A. More than 90% of persons with lung cancer will develop brain metastases.
    B. It is extremely rare for persons with lung cancer to develop brain metastases.
    C. The most common type of brain cancer metastases in women arises from breast cancer, not lung cancer.
    D. Metastases from lung cancer usually develop 2 to 3 years after diagnosis.

11. A 35-year-old patient has a tumor in the cerebellum, where the brainstem connects with the spinal cord. His fiancé reports that he has had symptoms over the past few months such as headache, blurry vision, and what they thought may have been a few seizures. When he developed a droopy eyelid, she brought him into the emergency department. Now he is scheduled to have a surgical resection. What is not an anticipated result of the surgery?
    A. Obtain a diagnostic tissue sample.
    B. Preserve neurologic functioning.
    C. Completely eliminate pain.
    D. Make treatment efficacious by decreasing tumor burden.

12. After surgical resection, CT or magnetic resonance imaging (MRI) is recommended in order to assess
    A. for development of hydrocephalus.
    B. tissue inflammation and infection.
    C. for postoperative intracranial bleeding.
    D. residual tumor burden and establish baseline.

13. J.M., a 14-year-old young woman with malignant melanoma, has been brought in for increased confusion, headache, and some upper extremity numbness. She is going to have a lumbar puncture to detect
    A. metastases to the central nervous system.
    B. bacterial meningitis.
    C. multiple sclerosis.
    D. Guillain-Barré syndrome.

14. When J.M. (from the previous question) first arrived in the emergency department, she was complaining of a severe headache, seemed drowsy, and was not answering questions appropriately. Her mother says these symptoms got worse over the past 12 hours. Which diagnostic tool would be used at initial presentation to evaluate these new neurologic symptoms? ⚠
    A. CT with contrast
    B. CT without contrast
    C. Radioisotope bone scan
    D. Plain radiographs

15. J.B. is a 35-year-old woman who has a recently diagnosed primary brain tumor, an oligodendroglioma. She received external-beam radiation therapy for a 6-week period. Initially, she did well; however, approximately 5 months later, her mother and husband are reporting that she seems to be drowsy all the time, more so than when she was first diagnosed. Although J.B.'s treatments have eradicated much of her tumor, she is having side effects caused by
    A. accumulated hydrocephalus.
    B. focal seizures.
    C. subacute effects of radiation.
    D. acute effects of radiation therapy.

16. Posttreatment side effects like those exhibited by J.B. (in the previous question) can be mistaken for tumor progression. This may result in essential treatments being withheld or discontinued. These symptoms usually occur 4 to 6 months after treatment is completed and are called
    A. radio-induced demyelination.
    B. radiation necrosis.
    C. global effects.
    D. pseudoprogression of the tumor.

17. Which of the following statements are true regarding high-grade astrocytomas?
    A. They metastasize frequently to the liver, lung, or both.
    B. They infiltrate into the surrounding brain tissue.
    C. They are frequently encapsulated.
    D. They respond well to chemotherapy.

18. A 54-year-old patient with a glioblastoma multiforme was diagnosed with a deep vein thrombosis 1 month ago and has been taking warfarin (Coumadin) since that time. He reports a headache for the past week that is not helped by OTC pain relievers. The nurse contacts his provider to order which of the following tests? ⚠
    A. MRI
    B. Non–contrast-enhanced CT
    C. Ultrasonography
    D. Myelogram

19. A patient presents with a left visual field cut, and the MRI shows a brain tumor on the right side. The nurse would expect which lobe of the brain to be affected?
    A. Parietal lobe
    B. Frontal lobe
    C. Temporal lobe
    D. Occipital lobe

20. J.S. is a 26-year-old woman who has had a primary brain tumor for 7 years. She has had increased difficulty with somnolence, her gait, and headaches over the past 4 weeks. She returns with her mother to the clinic today to discuss her third craniotomy. Her mother asks why this is necessary. The nurse responds by explaining that
    A. second or third craniotomies are often performed for restaging purposes because lower grade tumors often become more malignant over time.
    B. a repeat craniotomy is done as a last hope effort to remove all of the tumor.
    C. the craniotomy will prevent metastatic spread to the lung.
    D. the craniotomy is being performed to place a vascular access device.

21. In planning treatment for patients with primary brain tumors, chemotherapy agents have not been particularly effective because of inadequate delivery across the blood–brain barrier. Which first-line therapy alkylating agent can cross the blood–brain barrier?
   A. Temodar (temozolomide)
   B. Trileptal (oxcarbazepine)
   C. Tarceva (Erlotinib)
   D. Hycamtin (Topotecan)

22. S.S. is a 58-year-old woman admitted to the oncology ICU for complaints of radicular pain in the lumbar sacral region followed by a sudden onset of confusion, headache, and somnolence. She has non-Hodgkin lymphoma. She has been diagnosed with metastatic lymphoma with CNS involvement in the leptomeninges. In the ICU, she developed stridor, difficulty breathing, and was intubated. To quickly reduce her symptoms and control the new onset of intracranial pressure, she will receive
   A. temodar.
   B. glucocorticoids.
   C. a high-dose methotrexate regimen.
   D. mannitol.

23. Malignant tumors of the spinal cord tend to arise from intramedullary support cells, including
   A. astrocytes.
   B. epithelial cells.
   C. glial cells.
   D. mast cells

24. J.L. is a 67-year-old man with a history of lung cancer. He was treated with surgery and radiation therapy, and his disease has been stable for approximately 8 months. He is seen in the walk-in clinic complaining of a new onset of radicular pain of his left leg and spinal tenderness in his lower back. What nursing assessment is most critical for this patient?
   A. Pupil checks
   B. Bowel and bladder function
   C. Cranial nerve examination
   D. Upper extremity strength

25. Which of the following types of radiation therapy is delivered in a single high-dose fraction using a head frame?
   A. Standard conventional radiation
   B. Brachytherapy
   C. Stereotactic radiosurgery
   D. Fractionated stereotactic radiotherapy

15 Leukemia

1. Which statements are accurate regarding leukemia?
   A. The most common type of leukemia in children is acute lymphocytic leukemia (ALL), accounting for 75% of cases.
   B. Most leukemia is diagnosed in children. *90% in adults*
   C. The most common type of leukemia in children is chronic lymphocytic leukemia (CLL).
   D. The most common type of leukemia in adults is ~~ALL~~. *CLL + AML*

2. The most common risk factors for leukemia include
   A. exposure to gasoline, kerosene, and oil industry products.
   B. alcohol consumption.
   C. workplace chemicals such as benzene and formaldehyde.
   D. coal tar, paving black top, and cement powders.

3. One of the criteria used in diagnosing CLL is
   A. the presence of greater than 20% lymphoblasts in the marrow and the presence of the Philadelphia chromosome.
   B. bone marrow aspirate with cytogenetic assessment and positive for the Philadelphia chromosome.
   C. bone marrow aspirate and biopsy with cytogenetic results showing a presence of more than 20% blasts in the marrow.
   D. the presence of greater than 5×10^9/B lymphocytes (5000/μL) in the peripheral blood for at least 3 months.

4. What is a symptom related to bone marrow failure?
   A. Seizure
   B. Recurrent infections
   C. Lymphadenopathy
   D. Bone pain

5. M.F. has CLL. His lymphocytes are greater than 6000 B lymphocytes/μL. His laboratory study results also reveal thrombocytopenia with platelet count of 96,000. The patient reports he has noticed some swollen lymph nodes in the groin and the left axilla area. He has early satiety. Using the modified Rai staging system for CLL, the nurse determines that his extent of disease is
   A. low.
   B. medium.
   C. intermediate.
   D. high.

6. M.F. (from the previous question) reports he has had one cold after another over the past few weeks. Chest radiography reveals pneumonia. He thinks these illnesses are caused by the long cold winter. The nurse suspects these symptoms are related to
   A. a latent tuberculosis.
   B. recurrent infections caused by neutropenia.
   C. a history of chronic sinusitis.
   D. exposure to second hand smoke.

7. J.P. has immune thrombocytopenia, one of the autoimmune cytopenias. A decision has been made to start the patient on corticosteroids in an attempt to decrease the effects of the B lymphocytes and allow for the red blood cells to function properly. The teaching tips the nurse provides about the potential side effects of corticosteroids include
   A. weight loss.
   B. dehydration.
   C. hypokalemia.
   D. sodium and water retention.

8. E.C., a 25-year-old female patient, is being sent to the clinic from her primary care provider after laboratory results show she has WBC of greater than 23,000, low hemoglobin and hematocrit, and a low platelet count of 14,000. She has been given a preliminary diagnosis of acute myelocytic leukemia (AML). The symptoms the nurse most likely expects her to display include
   A. easy bruising, enlarged axillary lymph nodes, and fever.
   B. easy bruising, early satiety, fatigue, and nose and gingival bleeding.
   C. early satiety, enlarged lymph nodes, and recurrent infections not responsive to antibiotics.
   D. fever, night sweats, bony pain, and malaise.

9. Which tests would the nurse expect E.C. to have to clarify her clinical diagnosis?
   A. Bone marrow biopsy with cytogenetics
   B. Cytogenetic testing to determine the presence of Philadelphia chromosome
   C. Determining the immunophenotype for T-cell antigen CD5 and B-cell surface antigens
   D. Florescence in situ hybridization (FISH) if bone marrow collection is not feasible

10. E.C., according to her mother, has been complaining of headaches, which is unusual for her. The nurse is aware that a small percentage of patients can develop CNS involvement from this disease. This may be manifested as
    A. vomiting.
    B. neck pain.
    C. seizure activity.
    D. jaw and tooth discomfort.

11. Which statement accurately describes staging systems for different types of leukemia?
    A. The Rai staging system is used for ALL.
    B. CLL is staged using the Ann Arbor Staging system.
    C. CML is described in phases: chronic, accelerated, and blast phase.
    D. AML is staged using the international staging system.

12. J.B., an 11-year-old boy, has been diagnosed with ALL. On diagnosis, his white blood cell count is 62,000/µL, and his cytogenetics pointed to T-cell involvement. Which risk category would fit JB?
    A. Low risk
    B. Standard risk
    C. Intermediate risk
    D. High risk

13. J.B. is being considered for stem cell transplant, and his family members are being considered as potential donors. What type of transplant will be used, and which test will identify a matching donor?
    A. Autologous stem cell transplant and *BRCA1* testing
    B. Xenograft transplants and Scl-70 testing
    C. Allogeneic stem cell transplant and human leukocyte antigen (HLA) testing
    D. Syngeneic transplant and nucleic acid amplification testing (NAAT)

14. Tumor lysis syndrome (TLS) is a constellation of metabolic changes taking place because of the rapid lysis of malignant cells after initiation of therapy. These lysed cells then enter the bloodstream. If not treated promptly, TLS can become a life-threatening emergency. Which of the following hematologic malignancies are most closely associated with TLS?
    A. CML
    B. AML
    C. CLL
    D. ALL

15. A.B. is a 63-year-old man with a new diagnosis of CML. His laboratory work order includes complete blood cell count (CBC), complete metabolic profile, D-dimer, disseminated intravascular coagulation (DIC) panel, and prothrombin time (PT) and partial thromboplastin time (PTT). A fluorescence in situ hybridization (FISH) test is also ordered because ⚠
    A. there is a previous history of deep vein thrombosis and the test will help to better evaluate this history.
    B. the patient desires a venous access device to determine if it is contraindicated.
    C. collection of bone marrow is not feasible.
    D. the patient needs a transfusion of packed red blood cells and there needs to be a determination if the patient has antibodies.

16. In obtaining a patient history from A.B., he reports that he has had diabetes for almost 10 years and currently takes metformin. The nurse notes on his laboratory work that his WBC count is more than 20,000, creatinine is 3.0, his blood urea nitrogen (BUN) is 34, and his glomerular filtration rate (GFR) is 18. He is at risk for ⚠
    A. tumor lysis syndrome.
    B. deep vein thrombosis.
    C. central nervous system involvement from his AML.
    D. diabetic ketosis.

17. In patients who have AML, the goal of their initial treatment is to eradicate the leukemic cells and achieve a complete remission (CR). This is usually accomplished by administering large doses of chemotherapy, called
    A. salvage therapy.
    B. interleukin therapy.
    C. induction therapy.
    D. consolidation therapy.

16 Lymphoma and Multiple Myeloma

1. Mr. J presents at his physician's office with enlarged lymph nodes and a history of night sweats. Although the physician suspects Hodgkin disease, which of the following will be required to make a diagnosis of Hodgkin disease?
   A. Fever accompanying night sweats
   B. A history of infections within 3 months of presentation with enlarged lymph nodes
   C. An excisional biopsy with Reed-Sternberg cells noted by the pathologist
   D. Chest radiography and CT scan of the chest and abdomen

2. S.S. is a 19-year-old man who is scheduled to receive initial treatment for Hodgkin disease. After watching an educational video on chemotherapy, he makes the following comment to his nurse. "I guess taking chemotherapy means I will never have children." Which of the following is the most appropriate nursing intervention?
   A. The nurse states, "I wouldn't worry about it" and starts the chemotherapy.
   B. The nurse discusses sperm banking and provides the patient with information, notifies the physician that the patient has concerns, and delays the chemotherapy until the patient can make a decision.
   C. The nurse documents in her notes that the patient has concerns and may need a consultation for sperm banking after this admission and then proceeds with the chemotherapy.
   D. The nurse tells the client that some people have problems but that he may not and offers to call the physician to talk with him further if the patient wishes. When the patient makes no further comment, the nurse proceeds with the chemotherapy.

3. Mr. G is a 52-year-old man who was diagnosed with intermediate grade non-Hodgkin lymphoma 2 years ago. He received six courses of cyclophosphamide (Cytoxan), doxorubicin, vincristine (Oncovin), and prednisone (CHOP) chemotherapy and achieved a complete remission. He returns today to the outpatient unit for routine follow-up and complains of left leg swelling. Which action is most appropriate initially?
   A. Recommend he keep his leg elevated as much as possible and call if symptoms have not improved in a week.
   B. Assess for lymphadenopathy in all lymph node regions with special attention to the inguinal lymph nodes.
   C. Discuss with the physician the need for Doppler studies to rule out deep vein thrombosis.
   D. Determine a dietary history of sodium intake.

4. Upon examination, Mr. G is found to have an enlarged left inguinal lymph node chain approximately 3.8 cm. Mr. G is afebrile with stable vital signs. The physician will most likely order
   A. CHOP chemotherapy to begin immediately.
   B. antibiotics because enlarged lymph nodes may be a sign of infection.
   C. a peripheral vascular physician consult to evaluate left leg swelling.
   D. a CT scan of the abdomen, pelvis, and chest and a lymph node biopsy.

5. Pain in a patient with multiple myeloma commonly results from
   A. intestinal obstruction caused by enlarging soft tissue mass.
   B. neural infiltration of plasma cells.
   C. lytic bone lesions.
   D. marrow infiltration.

6. C.R. has a diagnosis of multiple myeloma and has been receiving oral melphalan (Alkeran) and prednisone over a period of several months. The nurse notes a weight loss of 10 lb in the past month. The patient states, "The doctor said my blood protein was high, so I was trying to avoid protein in my diet." The best nursing intervention is to
   A. tell the client that he is doing well to avoid protein and congratulate him on his weight loss.
   B. explain to the client that the high blood protein is not a problem but that he should avoid a high-fat diet.
   C. explain to the client that the protein in his blood is from the myeloma, not his diet, and encourage a well-balanced diet.
   D. give the client a pamphlet on the importance of nutrition for persons with cancer.

7. D.B. is a 55-year-old man who was treated 8 years ago for malignant melanoma with surgery and chemotherapy. He presents to the emergency department complaining of shortness of breath, a lump under his arm, and extreme fatigue. When obtaining his history, which of the following would not be a priority for initial assessment?
   A. Aggravating or alleviating factors
   B. Symptoms of fever, night sweats, or weight loss
   C. Symptoms of nausea, vomiting, or early satiety
   D. Lymphadenopathy in the lower extremities

8. D.B.'s chest radiography done in the emergency department reveals mediastinal widening. A chest CT is done, and a large mediastinal mass is detected. Upon axillary lymph node biopsy, a large cell follicular lymphoma is diagnosed. Which of the following diagnostic tests is not necessary to determine treatment options?
   A. Obtain a 24-hour urine.
   B. Determine whether the lymph node biopsy is CD 20+.
   C. Obtain a CT scan of the abdomen and pelvis.
   D. Perform a bilateral bone marrow biopsy and aspirate.

9. Twenty-year-old M.K. owns a small lawn care business. He presents to the outpatient oncology clinic for routine follow-up for Hodgkin disease. He complains of recent weight loss and night sweats. The nurse believes the most likely cause of this is
   A. recurrence of his Hodgkin disease.
   B. his occupation requiring hard work in the heat.
   C. a dietary change related to improved focus on his health.
   D. apprehension and anxiety about the appointment, resulting in a loss of appetite.

10. Mrs. C is 61 years old and is undergoing autologous peripheral blood stem cell transplant for multiple myeloma. When getting out of bed this morning, she leaned against the side rail and experienced a sudden sharp pain in her forearm. The most likely cause of the pain may be
    A. bruising caused by low platelet counts.
    B. fracture of the patient's forearm.
    C. early morning aches and pains.
    D. a pinched nerve in her neck.

11. W.F., a 68-year-old woman, was recently diagnosed with multiple myeloma. She is fiercely independent and is concerned about the appointments keeping her away from her dairy farm. The nurse reviews her plan of care and stresses the importance of receiving which of the following medications regularly?
    A. Bisphosphonates
    B. Herbal supplements for bone strength
    C. Multivitamins with calcium
    D. Aspirin as an anticoagulant

12. In using the CRAB criteria (measurement of calcium, renal, anemia, and bone), what is not something a multiple myeloma patient might exhibit?
    A. Bone lytic lesions
    B. Anemia with HGB less than 10 g/dL
    C. Increased serum calcium levels
    D. Creatinine levels between 0.6 and 1.3 mg/dL

13. J.H. is referred from his university health clinic. He discovered a lump in his neck above his left clavicle. Initially, he thought it was the result of being hit with a lacrosse stick, but it has remained there for at least 1 month. He did not think much of it because it did not hurt. About 2 weeks ago he noticed another lump under his left axilla. He mentions that he has been tired, but he attributed that to playing lacrosse. He also reports he eats like a horse but cannot gain any weight. He wakes up every night drenched in sweat. The nurse is concerned because his symptoms are
    A. B symptoms of nodular lymphocyte predominant Hodgkin lymphoma (NLPHL).
    B. indicative of mononucleosis.
    C. associated with polymyalgia rheumatica.
    D. classic symptoms of rheumatoid arthritis.

14. J.H. proceeds through the diagnostic process with excisional lymph node biopsy and CT scans of the chest, abdomen, and pelvis, which did not reveal any lesions below his diaphragm. Reed-Sternberg cells were found, and a diagnosis of NLPHL was made. How would the nurse stage J.H.'s illness?
    A. Stage I
    B. Stage II
    C. Stage III
    D. Stage IV

15. NLPHL has which of the following characteristics?
    A. Risk factors include a family history of leukemia and personal previous infection with chicken pox (varicella virus).
    B. Radiation alone is responsible for curing 35% to 40% of newly diagnosed patients.
    C. It has an earlier stage disease, longer survival, and fewer treatment failures compared with classic Hodgkin lymphoma (HL).
    D. The U.S. death rate for HL has been stable over the past 20 years.

16. The triage phone nurse at a private oncology practice receives a call regarding S.R., who was diagnosed with multiple myeloma after a fall resulting in a wrist fracture several months ago. His wife is on the phone and wants to know if her husband should continue his daily dose of baby aspirin. She mentions that he is due to come in soon for his "special MPT." The nurse advises to have her husband continue the aspirin ⚠
    A. because he has had a fairly recent wrist fracture, and the aspirin will help with residual aches and pains.
    B. because he is in his late 60s, and the aspirin will hopefully prevent any cardiac incidents.
    C. because it has been recently touted to aid in the prevention of cancer of the colon, esophagus, stomach, and rectum.
    D. to prevent deep venous thrombosis, which is a risk factor of the patient's MPT treatment.

17. M.W. is a 70-year-old woman who has had insulin-dependent diabetes for many years. She has a new diagnosis of multiple myeloma and will be receiving Velcade, Revlamid, and dexamethasone. The nurse is educating her regarding these drugs and possible toxicities. The nurse explains that most likely ⚠
    A. she will no longer need to take any insulin.
    B. she should check her blood sugars and adjust her insulin dosage.
    C. she may sleep more frequently and for longer intervals.
    D. she may notice significant but gradual weight loss.

18. Risk factors related to Non-Hodgkin lymphoma (NHL) include
    A. Immunodeficiency: inherited, acquired, or solid organ transplant
    B. Tobacco smoking, tobacco chewing, and high-fat diets
    C. Whooping cough or rheumatic fever as a child
    D. Barrett esophagus of the gastroesophageal junction

19. The International Prognostic Index (IPI) is a prognostic tool that assigns patients to a risk group and predicts outcomes. In aggressive NHL, five risk factors are identified and a numeric scale suggests a favorable or unfavorable status. Measurements include
    A. age >40 years old is an unfavorable risk factor.
    B. number of extranodal sites less than two is favorable.
    C. patient performance status (ECOG) of 2 or greater is unfavorable.
    D. Ann Arbor Staging of 3 or less is favorable.

20. J.C. is 74 years old and has been diagnosed with a follicular lymphoma. Since her retirement 4 years ago, she has traveled extensively both inside the United States and internationally. She is very shocked with this diagnosis and is more surprised to hear that she has probably had the lymphoma for years. Her treatment plan will likely consist of
    A. surgery and radiation therapy to the splenic area.
    B. chemotherapy MOPP protocol.
    C. monoclonal antibody therapy.
    D. regional and local radiation, CHOP, and Rituxan.

21. The nurse educator is preparing a short overview presentation for nursing students regarding cancers of the lymphoid system. Pertinent facts include
    A. some lymphoid cells migrate to the thymus and mature into T cells.
    B. there is a limited number of lymphoid cells, and they eventually become depleted.
    C. T cells produce immunoglobulins.
    D. B cells proliferate peripherally.

22. Statistics regarding multiple myeloma include
    A. that it is the second most common hematologic malignancy in the United States.
    B. that multiple myeloma constitutes 8% of all cancers in the United States.
    C. that there is a higher incidence of multiple myeloma among the Hispanic population.
    D. that it produces osteoporosis which contributes to fractures.

23. Which of the following is the best explanation for the mechanisms at work in multiple myeloma?
    A. The cells involved in multiple myeloma cause failure in the coagulation cascade, and immature platelets are responsible for thrombosis, stroke, and large vessel cardiac events.
    B. Multiple myeloma affects the marrow's ability to produce mature, functioning WBCs, and the patient experiences repeated infections.
    C. In multiple myeloma, the patient's malignant B-cell line produces abnormally high levels of M proteins in the blood, which do not provide immune function.
    D. Multiple myeloma causes a disruption in the production of insulin by the β cells in the pancreas and impacts glucose absorption.

17 Bone and Soft Tissue Cancers

1. Bone cancers are categorized by the tissue of origin, anatomical location, and age at occurrence. Which of the following bone cancers is accurately described?
   A. Ewing sarcoma arises from osteoid cells; usually occurs in the upper arms, legs, and rib cage; and occurs in persons from 10 to 25 years of age.
   B. Chondrosarcoma begins in immature nerve tissue, is usually located in the bone marrow, and occurs in persons 20 to 45 years of age.
   C. Osteosarcoma emerges from osteoid tissue; is usually located in the knees, upper legs, and upper arms; and affects people 10 to 25 years of age.
   D. Myoma arises from the myelin sheath of the nerve and develops into a cartilaginous tumor that occurs in the major joints and is usually found in persons 20 to 35 years of age.

2. Which occurrence sites and rates for the Ewing family of tumors listed below are correct?
   A. Lower extremities, 30%; pelvis, 33%; chest wall, 11%; upper extremities, 6%; skull, 7%; and spine, 13%
   B. Lower extremities, 56%; pelvis, 13%; chest wall, 1%; upper extremities, 12%; skull, 4%; and spine, 14%
   C. Lower extremities, 35%; pelvis, 30%; chest wall, 3%; upper extremities, 22%; skull, 2%; and spine, 8%
   D. Lower extremities, 41%; pelvis, 26%; chest wall, 16%; upper extremities, 9%; spine, 6%; and skull, 2%

3. J.T. was treated for Ewing sarcoma of the thigh area when he was 20 years old, approximately 15 years ago. He has been well for many years. Now he appears tired and has an unexplained 15 pound weight loss, has a constant nonproductive cough, and shallow respirations. The nurse suspects he has
   A. developed metastatic disease to the lungs.
   B. pneumonia.
   C. mononucleosis.
   D. gastric metastases.

4. In light of his symptoms and his history, which diagnostic test should be ordered for J.T. initially?
   A. Chest radiography
   B. Computed tomography (CT) of the chest
   C. Bone scan
   D. Sputum for cytology

5. Which statement accurately describes Ewing sarcoma?
   A. Ewing sarcoma is primarily a disease of the bone in the upper body and usually affects adults.
   B. An estimated 35% to 50% of these patients will eventually become disease-free survivors.
   C. Radiation therapy is the primary treatment modality for Ewing sarcoma.
   D. Approximately 20% to 30% of patients have metastases at diagnosis. Metastatic spread occurs via the aggressive "round" cancer cell with indistinct borders.

6. Rhabdomyosarcoma
   A. occurs in adolescents 15 to 19 years old.
   B. emerges from synovial tissue.
   C. regularly presents in the head, neck, genitourinary tract, arms, legs, and neck.
   D. presents most often in the trunk.

7. What are skip metastases, often seen in patients with osteosarcoma?
   A. A pattern in which metastatic disease areas appear initially and then disappear with treatment, only to reappear at the same site again
   B. *Skip metastasis* is the term used in patients who do not develop the lung lesions common to osteosarcoma patients.
   C. Smaller areas of the same tumor occurring in the same bone but anatomically separated from the primary lesion
   D. Punched-out areas of severe bone loss in osteolytic lesions

8. Which statement about chondrosarcomas in children is accurate?
   A. They most often occur in the upper body, neck, and skull areas.
   B. They are soft tissue sarcomas that involve vascular tissue.
   C. They often present as dull, aching pain.
   D. They most commonly occur in infants.

9. G.J. is a 44-year-old man who works in the oil industry as a field engineer. He is on his feet most of the day, walks significant distances, and often physically assists the rig drillers. He describes a new onset of right leg pain just below the knee cap. The pain is described as aching and steady. He has a swollen lump on his fibula, firm, with no exudate, that is warm to touch. He has been limping for over a week when he walks. The patient denies any recent injury or fall. His preliminary diagnosis is osteosarcoma. Based on this history and diagnosis, the nurse would expect
   A. the alkaline phosphatase level to be elevated.
   B. the long bone radiographs to definitely reveal the lesion.
   C. the pain to decrease at night.
   D. there would also be pain in his left leg.

10. G.J.'s definitive diagnosis is chondrosarcoma. Which of the following also applies to chondrosarcoma?
   A. It occurs most often between the ages of 30 and 60 years.
   B. The diagnostic workup includes Bence Jones urine.
   C. Metastases are commonly to the brain, other bones, and the prostate.
   D. It is treated with precision surgery with narrow margins.

11. Leiomyosarcoma is a type of soft tissue sarcoma arising from smooth muscle and would likely be found in the
   A. gastrocnemius muscle.
   B. uterus.
   C. bladder.
   D. bicep muscles.

12. A tumor described as being seen within the bone on long bone radiographs as a "moth-eaten pattern" is likely a high-grade
   A. fibrosarcoma.
   B. synovial sarcoma.
   C. chondrosarcoma.
   D. lymphangiosarcoma.

13. Ewing sarcoma is a malignant tumor usually originating in the bone, primarily the long bone. Occasionally, the tumor will manifest itself outside the bone, in the muscles and soft tissue. This is called
   A. extraskeletal Ewing sarcoma.
   B. extraosseous Ewing sarcoma.
   C. primitive neuroectodermal tumor (PNET).
   D. dermatofibrosarcoma.

14. S.W. is a 6-year-old boy who has been referred to the pediatric oncology clinic for ongoing flulike symptoms and fatigue. His mother reports he has complained of left leg pain, but she does not see any bumps or lumps on his legs, and she knows of no fall or injury. The nurse suspects he may have Ewing sarcoma and also expects that
   A. a complete blood cell count (CBC) would reveal thrombocytopenia.
   B. he may report feeling cool numbness over the area.
   C. he will likely experience swelling and pain in the affected area.
   D. a diagnosis of Ewing is the first choice diagnosis of all bone and soft tissue sarcomas.

15. In patients who have soft tissue tumors,
   A. more than 30% will be diagnosed in the early stages of disease.
   B. most present with a swollen mass (>5 cm) which is usually painful.
   C. the goal of treatment is to remove the tumor, avoid amputation, and preserve function.
   D. a diagnostic workup often includes a spinal tap.

16. In the past, soft tissue tumor subtypes have been classified by their anatomical location. Currently, the classification system is based on
   A. cell histology.
   B. radiography results.
   C. tissue of origin.
   D. the degree of intracompartmental involvement.

17. Soft tissue sarcomas arise from the mesodermal layer of cell origin. These tumors can originate from several cells types—fat, nerve, muscle, joints, or deep skin tissues. Which statement accurately lists the incidence for the corresponding sites?
   A. Extremities, 45%; trunk and retroperitoneum, 23%; and viscera, 18%
   B. Extremities, 40%; trunk and retroperitoneum, 35%; and head and neck, 15%
   C. Lower extremities, 35%; upper extremities, 20%; retroperitoneum and GI tract, 30%; and head and neck, 15%
   D. Lower extremities, 25%; upper extremities, 40%; head and neck, 15%; and retroperitoneum, 20%

18. K.C., a 16-year-old basketball player, has a new diagnosis of osteosarcoma in his left thigh. He has been scheduled for surgery in an attempt to remove the tumor and preserve function. His parents are distraught over this diagnosis because K.C. had plans to play basketball in college. K.C. does not say much. His oncology nurse's role would be to
    A. tell him to focus on the prospect of rehabilitation and assure him that he will likely play college basketball.
    B. tell the patient and his parents that the nurse will see that a psychiatric consult is requested so K.C. can deal with his feelings.
    C. tell the patient and his mother that before surgery, the nurse wants him to reduce his anxiety by keeping his shades pulled in the room and refusing any visitors.
    D. tell K.C. that the nurse has cared for several patients with his diagnosis, and the nurse knows this must be very upsetting for him.

19. Nursing care of patients undergoing amputations would include preoperative education regarding phantom limb pain. An explanation would include the following facts:
    A. symptoms of phantom limb pain usually last for up to 1 year after surgery.
    B. patients may experience fever, diaphoresis, nausea, and loss of appetite.
    C. phantom limb pain can be triggered by stress, emotional upset, and fatigue.
    D. the more distal the amputation, the more intense phantom limb pain will be.

20. The nurse working in an outpatient oncology clinic is caring for a 23-year-old young woman who is a dancer. She is to undergo an amputation of her lower left leg. The patient reports that she is fine with it and has resolved herself to the fact that she will not be dancing any longer. As she leaves the clinic however, she is wiping away tears. The nurses' best response is to
    A. approach her and ask to speak with her for a few minutes.
    B. do nothing. It is natural for her to be upset, and this is something she needs to deal with on her own.
    C. call the pastoral services department and ask that they meet with the patient at her next appointment.
    D. contact the patient at home and give her information regarding a support group for amputees in the local area.

21. Postoperative nursing care of the patient who has had a limb amputated includes ⚠️
    A. frequent wrapping of the stump with elastic bandages or stump shrinkers.
    B. assisting the patient into a flat supine position for 30 minutes per day.
    C. elevating the stump for the first 48 hours after surgery.
    D. assisting the patient to dangle at side of bed and transfer to a chair on third day after surgery.

22. What factor would not affect the decision to amputate versus perform limb salvage surgery in bone and soft tissue cancers?
    A. Age, especially in children younger than 10 years, because surgery will affect limb growth
    B. Whether chemotherapy will also be used
    C. The ability to obtain acceptable surgical margins
    D. The nature of the blood vessels and nerves involved with the tumor

23. A patient with an osteosarcoma will undergo many diagnostic tests that reveal a variety of results as the disease progresses. Which of the following does not describe patterns of tumor growth seen in radiographs?
    A. High-grade tumors possibly appearing soft and viscous
    B. Low-grade lesions with margins having a moth-eaten pattern
    C. Aggressive tumors seen as perpendicular striated tissue (sunburst pattern)
    D. Appear "radish-like" on radiographs because of multiple layers of subperiosteal bone

24. Soft tissue tumors can be radiosensitive and radioresponsive. Radiation therapy is most effective in tumors that
    A. have metastasized.
    B. are localized
    C. are located in the brain
    D. have recurred.

18 HIV-Related Cancers

1. Which of the following are true statements about human immunodeficiency virus (HIV)?
   A. HIV-2 is more virulent than HIV-1.
   B. HIV has a short incubation and gradual progression.
   C. The average time from HIV infection to acquired immunodeficiency syndrome (AIDS) is 5 to 7 years.
   D. The average life expectancy is 11 to 14 years.

2. An infectious and lifestyle factor that does not negatively affect HIV disease progression is
   A. hepatitis C virus.
   B. poor nutrition.
   C. smoking.
   D. circumcised males.

3. Which statement is true about HIV prevalence?
   A. Heterosexual women comprise 30% of HIV diagnoses per year.
   B. African Americans and Asians are disproportionately affected.
   C. Approximately 20% of patients are unaware of an HIV diagnosis.
   D. Patients younger than age 40 years are the fastest growing HIV-positive patients at increased risk for non–AIDS-defining diseases and cancers.

4. Which of the following is the most frequently diagnosed AIDS-defining malignancy?
   A. Kaposi sarcoma (KS)
   B. B-cell lymphoma
   C. Cervical cancer
   D. Head and neck cancer

5. Which statement is not true about malignancies associated with viral infection?
   A. Patients are more likely to present with distant metastasis.
   B. These cancers are more common in white patients.
   C. These patients are more likely to be female.
   D. These cancers have a more accelerated conversion to malignancy in HIV-infected patients.

6. Which of the following nononcologic medications do not adversely interact with antiretroviral agents?
   A. Anticonvulsants
   B. Benzodiazepines
   C. Antiemetics
   D. Dexamethasone

7. What factors are associated with shorter survival in patients with HIV-related lymphoma?
   A. Stage II disease only
   B. CD4 count less than 400 cells/mm^3
   C. Age younger than 35 years
   D. Elevated lactic dehydrogenase

8. According to Centers for Disease Control and Prevention (CDC) guidelines, when should universal precautions be used to decrease the nurse's risk of occupational exposure to HIV? When the nurse is
   A. wiping a patient's tears.
   B. using a washcloth to remove diaphoresis in a feverish patient.
   C. draining peritoneal fluid from a patient with ascites.
   D. applying lotion to dry skin.

9. Which of the following is false about the histopathology of HIV-related lymphoma?
   A. Small cell lymphomas are typically found in the gastrointestinal (GI) tract.
   B. Large cell lymphomas are more likely to involve the meninges.
   C. The majority of HIV-related lymphomas are intermediate or high-grade B-cell type.
   D. Lesions are painful and may be mistaken for KS.

10. Which treatments may be used to manage a patient diagnosed with primary central nervous system lymphoma (PCNSL) presenting with multiple lesions?
    A. Systemic bleomycin
    B. High-dose methotrexate and cytarabine
    C. High-dose Adriamycin
    D. Systemic chemotherapy with Cytoxan

11. In patients with HIV-related KS, the following are true about survival except
    A. shorter in patients with B symptoms.
    B. worse in patients with prior opportunistic infections.
    C. not improved in patients receiving combined antiretroviral therapy (cART).
    D. shorter in patients with GI tract lesions

12. J.D. is a 62-year-old gay man diagnosed with HIV and Hodgkin lymphoma. He is currently taking chemotherapy and has experienced low blood counts, fatigue, diarrhea, nausea, and vomiting. He has been in a monogamous relationship for the past 5 years and is concerned about transmitting HIV to his partner, who has tested negative. Which of the following strategies can be taught to J.D. and his partner to decrease the possibility of HIV transmission? ⚠

    A. When cleaning up J.D.'s body fluids, gloves do not need to be worn.

    B. Avoid sharing personal care items such as razors and toothbrushes.

    C. Recommend that it is important to use a condom of any kind during every episode of vaginal, rectal, or oral intercourse.

    D. Suggest abstaining from intercourse until chemotherapy has been completed because of the risk of infection.

13. Which of the following cancer screening techniques should be implemented in HIV-positive patients?

    A. Pap smear every 2 years for early detection of cervical cancer

    B. Periodic oral or dental examination to detect early oropharyngeal masses that can signal HPV-related squamous cell head and neck cancer

    C. Annual chest radiography to assess high-risk patients for lung cancer

    D. Annual screening with cytology or high-resolution colonoscopy for early detection of squamous cell cancer

14. What is a nursing intervention that can be used to maximize safety in patients undergoing treatment for HIV-related malignancies? ⚠

    A. Ask patients if they are experiencing any jaw pain or numbness or tingling in their fingers and toes; peripheral neuropathies are common in patients taking chemotherapy and antiretroviral agents.

    B. Instruct patients to stop any routine exercise program to preserve strength.

    C. Encourage patients to use aspirin for the management of malignancy-related pain.

    D. Counsel patients to increase caloric intake by eating three large meals daily.

15. Which of the following is true about other malignancies associated with HIV?

    A. Hepatitis B and HIV is more commonly associated with primary liver cancer than hepatitis C and HIV.

    B. Anal cancer has the highest incidence of death among HIV-related cancers.

    C. cART does not improve survival in patients with HIV infection and lung cancer.

    D. HIV infection increases the chance of cervical cancer recurrence after treatment.

16. A.M. is a 37-year-old Latina woman diagnosed with stage III cervical cancer and HIV infection. After a recent hysterectomy and lymph node dissection, she is going to start chemotherapy and cART. The nurse is concerned about her ability to understand the complex treatment regimen planned for her. Which of the following is true about health literacy that can inform a teaching strategy?

    A. Low health literacy issues are easily managed when a family caregiver is present and can translate for the patient.

    B. Low health literacy will not affect the patient's understanding of CD4 counts, viral load, and chemotherapy treatments.

    C. There are low rates of anti-retroviral medication adherence in patients with low health literacy.

    D. Low health literacy is associated with approximately 50% of patients maintaining regular medical care.

Questions 17 to 20 all discuss J.T.

17. J.T. is a 49-year-old man who visits his primary care physician with complaints of fever, chills, night sweats, and malaise. On history and physical examination, he has multiple enlarged lymph nodes and unexplained weight loss of approximately 15 lb over the past month. He has also had a cough for the past few weeks that has not gone away. He is gay, has multiple partners, smokes a pack of cigarettes a day, and drinks socially. He denies the current use of drugs but has had experience with cocaine in the past. His PCP explains that he would like to test him for HIV, order chest radiography, and send him for biopsy of one of the enlarged lymph nodes. Which of the following tests would not be helpful to confirm HIV positivity?

    A. ELISA (enzyme-linked immunosorbent assay) for antibody to HIV; if the result is positive, it should be repeated. A second positive test result is followed by a Western blot.

    B. Epstein-Barr virus test

    C. PCR (polymerase chain reaction)

    D. CD4 count

    E. Viral load test

18. J.T. has laboratory confirmation of HIV infection and a CD4 T-lymphocyte count of 180 cells/mm^3. Using CDC guidelines, what is his HIV staging?

    A. Stage I

    B. Stage II

    C. Stage III

    D. Stage IV

19. J.T.'s chest radiograph is positive for a pleural effusion, and the lymph node biopsy suggests non-Hodgkin lymphoma (NHL). A bone marrow biopsy is positive for NHL. Which of the following treatments might be started?
    A. cART therapy
    B. Chemotherapy using MBACOD
    C. Intrathecal administration of chemotherapy
    D. Stem cell transplant

20. J.T. has a limited support system. His parents are elderly and do not approve of his lifestyle. He does not have a consistent significant other but has many work colleagues. He does not want anyone to know about his diagnosis at this time. He has quite a few friends who have tested positive for HIV; some of his friends have died. At this time, which of the following nursing interventions is not appropriate to incorporate into the care plan to address his psychosocial needs?
    A. Determine J.T.'s past experience with illness.
    B. Explore his concerns about his diagnosis and treatment and his feelings about serious illness.
    C. Observe for signs of maladaptive coping strategies, especially because he has a history of substance use in the past; assist J.T. with learning alternative behaviors to manage stress and cope with his diagnosis.
    D. Include persons identified by the patient as significant others in teaching and care decisions.

21. What is not true about HIV-related KS?
    A. There is no causative association between Kaposi sarcoma herpesvirus (KSHV) and KS.
    B. Survival has increased with the use of cART.
    C. KS skin lesions range from purple to brown and are often painless.
    D. The incidence of KS in the United States is on the decline.

22. According to the Walter Reed Staging system for HIV, which of the following is true?
    A. If an opportunistic infection is present, the patient is in stage 6.
    B. If oral thrush is present, the patient is in stage 4.
    C. If chronic lymphadenopathy is present, the patient is in stage 1
    D. If patient has an abnormal skin test result, the patient is in stage 3.

24. What is not true regarding good- and poor-risk KS?
    A. Good-risk KS has a CD4 count less than 200/mcL.
    B. Poor-risk KS may have a history of oral thrush.
    C. Poor-risk KS has presence of B symptoms.
    D. Good-risk KS has a Karnofsky score greater than 70.

24. Which of the following statements is not true regarding anti-retroviral and chemotherapy agents that interact to cause toxicity?
    A. Zidovudine and gemcitabine can cause severe myelosuppression.
    B. Atazanavir and bevacizumab can cause hypotension.
    C. Tenofovir and Platinol can cause renal dysfunction.
    D. Stavudine and vinblastine can cause peripheral neuropathy.

25. Which of the following is an anti-retroviral inducer when administered with cyclophosphamide?
    A. Atazanavir
    B. Nelfinavir
    C. Nevirapine
    D. Zidovudine

26. Signs or symptoms related to a primary effusion lymphoma include which of the following?
    A. Cognitive changes and headaches
    B. Cough and dyspnea
    C. Malabsorption and diarrhea
    D. Epstein-Barr virus (EBV) titer positive

27. The nurse knows that in evaluating laboratory data of people with HIV-related cancers,
    A. chemotherapy will also cause a decrease in the CD4 count.
    B. CD4/T4 lymphocyte count increases in the absence of HAART.
    C. serum levels of B2 microglobulin will decrease in progressive infection.
    D. core antigen p24 serum levels will decrease with progressive infection.

19 Nursing Implications of Surgical Treatment

1. A patient describes her upcoming breast biopsy as using a fairly large needle to extract a piece of tissue. She is describing a(n)
   A. excisional biopsy.
   B. aspiration biopsy.
   C. core needle biopsy.
   D. incisional biopsy.

2. J.B., a 73-year-old man, has an increased risk for cholangiocarcinoma due to a history of primary sclerosing cholangitis. A few weeks ago, he became jaundiced, developed right upper quadrant discomfort, and experienced a decreased appetite. He has lost 14 lbs in a 2-week period. His liver enzymes are elevated, and a computed tomography (CT) scan reveals a common bile duct dilatation. The nurse expects him to be scheduled for
   A. multimodality treatment.
   B. endoscopic retrograde cholangiopancreatography (ERCP). → probably has a gallstone
   C. upper endoscopy.
   D. Swans-Ganz catheter placement.

3. Considering J.B.'s scenario above, which could also be considered as an option in his case?
   A. Placement of an Ommaya reservoir
   B. Placement of a Groshong catheter
   C. Stent placement by interventional radiology
   D. Brachytherapy with seed implant

4. M.B. is a 43-year-old woman who has been treated for colon cancer over the past 4 years and now has metastatic spread to the liver. She has many small tumors in her liver, scattered over both the right and left lobes. Which of the following would be a treatment option for her?
   A. Robotic surgery
   B. Preoperative radiation
   C. Carrier testing
   D. Ablation therapy

5. A patient is having his left leg amputated owing to sarcoma. He is in the operating room suite, and the lead operating room nurse is speaking to the surgeon, his assistant, and the staff. She reviews information about the operation (the patient, purpose, and site) and then asks if there are any questions. This process is called ⚠
   A. time out.
   B. review of systems.
   C. sign in.
   D. sign out.

6. B.C. is an 80-year-old woman with type 2 diabetes and chronic obstructive pulmonary disorder (COPD). She is scheduled to undergo exploratory laparotomy for suspected intestinal obstruction owing to colon cancer. She is in good health overall. Her diabetes is managed with oral agents. She smoked for 15 years but does not smoke any longer and does not require oxygen at home. According to the American Society of Anesthesiologists (ASA) classification system, which is B.C.'s status?
   A. ASA Physical Status 2
   B. ASA Physical Status 3
   C. ASA Physical Status 4
   D. ASA Physical Status 6

7. A peripheral nerve block is associated with which of the following?
   A. No sympathetic decrease in blood pressure
   B. Nausea, urinary retention, and itching
   C. Incompatibility with other forms of anesthesia
   D. Provides a short duration of pain relief (~4 hours)

8. C.G. underwent urgent abdominal laparotomy 3 days ago for a suspected bowel obstruction. A large cancerous mass was found in her descending colon. Today she is alert, but the nurse finds her slightly short of breath and somewhat listless. Her temperature is 100.8° F. When the nurse offered her some water, she appears too weak to sip it. What is the most important diagnostic test or intervention should C.G. have?
   A. An increase in her IV fluids to 150 cc/hr
   B. Tylenol 500 mg PO every 6 hours around the clock
   C. Blood cultures drawn stat
   D. Chest radiography stat

9. A patient just had breast reconstruction after a mastectomy and asks the nurse why she needs to have a drainage tube hanging out of her dressing. The nurse explains that drains are used to
   A. prevent the accumulation of fluid (e.g., pus, blood).
   B. allow for wound granulation.
   C. infusion of antibiotics to the wound, if necessary.
   D. allow for silicone injection into the breast.

10. A patient is undergoing lumpectomy for breast cancer followed by external beam radiation. She is asking for clarification of the rationale for the external beam. The nurse explains that
    A. this is called adjuvant therapy and is used to eliminate possible microscopic disease and decrease the risk of local recurrence.
    B. it is palliative therapy to improve her quality of life by decreasing the risk of local recurrence.
    C. the lumpectomy was performed to establish the type of cancer she has. This will be her primary treatment.
    D. today's cancer treatment always includes a combination of therapies, and there is no "primary" treatment.

11. Which factors are the most important overall considerations for wound healing?
    A. Recent transfusion and renal compromise or dialysis
    B. Poor circulation, age, and immune response
    C. Pain management, mobility, and timing of dressing changes
    D. Depth of the wound, dehiscence, and potassium deficiency

12. A patient recently underwent a wide excision and groin resection for synovial cell carcinoma. He calls the outpatient clinic complaining of swelling, redness at the incision site, and a low-grade fever. What should the nurse tell the patient?
    A. These are normal postoperative symptoms.
    B. Take your antidiuretic medication.
    C. Just call us back if your fever increases.
    D. You must come in and be seen.

13. A 45-year-old patient with a history of moderate ulcerative colitis is scheduled for a total colectomy with ileostomy creation. The surgeon says this is prophylactic cancer surgery, which is
    A. the reconstruction of anatomic defects to improve function and cosmetic appearance.
    B. surgery performed on an organ that has an extremely high risk of developing cancer.
    C. the insertion of various therapeutic hardware during active treatment periods to facilitate the delivery of treatment and increase patient comfort.
    D. to combat hormonal influence of the cancer.

14. The nurse is caring for a patient who has just returned from having a total laryngectomy. The nurse's immediate postoperative priority is
    A. pain management.
    B. maintaining an effective airway.
    C. maintaining effective communication.
    D. providing adequate nutrition.

15. An immediate educational priority for the patient who has had a total laryngectomy is
    A. a referral for speech therapy, functional swallowing assessment.
    B. a referral to a counselor for emotional issues surrounding his diagnosis.
    C. nutritional instruction that addresses wound healing.
    D. appropriate safety measures regarding the patient's life with a stoma.

16. The purpose of cytoreductive surgery is to
    A. establish tissue diagnosis.
    B. remove nonvital organs and tissues that have high risk or cancer regrowth.
    C. reduce tumor volume and improve the effect of other cancer treatment modalities.
    D. promote client comfort and quality of life without the aim of cure of disease.

17. Which of these surgical techniques involves the removal of bulky cancer with contiguous tissues, nodes, and vascular structures required to attain safe margins?
    A. Debulking resection
    B. Ablation
    C. En bloc resection
    D. Local excision

18. A patient underwent extensive surgery for stage IV ovarian cancer. Within 1 month of surgery, she began her chemotherapy. Now she presents with a partially dehisced incision and wound with continuous yellow-colored drainage. In managing her wound care, the nurse would anticipate
    A. using a method to protect the periwound area from drainage.
    B. cleaning the wound with closure at skin level using glue, staples, or stitches.
    C. consulting a social worker to explore the patient's feelings about an open wound.
    D. discussing the use of total parenteral nutrition with the physician.

19. Postoperatively, cancer patients are at greater risks for venous thromboembolism (VTE) in all of the following situations except
    A. been taking Rifampin or St. John's Wort.
    B. a previous history of cardiotoxic chemotherapy.
    C. used Thalidomide or Lenalidomide.
    D. had previous VTE.

20. Radiation therapy before cancer surgery can
    A. improve tumor resectability and alter the extent of surgery needed.
    B. affect the extent of surgery needed but also increase the functional disabilities after therapy.
    C. provide a more appealing option to patients but decrease treatment outcomes.
    D. improve treatment outcomes but increase the functional disabilities after therapy.

21. A.P. was diagnosed with colon cancer 7 years ago and underwent a left hemicolectomy. Over the past 5 years, he has been treated with both radiation treatments and chemotherapy, most recently with methotrexate and 5-FU. He has just returned to the nurse's unit from the recovery room after a right-sided colon resection for a circumferential mass lesion in his ascending colon. Knowing his history, which of the following conditions would not be considered a primary concern?
    A. Myocardial infarction
    B. Skin breakdown
    C. Diarrhea and dehydration
    D. Pulmonary fibrosis

22. Before the surgery, A.P. (from question 22) had right upper quadrant pain and an elevated carcinoembryonic antigen (CEA) of 14.0 ng/mL. An ileocecal malignancy was found, which caused persistent inflammation and abscess formation behind the cecum and the ascending colon. Because of the high potential for postoperative infections, perforations, wound contamination, and complications, the decision was made to leave the incision open for at least 2 days after surgery. This is called
    A. primary intention.
    B. laparoscopic approach.
    C. secondary intention.
    D. tertiary intention.

23. The patient's rehabilitation after cancer surgery is most positively affected by
    A. multidisciplinary discharge planning.
    B. referrals to support groups related to the patient's specific type of cancer.
    C. adequate pain management.
    D. specific instructions on any assistive or prosthetic device used after surgery.

20 Nursing Implications of Blood and Marrow Transplant

1. Which of the following is a basic principle of hematopoietic stem cell transplantation (HSCT)?
   A. The doses of antitumor treatment allow the rescuing of the hematopoietic system from the marrow-ablative effect of the treatment received.
   B. Stem cells are more effective for rescue of the recipient's hematopoietic system than cells from the marrow.
   C. Tumors that are resistant to chemotherapy can be treated effectively to increase the likelihood of a cure.
   D. Effective use of antimicrobials and carefully orchestrated preventative measures can decrease the risk of infections.

2. A patient is going to receive a stem cell transplant. Awareness of which of the following would guide the nurse in providing the client and family with supportive information?
   A. Syngeneic transplant provides the client with stem cells from a similar genetic match, drastically decreasing the risk for rejection.
   B. Allografting involves transplanting stem cells from a donor who is genetically different; thus the match is determined by blood typing.
   C. In allografting, the coexisting of donor and host stem cells in a mixed chimerism state can actually be beneficial.
   D. Autografting carries the risk of reinfusing malignant cells; thus, the cells must be treated before the infusion.

3. The family of B.C., who is scheduled for HSCT, questions why she requires additional radiation therapy as part of the conditioning for transplant when they had been told her disease was in remission. The nurse would respond by stating the purpose of the conditioning regimen is to
   A. prevent graft-versus-host disease (GVHD) for the recipient.
   B. eradicate malignant cells and decrease the risk of graft rejection.
   C. reduce the adverse effects during the acute phase of transplant
   D. mobilize HSCT cells from the bone marrow to the peripheral blood.

4. Sources of hematopoietic stem cells for transplantation can be derived from
   A. animal placenta and peripheral blood.
   B. whole blood previously collected for blood transfusions.
   C. bone marrow or blood circulating in the peripheral system of the donor.
   D. the blood cells pooled in the spleen of a donor.

5. A nonmyeloablative HSCT (mini-HSCT) is performed in clients who are
   A. young and newly diagnosed with disease involving the marrow, thus requiring an allogeneic transplant from an umbilical stem cell donor.
   B. scheduled for umbilical stem cell transplant with no current evidence of disease in the recipient's marrow.
   C. older with preexisting comorbid conditions who have disease that is likely to recur in the future.
   D. scheduled for autologous stem cell transplants but do not want to experience the intense side effects they have heard about.

6. Mr. O. has just been given the diagnosis of aplastic anemia. His family members are HLA typed for a possible match for a transplant. Unfortunately, there is no match. Mr. O asks his physician if he could be considered for an autologous HSCT. The physician tells the client that an autologous transplantation is not possible because
   A. autologous transplants for aplastic anemia are performed only on small children.
   B. aplastic anemia attacks and destroys the hematopoietic system, leaving diseased and insufficient cells to perform an autologous HSCT.
   C. the national marrow donor registry only recognizes unrelated transplants for clients with aplastic anemia.
   D. the cure rate for treating aplastic anemia with an autologous transplant is too risky because of his age.

7. The goal of pretransplant conditioning regimen is to
   A. reduce any remaining malignancy in the recipient to increase the likelihood of a cure.
   B. suppress the immune system of the recipient to allow for marrow engraftment (allografts only).
   C. decrease the risk of posttransplant complications especially life-threatening infections.
   D. combine high-dose chemotherapy with total lymph node or total body irradiation.

8. An allogeneic HSCT is one in which donor cells are derived from
   A. an HLA-matched donor.
   B. the client's own marrow.
   C. the client's identical twin.
   D. a cadaver of an individual who gave permission.

9. What is not a factor that may increase HSCT-related complications?
   A. Prior combination chemotherapy and radiation therapy
   B. Underlying kidney dysfunction
   C. Psychosocial dysfunction
   D. Previous infections

10. Common acute complications after HSCT are
    A. chronic graft-versus-host-disease.
    B. nausea, vomiting, and infection.   ] 80+ days
    C. herpes varicella zoster infection.
    D. impaired growth and development in children.

11. The target organs of acute graft-versus-host-disease (GVHD) are the
    A. skin, liver, and gastrointestinal (GI) tract.
    B. vagina, heart, and spleen.
    C. skin, pancreas, and brain.
    D. GI tract, eyes, and mouth.

12. Veno-occlusive disease (VOD) or Hepatic Sinusoidal Obstruction Syndrome (HSOS)
    A. occurs 100 days after HSCT.
    B. occurs only in recipients of allogeneic HSCT.
    C. occurs only in the stomach and heart.
    D. occurs between 3 to 21 days after HSCT.
       * both autos + allos

13. Mr. O. had an allogeneic HSCT 16 days ago. The nurse notes that Mr. O. has a weight gain of 5 lb since yesterday. He asks the nurse repeatedly what day it is. He also complains of upper right quadrant pain. The nurse suspects that Mr. O.
    A. may have acute gastrointestinal GVHD.
    B. is manifesting classic symptoms of VOD.
    C. needs a nonsteroidal antiinflammatory agent for pain.
    D. is not at risk for VOD because he has had an allogeneic HSCT.

14. A transplant center has a teaching program for all clients and their family members to prepare them for discharge. The nurse teaches the clients and family members that the most important method to avoid infections is to
    A. scrub the kitchen and bathrooms with bleach daily.
    B. wash their hands often and meticulously.
    C. stay at home except to come to the clinic.
    D. monitor temperatures every 2 hours.

15. Which of the following is an example of an intervention that demonstrates nurses' primary role in the outcomes of hematopoietic stem cell transplant (HSCT)? ⚠
    A. Reducing the risk for injury through teaching the client and family strategies to decrease risk of infection and bleeding during the period of aplasia
    B. Reducing the risk for anxiety as a complication by encouraging the client to rest and comply with protective isolation requirements
    C. Reducing the risk for complications from cyclophosphamide-induced hyponatremia by administering mesna as ordered
    D. Reducing the risk for veno-occlusive disease/hepatic sinusoidal obstruction syndrome by administering graft-versus-host-disease prophylaxis

16. Use of cryotherapy (ice chips) is an evidence-based mucositis prevention nursing intervention for clients receiving which chemotherapy agent?
    A. Etoposide infusion
    B. High dose melphalan
    C. Thiotepa intravenous
    D. Voriconazole prophylaxis

17. Which of the following is true regarding idiopathic pulmonary interstitial pneumonitis (infectious and noninfectious)?
    A. It occurs most frequently in younger clients who received busulfan and radiation therapy as part of the preparatory regimen.
    B. Interventions such as encouraging activity, turning, coughing, and deep breathing have little impact if the damage is interstitial.
    C. Intravenous and aerosolized antimicrobial therapy have demonstrated only minimal effectiveness if the client has hemorrhage.
    D. Clients with a history of chest irradiation or bleomycin therapy are at an increased risk for this complication.

21 Nursing Implications of Radiation Therapy

1. Which of the following is most accurate? Radiation therapy (RT) involves
   A. electromagnetic radiation in the form of energy waves; examples include protons, x-rays, and gamma rays.
   B. particulate radiation in the form of subatomic particles; examples include electrons, alpha particles, and photons.
   C. ionizing radiation in the form of x-rays, gamma rays, protons, and cosmic radiation.
   D. the ionizing radiation interacting with the atoms and molecules of the tumor cells, especially RNA.

2. Which of the following does not influence the biologic response to radiation?
   A. Level of DNA damage
   B. Oxygen effect
   C. Sensitivity of cell to radiation
   D. Ability of body to clear toxins

3. Which of the following are true about the "four Rs" of radiobiology?
   A. They include repair, redistribution, reoxygenation, and radiosensitivity
   B. Redistribution is the bringing of more cells into mitosis phase of the cell cycle.
   C. Repair occurs as decreased tumor burden allows better blood flow in the tumor.
   D. The time in which biologic changes appear and the severity of the effects of radiation are dependent on the four Rs.

4. As a nurse responsible for teaching a client and family members regarding cancer treatment for lung cancer, the goal would be for them to understand which of the following?
   A. Definitive RT is a primary cancer treatment with or without chemotherapy. The purpose is to kill all cells in a malignant tumor while limiting the dose to normal tissues.
   B. Neoadjuvant RT is given ~~after~~ *before* definitive treatment to ensure local control of disease remaining in the areas of the tumor.
   C. Adjuvant RT is given ~~before~~ *after* definitive treatment to shrink tumor and facilitate complete resection of the primary tumor.
   D. Control RT is given to high-risk areas to improve quality of life by preventing the future spread of disease in vulnerable areas. *at any point*

5. What is the purpose of total-body irradiation (TBI) as part of the preparatory regimen before allogeneic transplant? TBI is used to
   A. eliminate from the body any unwanted bacteria before an anticipated period of neutropenia.
   B. deplete T-cell levels in the transplant recipient, thereby decreasing the chance of graft-versus-host disease (GVHD).
   C. mobilize increased numbers of progenitor stem cells from the donor's bone marrow into peripheral circulation for collection.
   D. kill any residual malignant cells and immunosuppress the engraftment.

6. Mr. B. is scheduled to undergo external-beam radiotherapy to his lumbar spine for his metastatic prostate cancer. During the initial nursing assessment, his nurse notes that his baseline hemoglobin (Hgb) is 10 g/dL. The treatment plan includes evaluation of his energy level weekly because
   A. external-beam radiation to any field involving bone marrow will decrease the baseline Hgb by half within 1 week.
   B. Mr. B will likely be nauseated from his therapy and be unable to maintain an iron-rich diet.
   C. hematuria commonly occurs after this type of radiation therapy, resulting in an increase in his anemia.
   D. the standard of care during radiation therapy includes a weekly physical assessment to optimally manage all possible side effects of the therapy or underlying disease.

7. The most common and recommended measurement of radiation exposure is
   A. LDR. – *brachytherapy*
   B. Rads.
   C. Grays.
   D. HVL.

8. When preparing a teaching plan for a client and family regarding radiopharmaceutical therapy, how would the nurse differentiate it from other types of radiation therapy for cancer?
   A. The principles of time, distance, and shielding are not as critical because the source is sealed in a special container for treatment.
   B. It is delivered intravenously, orally, or into a body cavity; the radioactivity is distributed fairly evenly over the body.
   C. Because it is a pharmaceutical product, the regulation is less stringent than external source of radiation therapy.
   D. It allows uptake of radioactive exposure at a predetermined dose to a target organ or area of the body.

9. Which factor does not influence the side effects of radiation therapy? *not a factor*
   A. Time-dose-distance volume relationship
   B. Radiosensitivity for both acute and delayed effects
   C. Ability of client to maintain nutritional intake
   D. Radiation type, energy, and depth of treatment

10. To maximize radiation protection and safety based on the principles of time, distance, and shielding, safety measures include ⚠
   A. use of biohazardous containers to transport the linens to the laundry while a client is receiving radiation therapy via an unsealed source.
   B. restricting use of the toilet for body fluids while the client is receiving radiation therapy via an unsealed source.
   C. promptly replacing any dressings at the implant site that become displaced for the patient receiving therapy via a sealed radioactive source.
   D. measuring the exposure rate of all staff providing direct care as well as rates in uncontrolled areas such as the room next door.

11. Which of the following are identified as acute-responding tissues for radiation therapy?
   A. Testis, small bowel, and thyroid
   B. Oral mucosa, vagina, and larynx
   C. Salivary gland, liver, and lymph vessels
   D. Bone marrow, ovaries, and uterus

12. Individuals undergoing pelvic radiotherapy for colorectal cancer might experience which of the following secondary side effects?
   A. Hypokalemia
   B. Hypocalcemia
   C. Hyperphosphatemia
   D. Hypermagnesemia

diarrhea = primary
↳ lose K in dia

13. The delivery of radiation therapy is divided into small fractions for what reason?
   A. Delivering the same total dose of radiation at one time can only be done by use of brachytherapy technique.
   B. Fractionation allows for recovery of the surrounding nonmalignant tissues and in some tissues promotes recruitment of the malignant cells into the cell cycle for an improved cell kill.
   C. Daily treatments over several weeks allow for the development of a therapeutic relationship between the health care providers and the individual undergoing treatment.
   D. Fractionation helps to deoxygenate the malignant cells in the radiation field, making them more sensitive to the radiation.

14. Which of the following should be used when planning interventions related to knowledge deficit in patients?
   A. Determining who will be the learner (patient, family, significant other, or caregiver)
   B. Determining cultural influences on health education
   C. Providing teaching on potential side effects and side effect management based on an individual's learning style (written, verbal, audiovisual, presentation, or a combination of all of these)
   D. All of the above

22 Nursing Implications of Chemotherapy

1. Cancer chemotherapy is a systemic form of cancer treatment that is based on concepts of cellular kinetics, including the cell life cycle, cell cycle time, growth fraction, and tumor burden. Which statement correctly describes cellular kinetics?
   A. As the tumor burden increases, the growth rate quickens and the number of cells actively dividing increases.
   B. Tumor burden is the number of cells that are actively dividing in a tumor and responsive to treatment.
   C. Cell cycle time is the process of reproduction that occurs in normal as well as malignant cells.
   D. A shorter cell cycle time results in higher cell kill with exposure to cell cycle–specific agents.

2. The choice of agents to include in combination chemotherapy is guided by
   A. location of tumor.
   B. tumor burden and growth fraction.
   C. having different biologic effects.
   D. physical and psychosocial status of client.

3. Cardiac toxicity is most strongly associated with which chemotherapeutic agent?
   A. Fluorouracil (5FU)
   B. Doxorubicin (Adriamycin)
   C. Nitrogen mustard (Mustargen)
   D. Cisplatinum (Cisplatin)

4. When the goals of the current chemotherapy are to extend the length and improve quality of life, usually because a cure is not realistic, this is which type of therapy?
   A. Control
   B. Palliation
   C. Adjuvant
   D. Combination

5. Cell cycle–specific agents
   A. are dose dependent and must be administered as bolus doses.
   B. are schedule dependent and most effective if administered in divided doses or by continuous infusion.
   C. exert their major cytotoxic effects in all phases of the cell cycle.
   D. are most effective when administered as a short infusion.

6. Ms. J. complains of burning and pain at her peripheral intravenous (IV) site during vesicant administration. The nurse stops the infusion and aspirates for blood return. There is no blood return. What is indicated at this time? ⚠
   A. Stop the infusion, aspirate for residual medication, instill dexamethasone, remove the needle, and apply heat.
   B. Stop the infusion, instill sodium thiosulfate, remove the needle, and apply cold.
   C. Continue the infusion because there is no evidence of swelling or redness.
   D. Stop the infusion, aspirate for residual medication, remove the needle, and apply the recommended antidote.

7. Mr. P is receiving bleomycin as a systemic therapy. Which toxicity is most commonly associated with bleomycin (Blenoxane)?
   A. Renal toxicity with hemorrhagic cystitis
   B. Ototoxicity with tinnitus
   C. Pulmonary toxicity with pneumonitis
   D. Diarrhea beginning 24 hours after the completion of chemotherapy

8. Which of the following is not considered a chemoprotective agent?
   A. Dexrazoxane
   B. Amifostine
   C. Anthracycline
   D. Mesna

9. Which of the following statements is true about allergic reactions to chemotherapy?
   A. Reactions to paclitaxel occur most frequently after the third or fourth cycle.
   B. Reactions to platinum agents occur most often after the first or second infusion.
   C. Reactions to bleomycin are predictable based on skin testing.
   D. Any chemotherapy agent can cause an allergic reaction during any cycle.

10. Nursing responsibilities to foster client safety related to administration of antineoplastic agents include all of the following except
    A. ensuring the accuracy and completeness of chemotherapy orders.
    B. wearing required chemotherapy personal protective equipment (PPE).
    C. reviewing potential side effects and toxicities of agents to be administered.
    D. verifying previous and current laboratory test values for potential concerns.

11. The below established guidelines for the safe administration of chemotherapy and the safe handling of body wastes address safety for nurses, *except*
    A. occupational exposure to these agents include an increased risk for malignancies.
    B. the agents can cause embryofetal malformations/defects.
    C. the agents are associated with genotoxic effects schedule.
    D. administering the agents on the prescribed time.

12. Which of the following chemotherapy agents is considered a vesicant and requires dexrazoxane as an antidote?
    A. Idarubicin
    B. Carboplatin
    C. Cisplatin   *irritants*
    D. Ifosfamide
    → *sodium thiosulfate is the antidote*

13. All nurses involved in chemotherapy administration should know that
    A. surgical masks can be used to protect against vapors or aerosols.
    B. nurses who wear glasses can choose to opt out of wearing face shields.
    C. gowns should be disposable but can be reworn if only used by one nurse.
    D. double gloving is preferred for drug administration and handling body wastes.

14. When infusing vesicant chemotherapy agents through a central venous line, nurses should verify a blood return
    A. before the infusion.
    B. before, during, and after the administration.
    C. at the completion of the infusion.
    D. only if absolutely necessary.

15. Ms. S received her first cycle of intraperitoneal cisplatin yesterday via a Tenckhoff catheter for ovarian cancer. On assessment today, noted that she has a temperature of 101° F (38.3° C) and complains of abdominal pain. A potential cause of her symptoms is
    A. peritonitis caused by nonsterile access of the Tenckhoff catheter.
    B. that the tumor is responding to the intraperitoneal therapy.
    C. the chemotherapy was instilled too rapidly.
    D. that the drug was placed in an incorrect diluent.

16. The nurse has just begun the infusion of the first cycle of paclitaxel (Taxol) for Ms. T. She relates that she is feeling very uneasy and she is moving around in the chemotherapy chair. The nurse would suspect → *early sign of rxn*
    A. an impending hypersensitivity reaction.
    B. the client is overly anxious about getting chemotherapy.
    C. acting out to impress her husband about the seriousness of her illness.
    D. reacting to the prehydration fluids.

17. Ms. J. is being prepared for dismissal after chemotherapy administration of vincristine. Discharge medication instructions should include
    A. a bowel regimen to prevent constipation.
    B. a muscle relaxant to prevent foot drop. → *can also cause foot drop but would not prescribe relaxants for it*
    C. an anxiolytic to prevent hot flashes.
    D. loperamide (Imodium) to prevent diarrhea.

18. Ms. C. is midway through the infusion of her ninth cycle of carboplatin (Paraplatin) for ovarian cancer. She begins to complain of perioral and palmar itching and slight shortness of breath. Based on her symptoms, the nurse would suspect → *prodromal systems*
    A. paresthesia of her vagus nerve caused by carboplatin.
    B. palmar plantar erythrodysesthesia.
    C. an impending pulmonary embolus caused by abdominal carcinomatosis.
    D. an allergic reaction to the carboplatin.
    * *usually occur after le cycles, midway thru infusion*

19. Ms. A is ready to begin chemotherapy and is scheduled to receive cyclophosphamide (Cytoxan) and doxorubicin. Which results would necessitate a change in the proposed regimen?
    A. A lactate dehydrogenase (LDH) concentration of 135 international units/L
    B. A multiple gated acquisition (MUGA) of 30%
    C. A CA-125 level of 35 after surgical debulking
    D. A hematocrit of 34% according to recent laboratory work

20. Mr. T. is receiving irinotecan (Camptosar). Nursing considerations should include prophylaxis for
    A. stomatitis.
    B. constipation.
    C. pneumonitis.
    D. diarrhea. - *dose-limiting SE*

21. Which agent is considered an irritant?
    A. Doxil   - *liposomal doxirubicin*
    B. Idamycin
    C. Oncovin   *vesicants*
    E. Adriamycin

→ converted to 5-FU when metabolized

22. Capecitabine (Xeloda) would exhibit toxicities similar to
    A. vinblastine (Velban).
    B. tamoxifen (Nolvadex).
    C. 5-fluorouracil (5-FU).
    D. prednisone.

23. What is true regarding PPE guidelines?
    A. Powdered, disposable gloves should be worn at all times while preparing to administer chemotherapy.
    B. Double gloves should be worn during chemotherapy administration.
    C. Gowns can be reworn if it is the same staff member and it is not soiled.
    D. Surgical masks can be worn to reduce inhalation of chemotherapy during administration.

24. A potential long-term health risk that may develop as a result of exposure to antineoplastic agents is
    A. renal failure.
    B. hearing loss.
    C. an increased risk of cancer.
    D. liver failure.

25. Which of the following is a potential route for cytotoxic exposure for nurses administering antineoplastic agents?
    A. Flare reactions
    B. Hypersensitivity reactions
    C. Inhalation of aerosols
    D. Extravasation of drugs

26. A nurse is caring for a client receiving a continuous infusion of 5-fluorouracil (5-FU). The client puts the call light on and announces that the intravenous (IV) line has pulled apart and is leaking. After stopping the infusion, the nurse should
    A. reconnect the IV tubing.
    B. call the safety officer.
    C. locate a spill kit and cordon off the area.
    D. remove the client from the room.

27. Which of the following is not a recommended optimum quality for a biologic safety cabinet or a compounding aseptic isolator used when preparing antineoplastic agents?
    A. Hood that vents to the outside
    B. Vertical unidirectional airflow
    C. Continuously operating fan
    D. Housed in an area with positive pressure

    ↳ need negative

28. An example of a nursing intervention to minimize exposure during the disposal of antineoplastic agents is to
    A. clip or recap needles after administration.
    B. discard all unused portions of drug down a drain.
    C. dispose of biohazardous containers and contaminated equipment in a sealable polypropylene bag.
    D. dispose of gowns and gloves in regular trash bins.

29. Which of the following is a safety-related nursing intervention when working with chemotherapy agents? ⚠
    A. Create positive pressure within the vial by adding a volume of air.
    B. Clear all contents from the neck of the ampule before opening to access drug.
    C. Use double gloves for all handling, changing gloves every 30 minutes and whenever contamination occurs.
    D. Carefully remove the gown so that others may use it.

30. What would be the nurse's first action after direct contact with an antineoplastic agent?
    A. Complete an incident report.
    B. Remove contaminated personal protective equipment.
    C. Cleanse the area with soap and water.
    D. Seek medical attention.

31. When is aerosolization a problem in the preparation of antineoplastic agents?
    A. When spiking a bag
    B. When discontinuing an infusion
    C. When discarding contaminated materials
    D. When withdrawing needles from vials

23 Nursing Implications of Targeted Therapies and Biotherapy

1. The family of a client wants to know the differences between molecular kinase inhibitors from the monoclonal antibodies the client had previously. What are the key differences?
   A. Monoclonal antibodies are smaller than kinase inhibitors and have less of a potential for immune system activation.
   B. The kinase inhibitors are larger molecules that have less of a likelihood for drug–drug interactions.
   C. Monoclonal antibodies are smaller molecules with a much longer half-life.
   D. The kinase inhibitors are oral agents with shorter half-lives and have a greater potential for drug–drug interactions that require monitoring.

2. In addition to primary treatment in clients with cancer, biotherapies also play a treatment role in all of the following except
   A. diagnosis of cancer.
   B. to downstage a tumor.
   C. radiosensitization.
   D. capillary leak syndrome.

3. A monoclonal antibody that is made up primarily of mouse protein but has a human protein component is
   A. humanized.
   B. primatized.
   C. murine.
   D. chimeric.

4. Which of the following options apply to targeted therapies that have been approved for use in cancer therapy?
   A. Rituximab is a chimeric agent and trastuzumab is a humanized agent; thus they work together when used in breast cancer.
   B. There are no adverse events of antiangiogenesis agents.
   C. The mTOR agents target rapamycin pathways, thus regulating cell survival, proliferation, and growth.
   D. They are primarily used as conjugated agents attached to a chemotherapy drug or other agent or toxin.

5. When a client receives a monoclonal antibody, the factor that best predicts for an allergic type reaction during administration is
   A. a history of reactions to other antineoplastic agents.
   B. extent of tumor burden.
   C. percentage of murine protein in the antibody.
   D. exclusion of steroids in the premedication regimen.

6. Which of the following statements applies to the mTOR inhibitors?
   A. Noninfectious pneumonitis is a class effect of these inhibitors.
   B. Immunosuppression is seen primarily when conjugated with chemotherapy.
   C. Gastrointestinal perforation is seen with the occurrence of gut mucositis.
   D. They are less likely to contribute to problems related to CYP450 substrates.

7. A client receiving high-dose interferon therapy for stage 3 melanoma experiences a doubling of transaminases. This is generally associated with   ALT + AST
   A. anticipated side effects of treatment.
   B. previous exposure to hepatitis.
   C. improper dosing of interferon.
   D. hepatic metastasis.

8. The dosing of biotherapy agents is determined based on the
   A. optimal biologic dose.
   B. minimally toxic dose.
   C. lowest myelosuppressive dose.
   D. maximum tolerated dose.

9. Mr. J completed treatment for a B-cell non-Hodgkin lymphoma (NHL) 3 weeks ago with ibritumomab tiuxetan (Zevalin). He presents to the clinic today with complaints of increasing fatigue, dyspnea on exertion, and increasing bruising. His current symptoms are likely related to
   A. tumor lysis syndrome.
   B. pulmonary embolism.
   C. disease progression.
   D. myelosuppressive effects of therapy.

10. The greatest risk for allergic reactions exists when administering which of the following classifications of biotherapy agents?
    A. Monoclonal antibodies
    B. Interleukins ~rare
    C. Interferons
    D. Colony-stimulating factors

11. The two most difficult to manage side effects of interferon therapy are
    A. fatigue and diarrhea.
    B. flulike syndrome and headache.
    C. fatigue and central nervous system (CNS) alterations.
    D. skin reactions and flulike syndrome.

12. Evidence-based interventions to maintain skin integrity for clients receiving biotherapies and targeted therapies include
    A. using systemic antibiotics to treat papulopustular rashes.
    B. using decreasing severity of rashes through measures including sun protection, tetracycline, topical steroids, and skin moisturizers.
    C. decreasing the risk of bleeding by promotion of the control of hypertension in the client.
    D. decreasing the dose of the biotherapy and targeted therapies and encourage frequent warm showers.

13. A client shares that he is worried about receiving a biotherapy drug because he has heard about clients dying during this type of treatment. How should the nurse respond?
    A. Encourage the client to share his concerns with the physician before signing the informed consent document.
    B. Explain the strict regulatory processes now in place to safeguard clients against harm while on new pharmacologic agents.
    C. Review the drug data with the client and encourage him to ask questions.
    D. Assure the client that deaths are very rare with approved pharmacologic agents, but stress that the decision of whether or not to take the agent is voluntary.

24 Nursing Implications of Support Therapies and Procedures

1. The use of blood component therapy (BCT) in cancer care has increased primarily because of
   A. client awareness of benefit.
   B. abundant community donations.
   C. advancement of surgical oncology techniques.
   D. increasing cure rates resulting from BCT.

2. The spouse of a client is inquiring regarding approaches to increase the safety of his wife who may require blood products in conjunction with an elective surgery. The nurse should explain that blood received from an autologous donor is
   A. human leukocyte antigen (HLA) matched.
   B. collected during organ harvesting.
   C. collected from the intended recipient.
   D. collected and transfused within the same facility.

3. C.J. demonstrates gum bleeding related to severe mucositis. Her platelet count is 40,000/mm³ with the chemotherapy administered 2 weeks ago. Hemoglobin is 9 g/dL. The patient states that she is very tired. There is no indication of an infection, and her temperature is currently 99.6° F. What blood component therapy would the nurse anticipate as she plans nursing care?
   A. Random platelets to decrease the risk of bleeding
   B. Single-donor platelets to delay alloimmunization and decrease the risk of infection with exposure to only one donor
   C. Frozen pack red blood cells (RBCs) because of a history of severe reactions to blood products
   D. There is no real indication for blood component therapy at this time

4. The use of blood component therapy (BCT) has increased as a supportive therapy during cancer treatment. Which of the following is a treatment related factor that increases the likelihood that BCT will be needed?
   A. The presence of chronic bacterial infections and chronic or acute viral infections
   B. Radiation therapy to a significant portion of the client's bone marrow
   C. Comorbidities such as heart disease, diabetes, renal failure, and liver disease
   D. Malnutrition, including deficiencies in folate, vitamin B12, and iron

5. In addition to febrile complications of BCT, the nurse monitors the recipient's response for which of the following?
   A. Allergic reactions, hypothermia, and hemolytic reactions
   B. Fluid volume overload and deep vein thrombosis (DVT) caused by the platelet increase
   C. DVT and other coagulation problems
   D. Bone marrow reaction to the unrelated presence of unrelated stem cells

6. W.B. will be receiving blood component therapy for the first time since her diagnosis of multiple myeloma. Which of the following would the nurse prioritize as a cognitive outcome?
   A. The client believes the therapy will be helpful.
   B. The client understands the process of component infusion.
   C. The client describes signs and symptoms of reactions to therapy.
   D. The client relates to the need for blood component therapy.

7. A client receiving BCT is demonstrating uncontrolled shaking, chills, an elevated temperature, shortness of breath, dyspnea, wheezing, and a headache. How would the nurse prioritize her interventions?
   A. This is most likely an acute transfusion reaction; report it to the provider and the transfusion service or blood bank to obtain intervention orders.
   B. Stop the infusion immediately and keep the intravenous (IV) line open with normal saline solution.
   C. Administer 25 to 50 mg of diphenhydramine IV to decrease the severity of the reaction.
   D. Administer 24 to 50 mg of meperidine IV to treat the uncontrolled rigors and the shaking.

8. The nurse is preparing a BCT infusion. She knows that which of the following guidelines maximizes client safety? ⚠
   A. Using a gravity-flow infusion line
   B. Adding medications through the Y-port slowly
   C. Using the smallest gauge intravenous (IV) catheter available
   D. Together with a second RN, checking BCT product with client ID

9. J.B. is a 57-year-old client post radiation therapy for lung cancer who presented with a fever and productive cough. The family is asking about vascular access devices because the client has a needle phobia and a history of difficult IV access, and the physician indicates the plan is to administer the treatment twice a day for 2 weeks. The nurse will prepare to teach the client and family regarding which type of IV access device?
   A. Implanted ports
   B. Midline catheters
   C. Tunneled catheters
   D. Peripheral catheters

10. The nurse is teaching a client and the family about the option of a peripherally inserted central catheter (PICC). He knows the client needs more teaching when the client describes the catheter as
   A. a silicone connection to an artery.
   B. inserted above the antecubital fossa in a vein.
   C. having decreased risks for pneumothorax.
   D. decreasing the need for intravenous sticks.

11. A client will receive a vesicant medication as part of the chemotherapy protocol. The nurse's plan to maintain safety during the infusion includes ⚠
   A. using a computer-controlled infusion pump for accuracy.
   B. bringing the medication to body temperature before infusing.
   C. extending the time over which the medication slowly infuses.
   D. maintaining aseptic technique when establishing venous access.

12. A client returns from surgery, during which a tunneled catheter was implanted. The nurse finds the intravenous solution infusing at 30 mL/hr. The infusion rate can be increased to the ordered 125 mL/hr when which of the following tests confirms placement?
   A. Computed tomography (CT) scan
   B. Endoscopic confirmation
   C. Blood return on aspiration
   D. Radiographic validation

13. The oncology nurse is evaluating the potential for a client to receive an implanted venous access device. Which of the following best supports the decision for the individual to have this type of device?
   A. The client demonstrates the ability to care for the device.
   B. The client needs chemotherapy infusions and blood samples.
   C. The client expresses concerns about implantation of the device.
   D. The client and family are reluctant to care for an external device.

14. When changing the dressing on a cannulated implanted port, which principle would guide nursing care during the procedure?
   A. The procedure requires strict aseptic technique.
   B. The insertion site must be covered with opaque dressing.
   C. It is a clean procedure because risk for infection is low.
   D. The client should hold his or her breath while the needle is inserted.

15. K.K. is being discharged from the ambulatory infusion center with an infusion system for continuous chemotherapy infusion. What would indicate that client and family are adequately prepared for use of the infusion system if they know how to
   A. flush the line with sterile water every 12 hours.
   B. monitor the infusion system for proper functioning.
   C. attach a second line to the infusion for pain control.
   D. change the dose of the drug whenever the client sleeps.

16. J.B. has had a tunneled catheter for chemotherapy over the past 6 months. He comes into the infusion center on a monthly basis. During this visit, the client indicates the local clinic staff has been experiencing difficulty obtaining blood for laboratory tests. This type of problem can occur secondary to
   A. applying too much pressure during an infusion, causing a ruptured line.
   B. inadequate flushing after blood draws, causing an infectious clot.
   C. inconsistent use of the push-stop method during routine flushing.
   D. a line that was not properly secured and has been partially pulled out.

17. Damage to implanted venous access catheters may occur as a result of
   A. nonsteroidal antiinflammatory drug (NSAID) use.
   B. bathing with the access device in place.
   C. excessive pressure with infusions.
   D. lack of use for greater than 96 hours.

25 Pharmacologic Interventions

1. Which statement made by family members indicates the need for additional teaching regarding risk factors for infection during cancer treatment?
   A. I am concerned about him not doing his mouth care. He just keeps saying his dentist says he has always taken good care of his teeth.
   B. When I asked about his kidneys, I was told his BUN and creatinine are rising. Will that increase his risk of getting an infection?
   C. I know that his incision from his surgery is not quite healed. How soon can we start getting him in the shower?
   D. When he received his rituximab, we were told that it can affect the cells that normally fight infections.

2. Of the classifications of antimicrobials, which drugs are commonly used as first-line therapy to treat neutropenic fever?
   A. Penicillins, cefepime, and meropenem
   B. Penicillins, voriconazole, and meropenem
   C. Penicillins, cefepime, and echinocandins
   D. Penicillins and meropenem

3. How would the nurse respond to a family member who is concerned about infection risk for a client receiving dose intense therapy because her father died of an infection?
   A. Infections are almost a given in severely immune-suppressed individuals receiving cancer therapy.
   B. Although we can't prevent every infection, two important things to do are handwashing and temperature monitoring.
   C. We have so many newer medications to fight infections today than the past, how long ago did he die?
   D. With your experience, you will be able to know when an infection might be causing a problem, and you can contact us.

4. Mrs. T reports that she is pleased that her husband finally seems more hopeful now that his mother has arrived from their homeland. Mr. T's mother always knew what to give him when he was not feeling well—usually a home remedy she made herself. How would the nurse respond to this comment?
   A. Adults of all ages perk up when their mother arrives to care for them; it is that "desire to be mothered."
   B. Encourage them to have his mother come to the clinic for personalized teaching.
   C. Hope his mother's presence may increase his motivation to become active.
   D. Acknowledge that some cultures use alternative therapies which are not closely regulated and may actually contain sources of contamination that could put her husband at risk for an infection or interact with other medications the patient is receiving increasing the risk of a drug reaction.

5. G.H. has just been diagnosed as having a *Candida* infection. Which medication does the nurse expect the primary practitioner to order?
   A. Amphotericin B or fluconazole (Diflucan)
   B. Caspofungin (Cancidas) or ciprofloxacin (Cipro)
   C. Voriconazole (Vfend) or imipenem
   D. Cidofovir (Vistide) or fluconazole (Diflucan)

6. Aminoglycosides are used in conjunction with other antimicrobials to treat infections in clients with cancer. The major toxicity of aminoglycosides is
   A. hepatotoxicity.
   B. cardiac toxicity.
   C. nephrotoxicity.
   D. neurotoxicity.

7. Mrs. C is receiving cefepime (Maxipime) for an infection. The nurse teaching Mrs. C and her family regarding signs and symptoms of hypersensitivity reactions would instruct them to observe for which of the following?
   A. Shortness of breath, hives, and itchiness
   B. Increased thirst
   C. Decreased urine output
   D. Increased urine output

8. The physician has indicated empiric antimicrobial therapy will be initiated on T.Z. because of an elevated temperature. The nurse knows that
   A. oral agents provide for ease of administration and decreased cost, so they are usually indicated.
   B. a gram-negative spectrum of coverage is vital to cover for common infectious organisms among individuals with cancer.
   C. if the fever does not respond to initial therapy, a nonbacterial cause or inadequate serum and tissue levels should be considered.
   D. antifungal therapy should be considered if the patient has a past history of an outbreak during chemotherapy.

9. Guidelines for acyclovir include
   A. to ensure adequate blood levels, doses should be based on actual body weight.
   B. it is effective preemptive therapy for cytomegalovirus (CMV) in high-risk clients with cancer.
   C. probenecid is given to prevent renal reabsorption and related toxicities.
   D. fluid hydration is necessary if therapeutic IV doses are used.

10. Which of the following presents the rationale for how nonsteroidal antiinfammatory drugs (NSAIDs) suppress the inflammatory response?
    A. Inhibit cyclooxygenase and the production of prostaglandins
    B. Block opiate neurotransmitters thus decreasing neuropathic pain
    C. Suppress prostaglandins which mediate the transmission of neuropathic pain
    D. Increase macrophage migration to the injury thus decreasing inflammation

11. Mr. P has coronary artery disease and takes one aspirin daily. He was recently diagnosed with metastatic lung cancer, and the physician has prescribed naproxen and dexamethasone for bone pain. Instruction should include awareness of which of the following complications?
    A. Gastrointestinal ulceration, fluid retention, and renal insufficiency
    B. Bleeding and changes in normal bowel function toward constipation
    C. Fluid retention, renal insufficiency, and immune suppression
    D. Constipation, leading to gastrointestinal ulceration and bleeding

12. An important factor to consider regarding potential drug interactions with NSAIDs is that they can
    A. decrease the effects of phenytoin and warfarin.
    B. increase renal clearance of methotrexate.
    C. decrease the effectiveness of warfarin.
    D. increase the effects of phenytoin, sulfonamide, and warfarin.

13. A 16-year-old young woman has osteosarcoma with bone pain. She is taking an NSAID and will be receiving a corticosteroid indefinitely. Which of the following would be the nurse's greatest concerns for discussion?
    A. Dizziness, drowsiness, and mental confusion
    B. Headache, abdominal pain, and bleeding
    C. Altered renal function and potential mental changes
    D. Acne, weight gain, and moon face → *body image*

14. Mrs. T is a 74-year-old woman who has metastatic lung cancer and complains of bone pain. Her cancer is being treated with docetaxel and irinotecan chemotherapy. Her pain is being treated with oxycodone hydrochloride (OxyContin) 30 mg twice daily, ibuprofen 600 mg orally three times daily, and amitriptyline 25 mg orally at bedtime for the past 4 weeks. She also complains of weight gain of 5 lb and worsening constipation. The most likely explanation for this client's complaints is
    A. amitriptyline weight gain and ibuprofen-induced constipation.
    B. ibuprofen weight gain and OxyContin-induced constipation.
    C. OxyContin weight gain and docetaxel-induced constipation.
    D. amitriptyline weight gain and irinotecan-induced constipation.

15. Which of the following unique teaching components should be emphasized for clients and their family members regarding naproxen?
    A. It is a prescription-only NSAID.
    B. Do not crush the tablet; it is a long-acting medication.
    C. Always take this medication with food.
    D. There is a potential for drug interaction with warfarin.

16. Principles of pain management with antiinfammatory agents include that
    A. in addition to pain management, they are indicated in the symptomatic management of tumor lysis fever.
    B. when clients need opioids, discontinuation of the NSAIDs is recommended to avoid drug interactions.
    C. they provide adequate pain control throughout the course of the disease for most clients with cancer.
    D. potential adverse effects include cardiac toxicity and confusion, especially in young adults.

17. A beneficial nursing implication of the salicylates choline magnesium trisalicylate and salsalate is they
    A. have demonstrated gastrointestinal (GI) safety.
    B. are less likely to cause liver problems.
    C. have a long half-life that allows for once-daily dosing.
    D. do not have antiplatelet effects.

18. A major difference between the short-acting corticosteroids and the intermediate- and long-acting ones is that
    A. short-acting corticosteroids have greater sodium and water retention activity.
    B. intermediate-acting corticosteroids cause fewer sleep disturbances.
    C. short-acting corticosteroids can be given in smaller total doses.
    D. short-acting corticosteroids cause fewer gastrointestinal side effects.

19. The nursing intervention related to neuromuscular and skeletal effects of corticosteroids is to
    A. administer pain medication as needed.
    B. limit activity to avoid fatigue.
    C. assess for signs and symptoms of edema.
    D. monitor bowel function for constipation.

20. Which of the following places anticancer drugs appropriately in terms of emetogenic potential?
    A. Paclitaxel, ifosfamide greater than 2 g/m^2, and busulfan—moderate (30%-90%)
    B. Vinorelbine, vincristine, and etoposide—low (10%-30%)
    C. Bleomycin, docetaxel, and melphalan—very low (<10%)
    D. Dacarbazine and cyclophosphamide—high (>90%)

21. One reason for administering 20 mg of IV dexamethasone before a chemotherapy regimen containing paclitaxel and carboplatin is to
    A. prevent allergic reactions to cisplatin.
    B. stimulate appetite after chemotherapy.
    C. improve antiemetic efficacy.
    D. decrease the chance of chemotherapy-induced diarrhea.

22. Mr. D is to receive doxorubicin (Adriamycin) 60 mg/m^2 and cisplatin 100 mg/m^2 IV on day 1 of his treatment protocol. An effective antiemetic regimen for this combination regimen is
    A. a 5-HT3 antagonist plus metoclopramide and lorazepam.
    B. metoclopramide plus dexamethasone and lorazepam.
    C. a neurokinin 1 inhibitor plus 5-HT3 antagonist plus dexamethasone.
    D. a phenothiazine (e.g., prochlorperazine) plus a 5-HT3 antagonist.

23. Which places a client at greatest risk for nausea and vomiting with equivalent emetogenic chemotherapy?
    A. Chemotherapy-induced nausea and vomiting in a 60-year-old man
    B. Chemotherapy-induced nausea and vomiting in a 45-year-old woman
    C. Increased alcohol intake in a 65-year-old man with lung cancer
    D. Delayed nausea and vomiting in a 60-year-old patient with gastric cancer

24. Mr. D has two episodes of vomiting on day 3 after his cisplatin. Which antiemetic is appropriate for treating his emesis?
    A. Granisetron 1 mg IV
    B. Prochlorperazine 10 mg PO
    C. Lorazepam 0.5 mg sublingually
    D. Diphenhydramine 25 mg PO/IV

25. Mr. D returns to the clinic for the next cycle of high-dose cisplatin. On the previous cycle of cisplatin, he had received granisetron 1 mg IV before cisplatin. He had two emetic episodes on day 1 and two emetic episodes on day 3. What would be the most rational therapy for this client?
    A. Administer granisetron 1 mg IV + dexamethasone 20 IV, both 30 minutes before chemotherapy followed by granisetron 1 mg PO qd and dexamethasone 8 mg PO bid for 3 days.
    B. Add prochlorperazine 10 mg IV on days 2 and 3 to the granisetron and dexamethasone to improve coverage.
    C. Add lorazepam 1 mg IV or PO on days 2 and 3 to the regularly indicated antiemetic to enhance the long-term benefit.
    D. Switch to aprepitant (Emend), 125 mg PO on day 1 and 80 mg PO on days 2 and 3.

26. Nursing actions when selective serotonin antagonists (5-HT3 antagonists such as ondansetron or granisetron) are prescribed include
    A. administering diphenhydramine to prevent extrapyramidal symptoms (EPSs).
    B. monitoring vital signs for hypertension.
    C. administering acetaminophen for headache.
    D. teaching clients to take only as needed for nausea and vomiting.

27. The advantage of selective serotonin antagonists over metoclopramide or a phenothiazine is the
    A. lower cost of the medications.
    B. absence of extrapyramidal side effects.
    C. absence of sedation with the medications.
    D. absence of anticholinergic effects.

28. Which of the following drugs is not regarded as a potential augmenter for antiemetics?
    A. Diphenhydramine
    B. Dexamethasone
    C. Lorazepam
    D. Cimetidine

29. A client reports to the infusion center with an emesis basin and complaining of two episodes of vomiting. What is indicated?
    A. This is strictly emotional. Teaching should focus on improved coping.
    B. It is not associated with prior episodes of poorly controlled nausea and vomiting.
    C. Teaching should focus on the identification of cues that trigger the reaction.
    D. This nausea and vomiting arises from the frontal region of the brain.

30. Antiemetics that belong to the same class as Zofran affect nausea and vomiting by acting as
    A. 5 HT3 agonists.
    B. D2 antagonists.
    C. NK-1 agonists.
    D. 5HT3 antagonists.

31. What is a true statement regarding the classification of nausea and vomiting?
    A. Acute—mediated release of serotonin from enterochromaffin cells
    B. Late—occurs within 24 hours of chemotherapy administration
    C. Breakthough—arises from the cortex and limbic regions of the brain
    D. Refractory—a classic Pavlovian-conditioned response

32. Which principle is most important for the nurse to teach clients and family members regarding management of chemotherapy-induced nausea and vomiting during the first round of treatment?
    A. Delayed emesis has been identified as a common problem and should be treated during future rounds.
    B. Selection of appropriate antiemetics should be based primarily on the cost of the agents.
    C. A complete follow-up assessment of outcomes 48 to 72 hours after chemotherapy is important.
    D. The primary goal is prevention of nausea and vomiting because this will influence side effects during future rounds.

33. Which statement made by family members indicates a need for additional teaching focused on safety? ⚠
    A. I am glad there are so many different options for the prevention of nausea and vomiting for when we go home; D.F. did so well last time.
    B. Because D.F. had quite a bit of problems with side effects, I heard it is an indication that the chemotherapy was working.
    C. D.F. really slept most of the day after the chemotherapy; I think I will just plan to go to work so I don't miss so much time.
    D. We really need to watch the expenses with the medications that were ordered. Is there any assistance available?

34. Which statements place antiemetics with the appropriate neurotransmitter target?
    A. Serotonin—aprepitant
    B. Cannabinoid agonist—dronabinol
    C. Histamine H1 antagonist—prochlorperazine
    D. Dopamine D2 antagonist—promethazine

35. When comparing prophylaxis of nausea and vomiting for highly and moderately emetogenic agents, what additional medication is recommended?
    A. Metoclopramide
    B. Prochlorperazine
    C. Neurokinin-1 inhibitor
    D. 5 HT2 antagonist

36. Family caregivers of T.D. reported that they noticed what almost appeared to be perpetual motion after his most recent chemotherapy treatment. What would be a nursing priority to consider? ⚠
    A. Inquire regarding known allergies to medications and report them to the ordering practitioner.
    B. Determine if the antiemetic protocol included prochlorperazine and consider diphenhydramine for the akathisia.
    C. Determine if T.D. has a history of psychiatric problems or the occurrence of similar response in the past.
    D. Review the chemotherapy medications for potential side effects that could have caused this problem.

37. What accurately describes current understanding of cancer-related pain?
    A. Accurate evaluation should be able to identify a cause of the pain described by the client.
    B. It is extremely difficult to control all cancer pain without causing extensive amount of sedation.
    C. Pain is caused by the tumor itself about 70% of the time and diagnostic or therapeutic approaches about 20% of the time.
    D. Analgesics work by interfering with pain transduction, transmission or nociception, or perception.

38. What articulates essential principles of cancer pain management?
    A. Selection of the appropriate analgesia should be based primarily on the known cause of the pain, such as bone versus tissue pain.
    B. The most appropriate dose of pain medication is the lowest recommended starting dose based on pharmacology.
    C. The breakthrough dose of pain medication in a client receiving around the clock medications should be 10% to 20% of the 24-hour long-acting dose.
    D. Tolerance is usually an indication that the client has developed psychological dependence to the pain medication.

39. Which of the following statements does not appropriately address pain medication–related adverse effects caused by compromised organ systems?
    A. Renal insufficiency may slow the rate of elimination of morphine, codeine, and tramadol or their metabolites, leading to increased potential for toxicities.
    B. Hepatic insufficiency decreases the amount of fentanyl, morphine, and oxycodone available because of decreased first-pass effect and altered enzyme pathways.
    C. Underlying restrictive or obstructive respiratory or lung disease may potentiate respiratory compromise from opioids administered for pain relief.
    D. Brain involvement with metastasis and underlying seizure disorders may predispose to central nervous system–related toxicity with opioids.

40. T.R. contacted the nurse with complaints of increased pain and diarrhea. Treatment plan at this time includes a feeding tube for nutritional support and metoclopramide for chemotherapy-induced nausea and vomiting. What would the nurse's assessment be?
    A. The pain is most likely an indication that the tumor is responding to the chemotherapy; treatment will need to be modified.
    B. If the diarrhea is adequately treated and becomes better controlled, pain management will likely improve.
    C. The progression of disease probably warrants an increase in pain medications for better management.
    D. Altered gastrointestinal function, including use of tube feedings and metoclopramide, will change pain medication transit time and absorption.

41. Which opioid analgesic is more likely to cause respiratory depression?
    A. Meperidine
    B. Acetaminophen
    C. Methadone
    D. Morphine

42. When caring for a client with a feeding tube who has a new order for morphine sustained-release (SR) tablets, the nurse should ▲
    A. crush the tablets and administer it concurrently with the tube feeding.
    B. clamp the tube for 30 minutes, crush the tablets, and then administer.
    C. find an alternative route of administration (e.g., intrarectally or vaginally).
    D. crush the tablets and add to tube feeding solution.

43. J.C. is taking aspirin for rheumatoid arthritis and is also receiving 5-FU, doxorubicin, and methotrexate for colon cancer. What risk may be increased significantly as a result of drug interaction? ▲
    A. Cardiac toxicity
    B. Methotrexate toxicity
    C. Diarrhea
    D. Aspirin toxicity

44. Mr. C is being discharged on SR morphine and acetaminophen. Which instruction would the nurse question?
    A. Take both morphine and acetaminophen around the clock.
    B. Increase fluid and fiber intake to prevent constipation.
    C. Use SR morphine for breakthrough pain.
    D. Avoid driving hazardous vehicles that require mental alertness.

45. What is seen with a meperidine–phenytoin drug interaction?
    A. Decreased renal clearance of phenytoin
    B. Reduced plasma levels of meperidine
    C. Enhanced CNS depressant effects
    D. Increased risk of allergic reaction

46. How do the CNS effects of opioid analgesics influence the nursing interventions for client safety? ▲
    A. The level of sedation may indicate the degree of respiratory depression.
    B. Gastric upset may indicate increased risk of a GI bleed.
    C. Monitor orthostatic hypotension for fall risk.
    D. Increase fluid and dietary fiber intake for constipation.

47. Which principle is most important for the nurse to teach clients and family members regarding management of chemotherapy-induced nausea and vomiting during the first round of treatment?
    A. Use of too much medication will potentially contribute to sedation with little additional antiemetic effect.
    B. The goal should be prevention of nausea and vomiting; waiting to see if there is a problem contributes to future problems.
    C. If acute nausea and vomiting are controlled, the individual will not experience delayed nausea and vomiting.
    D. Breakthrough nausea and vomiting should be treated with the use of an antianxiety agent.

48. Which statement made by family members indicates a need for additional teaching focused on safety? ⚠
    A. The constipation that comes with pain meds is almost worse than the pain.
    B. How do we determine when she or he is really having pain?
    C. I don't want my mother to suffer like my father; I want her totally pain free.
    D. What do we do when the pain medications cause nausea and vomiting?

49. Which of the following is true related to the onset of action for fentanyl?
    A. IV 2 to 3 minutes
    B. IV 5 to 6 minutes
    C. Patch 8 to 10 hours
    D. Buccal 15 to 30 minutes

50. Which statements apply to our nursing understanding regarding anxiety?
    A. Anxiety is an unpleasant, multifactorial experience that interferes with the ability to cope with cancer and cancer treatment.
    B. Anxiety is present in an estimated half of all clients with cancer and has psychosocial, emotional, and spiritual components.
    C. Anxiety is most likely to be present during a new diagnosis, disease status change, and end of life, but not ongoing treatment.
    D. There are no risk factors for anxiety.

51. In addition to anxiety, anxiolytics are also used as a supportive pharmacologic intervention in clients with cancer to do all of the following except
    A. manage depression and seizures.
    B. decrease pain related to anxiety.
    C. decrease food aversions.
    D. aid in alcohol and narcotic withdrawal.

52. A sedative hypnotic agent with minimal daytime hangover is
    A. triazolam.
    B. phenobarbital.
    C. chlordiazepoxide.
    D. diazepam.

53. A major disadvantage of using a barbiturate as a sedative–hypnotic agent is
    A. rebound anxiety.
    B. loss of concentration and depression of affect.
    C. tolerance builds quickly.
    D. high incidence of Stevens-Johnson syndrome.

54. In a client with brain metastases, phenytoin (Dilantin) may be a necessary prophylactic medication if the client is receiving which of the following drugs?
    A. Granisetron and dexamethasone
    B. Prochlorperazine and meperidine
    C. Acetaminophen and codeine
    D. Naproxen and dexamethasone

55. G.R. is complaining about anxiolytic side effects and wants to stop them at this time. Why would immediate discontinuation not be advisable? There is a risk of
    A. an acute relapse of anxiety symptoms.
    B. psychosis, seizures, and coma.
    C. increased problems with chemotherapy-related nausea and vomiting.
    D. abrupt change in tolerance of pain medications.

56. What statement from the family of a 67-year-old client with a history of alcohol use and chronic obstructive pulmonary disease (COPD) who has lung cancer and is receiving a benzodiazepine for anxiety would indicate a critical need for additional teaching? ⚠
    A. We seem to be doing better, although he is a little sleepy in the morning; at least he sleeps during the night, and so can we.
    B. The pain he had been complaining about in his abdomen seems to be getting worse; could that be spread of disease?
    C. It is so much easier now that the anxiety is under control because we can at least leave him alone when we have to.
    D. Our grandchildren are coming for the holiday. One of them has been ill with respiratory symptoms; can they still come?

57. What would be an advantage of having a client on buspirone compared with chlordiazepoxide?
    A. Decreased cost for the client
    B. Reduced incidence and severity of side effects
    C. Fewer drug–drug interactions
    D. Fewer food–drug interactions

58. What is a common side effect of concern for clients receiving serotonin reuptake inhibitors?
    A. Hot flashes
    B. Neuropathy
    C. Sexual dysfunction
    D. Increased appetite

59. Seizure-related safety is a potential concern in individuals receiving which of the following antineoplastic agents? ⚠
    A. Ifosfamide, bleomycin, and busulfan
    B. High dose methotrexate, carmustine, and gemcitabine
    C. Busulfan, cyclophosphamide, and dacarbazine
    D. Ifosfamide, high-dose methotrexate, and busulfan

60. Agents such as phenobarbital, carbamazepine, and phenytoin are less likely to be used for seizure control because
    A. their enzyme induction characteristics contribute to a risk for drug interactions.
    B. consistent and adequate blood levels are difficult to accomplish.
    C. they are more likely to cause safety concerns because of a risk of falls. ⚠
    D. secondary fatigue and tremor contribute to decreased quality of life for clients.

61. What would be required as part of the assessment for a client whose seizures had been previously well controlled but who has now experienced seizures at home?
    A. Plan for an additional workup because this is most likely an indication the tumor is progressing and therapy will need to be changed.
    B. Assess the client for sleep disturbances.
    C. Assess the client for recent history of trauma such as a fall resulting in a head injury.
    D. Explore a list of the at-home medications for drugs that may have lowered the seizure threshold.

62. Which principles of medical management of seizures should guide care of a client newly identified as experiencing a seizure?
    A. Understanding the etiology of the seizure is important; a neurology consult may be necessary.
    B. The client will most likely get started on dual therapy because it has been shown to be more effective.
    C. The seizures are most likely an indication the client's disease has spread to the brain.
    D. Phenytoin and phenobarbital are the gold standard for therapy and thus the most likely agents to be ordered.

63. R.T. has been admitted recently and is taking multiple medications, including gabapentin. There is no indication of a history of brain involvement or suspicion of the same. How would the nurse address this?
    A. Determine if the client has neuropathic pain perhaps related to past chemotherapy agents.
    B. Ask the client about management of the gabapentin-induced sedation and implement fall precautions.
    C. Review all current medications to assess for the potential of drug–drug interactions.
    D. Ask the client and family if they have noticed any weight gain related to the gabapentin.

64. How would the nurse respond to a family member who states he has heard a lot about the use of growth factors, such as oprelvekin, in cancer care. He wants to know if this is an option for his father, who is having problems with bleeding from a low platelet count. Why would oprelvekin not be indicated?
    A. High cost and significant toxicity limit its use.
    B. It is not FDA approved for bleeding because of low platelet nadirs.
    C. Thrombocytopenia typically does not require medical intervention.
    D. The risk of allergies to the product is too great at this time.

65. Which hematopoietic growth factor is a multi-lineage factor that stimulates secondary cytokines such as tumor necrosis factor (TNF) and interleukin-1?
    A. Pegfilgrastim
    B. Darbepoetin
    C. Oprelvekin
    D. Sargramostin

66. Which principles apply to the management of myeloid growth factors?
    A. Treatment of febrile neutropenia with G-CSF or GM-CSF is more effective than prevention of febrile neutropenia with G-CSF or GM-CSF.
    B. Risk of neutropenia is influenced by treatment protocol myelotoxicity and patient-related factors.
    C. Erythropoietin (EPO) has been shown to decrease the number of red blood cell transfusions to treat anemia.
    D. Oprelvekin has been shown to decrease mortality rates in clients with low platelet nadirs.

67. What assessment findings would lead to consideration for initiation of hematopoietic growth factors?
    A. Neutropenia—absolute neutrophil count less than 1000/mm3
    B. Anemia—hemoglobin level less than 10 g/dL
    C. Thrombocytopenia platelet count less than 40,000 cells/mm
    D. Fever not responding to antimicrobials

68. The following is true about hematopoietic growth factors.
    A. They exert biologic effects such as enhancing differentiation or maturation of immunologic cell lines.
    B. They promote tumor activity by stimulating bone marrow stem cells.
    C. They are used for primary treatment of breast cancer.
    D. They do not affect the duration of neutropenia.

69. Which nursing action is recommended when administering a hematopoietic growth factor (HGF)?
    A. Add albumin in the carrier solution.
    B. Instruct the client to use acetaminophen for bone pain.
    C. Shake the vial vigorously during reconstitution.
    D. Administer the HGF before chemotherapy.

70. Granulocyte colony-stimulating factor (G-CSF) acts by
    A. decreasing phagocytic activity.
    B. stimulating precursors committed to neutrophil lineage.
    C. interacting with specific receptors on erythroid burst-forming units.
    D. regulating megakaryocytopoiesis.

71. A common side effect of filgrastim (G-CSF) is
    A. sedation.
    B. liver dysfunction.
    C. constipation.
    D. bone pain.

26 Complementary and Integrative Modalities

1. Complementary and alternative medicine (CAM) is a complex field that
   - A. uses alternative therapies, which are evidence-based nontraditional approaches used in place of conventional treatments.
   - B. often includes integrative medicine, an approach that takes into account each client's unique circumstances to customize treatment.
   - C. uses holistic health care, an entire domain of therapies that fall outside of conventional medicine.
   - D. only uses approaches that lack adequate evidence and should be discouraged because they place clients at increased risk for problems.

2. Whole medical systems involve a focus on the relationship between the structure and function of the body. This is a part of
   - A. traditional Chinese medicine.
   - B. chiropractic medicine.
   - C. homeopathy.
   - D. osteopathic medicine.

3. How are complementary and alternative medicine (CAM) treatments and methods categorized?
   - A. The clearest delineation is to understand CAM as anything that is not FDA approved for traditional medicine.
   - B. There is universal agreement to use two categories: natural products and mind–body practices.
   - C. The National Center for CAM distinguishes it as involving the two broad categories of natural products and mind–body practices.
   - D. Ayurveda differentiates the therapies as those that focus on balance and those that focus on energy flow.

4. Which of the following is a safety issue when using aromatherapy? ⚠
   - A. Standardization of the preparation of the essential oils used in practice is lacking.
   - B. Use of aromatherapy can trigger depression; these agents target psychological well-being.
   - C. Agents have a very narrow range of safe applicability.
   - D. Clients frequently develop an allergy to the transporter.

5. The term Feldenkrais refers to
   - A. gentle manipulation of the skull to reestablish natural configuration and movement.
   - B. the use of vigorous massage to stimulate the flow of lymphatic fluid out of an area of the body.
   - C. a somatic education system that teaches movement and gentle manipulation to increase body awareness and function.
   - D. a technique that uses movement and touch to restore balance in the body.

6. Which answer best describes manipulative and body-based practices?
   - A. Dance therapy and Qigong
   - B. Physical therapy, Qigong, and mindfulness
   - C. Only eye movement desensitization
   - D. Mindfulness and eye movement desensitization

7. Which statement does not apply to meditation?
   - A. It is a mind–body modality of CAM.
   - B. Evidence has shown it can enhance sense of well-being.
   - C. Meditation involves training clients to develop awareness of experiences moment by moment and in the context of all senses.
   - D. Techniques require the use of a coach who can narrate the activity.

8. Neurolinguistics programming (NLP)
   - A. has evolved into mainstream practice with multiple variations ranging from restorative to high power levels.
   - B. enhances coordination and balance and promotes physical, emotional, and spiritual well-being.
   - C. is a systematic approach to changing thought patterns, thereby changing feelings or perceptions.
   - D. has a meditative component that brings harmony to the body, mind, and spirit of the individual.

9. Herbal therapy
   - A. can be safely taken with any combination of OTC medicine or doctor-prescribed drug.
   - B. can be taken internally, inhaled, or applied directly to the body with the aim of restoring health.
   - C. focuses primarily on the use of water baths, steam baths, and the application of hot or cold compresses to enhance absorption.
   - D. involves the use of herbs that are carefully regulated by the Food and Drug Administration (FDA) to ensure the safety of the product.

10. Reiki is
    A. a technique for balancing the flow of energy in the body through the transfer of human energy.
    B. an energy healing technique that uses nursing process and specific protocols.
    C. the use of magnetic fields to positively impact the body to stimulate healing.
    D. an energy healing modality in which the practitioner directs the flow of energy to various parts of the body to facilitate healing and relaxation.

11. For clients using complementary therapies, nurses should assess for all except
    A. disturbances in psychosocial status.
    B. disturbances in age-related developmental issues.
    C. client and family preferences related to cultural practices.
    D. the ability of the individual to cover the cost of complementary therapy.

12. There are many valid reasons why some people with cancer seek alternative regimens, including
    A. possible improvement in quality of life during cancer treatment.
    B. mistrust of conventional medicine practice.
    C. evidence-based practices that are widely accepted and result in frequent cancer remissions.
    D. research that demonstrates CAM therapies can replace conventional medical treatment.

13. A client is curious about a nontraditional regimen and is asking multiple questions. Which question would concern a nurse the most?
    A. What are the benefits and risks associated with this type of complementary therapy?
    B. Will this specific type of therapy interfere with my conventional cancer treatment?
    C. Is this therapy part of a clinical trial? If so, who is sponsoring the trial?
    D. Because there is so much information about this regimen, it must be effective for my type of cancer, right?

14. What is the guiding principle behind Ayurveda?
    A. Maintaining balance in the body, mind, and consciousness is used to preserve health and treat illness.
    B. It is based on the precept of healing through the administration of specific substances.
    C. It focuses on the relationship between the structure and the function of the body.
    D. It combines five elements, fire, earth, metal, water, and word, which correspond to various organs and tissues in the body.

15. Acupuncture is often successful in alleviating pain because of
    A. the placebo effect; patients expect pain relief and therefore feel less pain.
    B. the introduction of pain at the insertion site allows the client to refocus his or her perception of the original site of pain.
    C. the stimulation of the nerve fibers entering the dorsal horn of the spinal cord, which mediates the impulses at other parts of the body and allows the client to experience less pain at the original site.
    D. the pressure applied by exerting a finger and thumb on specific points on the surface of the skin acts as an entrance and exit for an internal healing force, thereby eliminating the overall sensation of pain.

16. Homeopathy is a system of healing that uses
    A. diluted substances to alleviate disease or symptoms of disease.
    B. extracts of crude products to alleviate a variety of diseases.
    C. large doses of herbal products given over a period of weeks for symptom relief.
    D. small amounts of a raw herb in a cup of water steeped or soaked for several minutes into a drink for daily consumption.

27 Alterations in Hematologic and Immune Function

1. During the nadir period after chemotherapy, the patient should be instructed to avoid all drugs that alter platelet development. These include
   A. aspirin, clopidogrel, and sulfonamides.
   B. aspirin, iron supplements, and vitamins.
   C. aspirin, vitamins, and morphine.
   D. aspirin, iron supplements, and sulfonamides.

2. When implementing a care plan for an inpatient with a low absolute neutrophil count (ANC), the nurse should ⚠
   A. remove water pitchers from the room.
   B. follow infection precautions.
   C. allow fresh flowers and plants in the room.
   D. use clean technique when caring for all indwelling catheters (e.g., urinary, central lines, feeding tubes).

3. What would not be considered a risk factor for becoming neutropenic?
   A. Tumor invasion of the bone marrow
   B. Malnutrition
   C. Received radiation therapy to the pelvis
   D. Hyperalbuminemia

4. Colony-stimulating growth factor administration is initiated prophylactically when
   A. a chemotherapy dose has been reduced.
   B. a patient has experienced a previous anemia with chemotherapy administration.
   C. a patient undergoing radiation therapy for cancer treatment.
   D. a patient is at risk of grade 3/4 chemotherapy-induced neutropenia or febrile neutropenia and dose intensity is necessary for optimal outcomes.

5. Patients at high risk for development of thrombocytopenia include those
   A. undergoing treatment using high doses of interferon.
   B. with normal bone marrow function.
   C. with hypercoagulation disorders such as paraneoplastic syndromes.
   D. who have been administered growth factor.

6. Risk factors for infection include
   A. altered mucosal barriers.
   B. trimming fingernails and toenails.
   C. daily bathing.
   D. strict handwashing.

7. Hemorrhage can result from
   A. chemotherapy administration.
   B. platelet count of 120,000/mm^3.
   C. hematocrit of 30%.
   D. disseminated intravascular coagulation (DIC).

8. Patients who experience which of the following are at a high risk for fever?
   A. An ANC of 2000/mm^3
   B. A platelet count of 100,000/mm^3
   C. Are three weeks post-surgical procedure
   D. Have hepatic metastasis

9. What is the definition of febrile neutropenia (FN)?
   A. ANC less than 1000/mm^3 and sustained temperature of 38° C (100.4° F)
   B. Sustained temperature of 38.3° C (101° F) or higher for more than 1 hour
   C. ANC less than 1500/mm^3 and a single temperature higher than 38° C (100.4° F)
   D. ANC greater than 1500/mm^3 and a single temperature higher than 38.3° C (101° F)

10. Which of the following places the patient at risk for opportunistic infection?
    A. Neutropenia
    B. Lymphopenia
    C. Thrombocytopenia
    D. Anemia

11. A.C. calls the clinic and reports a fever of 101° F (38.3° C) for the past 24 hours. This fever would not be uncommon if the patient received any of the following except
    A. bleomycin (Blenoxane) administration.
    B. acetaminophen for headache.
    C. interferon administration.
    D. vancomycin administration.

12. How is an ANC calculated?
    A. % neutrophils (segs + bands) divided by total WBC
    B. Total WBC divided by % neutrophils (segs + bands)
    C. % neutrophils (segs + bands) multiplied by WBC
    D. Actual number of neutrophils (segs + bands) multiplied by WBC

13. From which stem cells do platelets arise?
    A. Lymphoid stem cells
    B. Megakaryocyte stem cells
    C. Myeloid stem cells
    D. Epithelial stem cells

14. J.B. presents to the clinic 20 days after treatment for a follow-up complete blood count (CBC). Her ANC remains below 500/mm^3. The nurse is concerned that J.B.'s prolonged neutropenia could lead to
    A. thrombocytopenia.
    B. disseminated intravascular coagulation.
    C. tumor lysis syndrome.
    D. sepsis.

15. Which of the following chemotherapy regimens are associated with an intermediate risk of myelotoxicity?
    A. MVAC (methotrexate, vinblastine, doxorubicin, cisplatin)
    B. FOLFOX (folinic acid [leucovorin], 5-fluoruracil, oxaliplatin)
    C. AT (doxorubicin, paclitaxel)
    D. ICE (ifosfamide, carboplatin, etoposide)

16. The normal life span of red blood cells is
    A. 1 to 3 days.
    B. 4 to 6 days.
    C. 10 to 12 days.
    D. 120 days.

17. The following bleeding precaution orders have been written for a patient with a platelet count of 10,000/mm^3. Which of the orders should the nurse question? ⚠
    A. Avoid using a blood pressure cuff or tourniquet.
    B. Administer rectal acetaminophen for fever of 101° F (38.3° C).
    C. Apply firm pressure to venipuncture sites for 5 minutes.
    D. Administer stool softener twice a day.

18. One of the most important physical barriers against invasion of organisms is
    A. presence of a venous access device.
    B. intact intestinal mucosal barrier.
    C. presence of an indwelling urinary catheter.
    D. altered immune system.

19. F.N. presents to the clinic with fever, fatigue, sore throat, and bruising. She was recently diagnosed with acute myelogenous leukemia (AML) and has finished a course of induction chemotherapy. Her CBC with differential shows the following:
    White blood cell count (WBC) = 1.7 K/uL
    Segs = 22%
    Bands = 4%
    Lymphocytes = 45%
    Monos = 25%
    Eosinophils = 3%
    Basophils = 0%
    Myelos = 1%
    Red blood cell count (RBC) = 3.34 M/uL
    Hgb = 11.0 g/dL
    Hct = 31.5%
    Platelets = 26,000/mm^3
    What is the patient's absolute neutrophil count?
    A. 546
    B. 5460
    C. 442
    D. 44.2

20. On presentation, her vital signs are blood pressure (BP) of 94/50 mmHg, temperature of 102° F (38.9° C), heart rate 116, and respiratory rate of 24 breaths/min. On physical examination, her oral mucosa, vascular access device, heart, lungs, and abdomen are all normal. In addition to blood cultures, all except what additional tests would be appropriate to obtain before starting IV antibiotics?
    A. Chest radiography, PA and lateral
    B. Urine culture and sensitivity
    C. Computed tomography (CT) of abdomen
    D. Vancomycin-resistant enterococcus (VRE) swab

21. Potential complications associated with prolonged hemorrhage include all the following except
    A. blood clots.
    B. viral disease from numerous blood transfusions.
    C. shock.
    D. transfusion reaction.

22. Granulocytes collectively include
    A. basophils, eosinophils, and neutrophils.
    B. basophils, lymphocytes, and neutrophils.
    C. eosinophils, lymphocytes, and monocytes.
    D. basophils, lymphocytes, and monocytes.

23. S.L. presents to the clinic for her fourth course of chemotherapy for breast cancer. Her WBC is 2.1 K/uL and ANC is 1000/mm^3. She is asymptomatic. What would be the next step?
    A. Proceed with planned chemotherapy.
    B. Admit S.L. to the hospital for hydration.
    C. Begin antibiotics immediately.
    D. Teach S.L. infection precautions and what symptoms should prompt her to call the physician or nurse.

24. Patients are at a severe risk of bleeding when
    A. neutrophils are 50%.
    B. lymphocytes are 30%.
    C. platelets are less than 20,000 mm³.
    D. erythrocytes are 20%.

25. A.H. returns to the clinic to receive his sixth course of etoposide (VP-16) and cisplatin (Platinol) for small cell lung cancer. After obtaining his blood counts, the platelet level is reported to be 30,000 mm³. What would be the next step?
    A. Administer platelets immediately.
    B. Teach A.H. about bleeding precautions and what symptoms should prompt him to seek medical attention.
    C. Proceed with chemotherapy.
    D. Call hospice for placement.

26. Which statement is true about nadir?
    A. Nadir is the highest point the WBCs reach after cancer treatment and occurs 7 to 14 days after treatment.
    B. Nadir is WBC lysis related to chemotherapy administration.
    C. Nadir is the lowest point blood cells reach after a cancer treatment and occurs 7 to 14 days after treatment.
    D. Nadir regularly occurs after biotherapy administration.

27. L.J. has just received chemotherapy for non-Hodgkin lymphoma and has been discharged from the clinic. The nurse should instruct L.J. to contact the physician immediately if which of the following side effects occurs?
    A. Nosebleed that will not stop after applying pressure
    B. Temperature of 100° F (37.7° C)
    C. One episode of nausea without vomiting after chemotherapy
    D. Excessive fatigue after chemotherapy

28. Which of the following drugs can cause a fever?
    A. Interferon, methotrexate, and doxorubicin
    B. Interferon, interleukin-2, and vancomycin
    C. Interleukin-2, penicillin, and amphotericin B
    D. Tumor necrosis factor, gentamicin, and vancomycin

29. Radiation to which of the following areas can result in prolonged cytopenia?
    A. Skull, sternum, and long bones
    B. Tibia, ribs, and skull
    C. Ulna, sternum, and vertebrae
    D. Skull, ribs, and colon

30. Z.S. presents to the clinic with a temperature of 102° F (38.9° C). What initial question should be asked in taking his history to determine risk for infection?
    A. Have you recently been treated for your cancer with chemotherapy, radiation, or biotherapy?
    B. Have you recently traveled outside the United States?
    C. Are you still taking your Coumadin every day?
    D. Have you been experiencing dizziness, fatigue, or shortness of breath?

31. Myelosuppression is defined as the reduction in bone marrow function that results in a reduced release of which cells into the peripheral circulation?
    A. RBCs, megakaryocytes, and tumor necrosis factor
    B. RBCs, WBCs, and platelets
    C. WBCs, erythroblasts, and colony-stimulating factors
    D. Platelets, RBCs, and interleukin

32. What is the most common dose-limiting toxicity of chemotherapy?
    A. Constipation
    B. Nausea and vomiting
    C. Diarrhea
    D. Myelosuppression

33. Which of the following is true about administering colony-stimulating factors?
    A. Filgrastim is administered as a single dose of 10 mcg/kg the day before treatment to stimulate neutrophils.
    B. Pegfilgrastim is administered 24 hours after treatment and up to 4 days after treatment.
    C. Pegfilgrastim is administered as a single dose of 6 mg per cycle on the day after treatment.
    D. Sargramostim is administered at a dose of 500 mcg/m²/week.

34. Neutrophils are the first line of the body's defense and work by destroying
    A. viruses that invade the body.
    B. fungal infection.
    C. bacterial infection.
    D. parasites.

35. In which patient population is prophylactic antibiotic use considered?
    A. A patient diagnosed with AML who has recently undergone chemotherapy
    B. A pediatric cancer patient receiving combination chemotherapy and radiation therapy for osteosarcoma
    C. A patient diagnosed with aggressive breast cancer on adjuvant therapy
    D. A patient at extreme risk for febrile neutropenia
    E. An elderly cancer patient with shingles

36. All except which of the following statements accurately describes effects and uses of erythropoiesis-stimulating agents (ESAs)?
    A. Anemia prevention
    B. Promote proliferation and differentiation of progenitor cells along multiple cell pathways
    C. May cause an increased risk of thrombosis
    D. May cause hypertension and seizures

37. Thrombocytopenia describes a decrease in the circulating
    A. platelets below 100,000/mm^3.
    B. WBCs below 1500/mm^3.
    C. neutrophils below 1000/mm^3.
    D. RBCs below 1000/mm^3.

38. Which of the following vital signs would not put the patient at high risk for clinical deterioration associated with infection and fever?
    A. Hypertension (systolic BP >160 mm Hg)
    B. Hypotension (systolic BP <90 mm Hg)
    C. Respiratory rate >24 breaths/min
    D. Pulse rate = 126 beats/min

39. Patients are at a severe risk of infection when the
    A. hemoglobin value is less than 10 g/dL.
    B. platelet count is less than 20,000/mm^3.
    C. ANC is less than 1500/mm^3.
    D. ANC is less than 500/mm^3.

40. Which is not a contributing factor for anemia?
    A. Myelodysplastic syndrome
    B. Excess folate
    C. Vitamin B12 deficiency
    D. Chronic renal insufficiency

41. K.F. received interleukin-2 for the treatment of metastatic malignant melanoma. During her treatment course, she experienced fever and chills that lasted for a number of days. Which of the following side effects are associated with prolonged fever and chills?
    A. Decreased fatigue
    B. Decrease in circulating cancer cells
    C. Increase in activity
    D. Increased muscle weakness

28 Alterations in Gastrointestinal Function

1. A patient complains of a dry mouth after treatment and within several weeks develops thick, ropy saliva. She also has trouble chewing her food. She has
   A. dysphagia.
   B. xerostomia.
   C. mucositis.
   D. trismus.

2. Large bowel obstructions most often occur in the
   A. sigmoid colon.
   B. transverse colon.
   C. ascending colon.
   D. descending colon.

3. A critical change in the condition of a client with constipation that should be immediately reported to the physician is
   A. inadequate fluid intake.
   B. absence of bowel sounds.
   C. abdominal cramping associated with laxative use.
   D. failure to evacuate daily.

4. Which of the following statements about xerostomia is accurate?
   A. It is not related to cumulative radiation therapy (RT) dose; it is only related to the volume of salivary gland tissue included in the treatment portals.
   B. Older people are more likely to recover salivary flow than younger adults.
   C. It can occur with the use of antihistamines, opioids, and phenothiazines.
   D. Salivary substitutes are more beneficial than salivary stimulation in patients who have some salivary function.
   E. Methylcellulose-based products are better tolerated and have a longer duration of action than mucin-based preparations.

5. An elderly woman presents with an esophageal mass and symptoms of dyspnea and dysphagia. A biopsy is positive for squamous cell carcinoma of the esophagus with metastases to the lung. Her symptoms of dyspnea and dysphagia are most likely the result of
   A. infection caused by irritation of the oral mucosa.
   B. compressive effects of the tumor on the esophagus.
   C. anxiety associated with a new cancer diagnosis and metastatic disease.
   D. anorexia associated with cancer.

6. Which of the following interventions are appropriate for patients with xerostomia?
   A. Decrease intake of liquids.
   B. Encourage the patient to eat popsicles.
   C. Encourage the patient to eat dry and spicy foods.
   D. Rinse with commercial mouthwashes frequently to increase moisture.

7. Which of the following interventions helps to relieve nausea?
   A. Eating fatty or fried foods
   B. Drinking caffeinated beverages
   C. Medicating with an antiemetic each time vomiting is experienced
   D. Medicating with an antiemetic on an around-the-clock basis until nausea subsides

8. A patient has completed 2 weeks of RT and concomitant chemotherapy for carcinoma of the trachea. He complains of "a lump in his throat," dysphagia, odynophagia, and occasional epigastric pain. What is he probably experiencing?
   A. Reflux
   B. Tracheitis
   C. Esophagitis
   D. Bronchitis

9. Which of the following can be used to dissolve and break up thick saliva?
   A. Papain and amylase
   B. Commercial toothpastes
   C. Caffeine-containing products such as coffee, tea, colas, and chocolate
   D. Corn or vegetable oil

10. Ascites is mostly linked with which cancer type?
    A. Cervical cancer
    B. Ovarian cancer
    C. Malignant melanoma
    D. Head and neck cancer

11. Which factor is the most important in determining the consistency and volume of colostomy output?
    A. Amount of food eaten
    B. Amount of fluid intake
    C. Location of colostomy
    D. Type of food eaten

12. In addition to radiotherapy to the head and neck area, which of the following comorbidities may cause xerostomia?
    A. Gum disease
    B. Liver cirrhosis
    C. Heart failure
    D. Diabetes

13. Diarrhea can lead to fluid and electrolyte imbalance. Which of the following imbalances is of particular concern?
    A. Hypokalemia
    B. Hypercalcemia
    C. Hypophosphatemia
    D. Hyperkalemia

14. Which would be correct nutritional advice for a client prone to constipation?
    A. Include foods low in fiber but high in roughage in the daily diet.
    B. Take all opioids with milk to reduce the incidence of gastrointestinal upset.
    C. Maintain fluid intake of 1000 mL/day to prevent dehydration.
    D. Include foods high in fiber and roughage in the daily diet.

15. Which of the following statements about the use of corticosteroids in the management of vomiting are true?
    A. Beware of classic steroid side effects even when used for a short time.
    B. Corticosteroids work well in combination with other antiemetics when highly emetogenic chemotherapy drugs are administered.
    C. The use of corticosteroids can cause a decrease in appetite.
    D. The use of corticosteroids can lead to dysphagia.

16. A patient is having RT as primary treatment for a piriform sinus lesion. How might the nurse describe xerostomia to the patient?
    A. Xerostomia is a side effect that is likely to be permanent.
    B. You can expect excessive saliva formation for at least 4 months after radiation.
    C. Multiple medications can be used to prevent and eliminate xerostomia.
    D. Receiving chemotherapy will only worsen xerostomia.

17. Which of the following is true about dysphagia?
    A. Typically a fast onset
    B. May be caused by candidiasis
    C. Associated with a diagnosis of stomach cancer
    D. Managed with anticholinergic agents

18. The tumors that most commonly obstruct the bowel are
    A. hepatic and colorectal.
    B. ovarian and colorectal.
    C. gall bladder and endometrial.
    D. pancreatic and ovarian.

19. A 64-year-old Vietnamese patient diagnosed with recurrent hepatocellular cancer and ascites has not responded to chemotherapy. She complains of diffuse abdominal pain and distention, cramping, nausea, and dyspnea. She has had multiple paracenteses in the past, but the fluid continues to accumulate. She desires a palliative care consultation. Of the nursing measures below, which should be used immediately?
    A. Provide comfort (pain medication and nonpharmacologic approaches).
    B. Teach the patient and her family about dietary changes to help control fluid development, such as salt and water restrictions.
    C. Weigh the patient daily.
    D. Educate about signs and symptoms of dehydration, infection, respiratory distress, and malnutrition, which may be associated with ascites.

20. What is not a correct nursing intervention that should be instituted to prevent aspiration associated with dysphagia? ⚠
    A. Elevate head of bed 45 to 90 degrees, with the head slightly forward while eating; maintain position for at least 4 hours after oral intake.
    B. Use thickening agents to lessen the risk for flow of liquids into the airway.
    C. Assist with moving food from front of the tongue to a posterior area using a long-handled spoon as needed.
    D. Avoid small pieces of solid foods that can become lost in the mouth.

21. Which of the following medications can cause mucositis and esophagitis?
    A. 5-Fluorouracil, cytosine arabinoside, and etoposide
    B. Busulfan, cyclophosphamide, and vinblastine
    C. Docetaxel, methotrexate, and capecitabine
    D. Carboplatin, cisplatin, and irinotecan

22. Which of the following medications does not include constipation as a side effect?
    A. 5-HT3 antagonists
    B. Morphine
    C. 5-Fluorouracil (5-FU)
    D. Vinblastine (Velban)

23. Which of the following is a risk factor associated with nausea and vomiting incidence?
   A. Hypocalcemia
   B. Men older than 50 years
   C. Increased gastric emptying
   D. Primary or metastatic tumor of the central nervous system (CNS)

24. Which of the following is a type of mucositis?
   A. Gingivitis
   B. Stomatitis
   C. Dysphagia
   D. Xerostomia

25. A patient is receiving a combination therapy of 5-FU and radiation for colorectal cancer. Which of the following side effects is he most likely to experience?
   A. Peripheral neuropathy
   B. Constipation
   C. Thrombocytopenia
   D. Diarrhea

26. When choosing an ostomy appliance for the patient, which of the following should be considered?
   A. Size of appliance
   B. Location of stoma
   C. Color of stoma
   D. Preference of the ostomy nurse

27. Which of the following is true about risk factors related to mucositis?
   A. Elderly patients have a higher risk of developing mucositis.
   B. Mucositis severity is correlated with the daily RT dose, not the total cumulative dose.
   C. Continuous chemotherapy infusion schedules have greater negative effect on mucositis than short infusions.
   D. The large intestine will show damage within a few days of cytotoxic exposure and the small intestine a short while later.

28. A 48-year-old woman with advanced ovarian cancer presents to the clinic with complaints of abdominal distention, persistent cramping pain in the lower abdomen after eating, nausea, and no bowel movement for 3 days. On assessment, she has hypoactive bowel sounds. Which of the following does the patient most likely have?
   A. Partial bowel obstruction
   B. Gastric outlet obstruction
   C. Proximal small intestine obstruction
   D. Bowel perforation with peritonitis

29. M.R. is 30 years old and is receiving doxorubicin and cyclophosphamide every 3 weeks for breast cancer. She feels jittery and nervous after her chemotherapy. She is taking ondansetron (Zofran) 4 mg, dexamethasone (Decadron) 10 mg, and prochlorperazine (Compazine) 15 mg according to her schedule. Which of the following actions would be most appropriate?
   A. Eliminate the dexamethasone from her protocol because it is making her jittery.
   B. Stop everything and start her on dronabinol (Marinol).
   C. Administer diphenhydramine (Benadryl) with the prochlorperazine because she is young and may be sensitive to prochlorperazine's effects.
   D. Discontinue both the dexamethasone and the prochlorperazine because either one can cause jitteriness and a hypersensitivity reaction.

30. A patient complains of pain in his throat and difficulty swallowing. The nurse practitioner suggests Orabase gel. The Orabase is intended to accomplish which of the following?
   A. Pain control only
   B. Protect, coat, and soothe any sore and painful areas in the mouth or on the gums
   C. Promote healing by reducing infection
   D. Prevent chemotherapy drug exposure to the oral mucosa

31. Mucositis is more likely to occur in which of the following malignant conditions?
   A. Malignant melanoma
   B. Bladder cancer
   C. Breast cancer
   D. Leukemia

32. A patient complains of abdominal bloating and cramping with no bowel movement for the past 5 days. She usually has a bowel movement every day. Bowel sounds are present. She completed her last dose of chemotherapy (doxorubicin and cyclophosphamide) approximately 10 days ago. What action should be recommended to alleviate her constipation?
   A. A glycerin suppository
   B. A Fleet enema to stimulate peristalsis
   C. A stimulant laxative until bowel movement; then evaluate the need for daily stool softeners or lubricant laxatives
   D. Begin bulk-forming laxatives for constipation and a mild narcotic for abdominal pain.

33. In which of these situations would a patient be a candidate to learn colostomy irrigation to avoid wearing a pouch?
    A. The patient has an ostomy and is to receive abdominal radiation.
    B. The patient has a temporary colostomy.
    C. The patient has a cecostomy.
    D. The patient has a sigmoid colostomy that produces formed stool.

34. According to the National Cancer Institute (NCI) Common Toxicity Criteria scale, grade 2 mucositis is defined by
    A. mild symptoms, erythema of oral mucosa only.
    B. severe pain interfering with oral intake.
    C. confluent ulcerations covering less than 25% of oral mucosa.
    D. moderate pain not interfering with oral intake.

35. A 63-year-old patient has metastatic colon cancer. His disease is refractory to 5-FU. He received his first dose of irinotecan (Camptosar) 2 days ago. He began having diarrhea 36 hours after his therapy. Which of the following is an appropriate intervention for management of diarrhea in this patient?
    A. Administer atropine to manage his diarrhea.
    B. Administer loperamide (Imodium-AD) and monitor closely for dehydration and fluid–electrolyte imbalance.
    C. Premedicate with dexamethasone before the next dose of irinotecan to prevent diarrhea.
    D. Modify his diet by decreasing fiber and roughage as diarrhea is an expected side effect.

36. Which of the following herbal products may be helpful for patients with nausea and vomiting?
    A. Ginger
    B. Echinacea
    C. Milk thistle
    D. Essiac

37. What are potential complications of bowel obstruction?
    A. Hyperkalemia
    B. Dyspepsia
    C. Fluid overload
    D. Bowel perforation

38. A 54-year-old patient is undergoing a stem cell transplant for a diagnosis of multiple myeloma. Which of the following interventions should be integrated into a plan of care for her?
    A. Administer Palifermin IV before stem cell transplant.
    B. Administer Palifermin IV the day after stem cell transplant.
    C. Administer amifostine IV prior to chemotherapy administration.
    D. Administer amifostine IV the day after stem cell transplant.

39. How does ondansetron work to alleviate nausea and vomiting?
    A. Blocks the action of serotonin, a natural substance that may cause nausea and vomiting.
    B. Acts directly on the vomiting center located in the brainstem.
    C. Decreases stimulation of the receptors of the labyrinth in the inner ear.
    D. Increases gastric emptying by stimulating the gastrointestinal (GI) tract through vagal visceral afferent pathways.

40. A 72-year-old patient has stage IIIC colon cancer. He had a colon resection and has been receiving FOLFOX for several weeks. He calls the cancer center and reports to the nurse that he has experienced constipation for the past 2 weeks despite taking laxatives. His last bowel movement was 4 days ago. He complains of abdominal discomfort and distention, nausea, and onset of rectal bleeding this morning. He is instructed to come to the clinic. What is the most likely cause of this patient's symptoms?
    A. Impaction from the constipating effects of 5-FU and oxaliplatin
    B. Bowel obstruction, possibly from recurrent colorectal cancer
    C. Change in dietary fiber intake and exercise
    D. Chronic use of laxatives and enemas, which are no longer effective

41. A patient is receiving radiation therapy to her abdomen and asks for dietary instructions to decrease her diarrhea. What would the nurse not include in the client's dietary teaching?
    A. Eat a high-fiber diet that is high in protein.
    B. Begin a low-residue diet that is high in protein.
    C. Avoid spicy, fried, and fatty foods.
    D. If you have a known or temporary lactose intolerance, stick to a low-lactose diet.

42. A patient had an abdominal perineal resection for rectal cancer and is getting ready for discharge to home. He and his wife have numerous questions about colostomy care. Which of the following should not be included in stoma teaching? ⚠
    A. Protect the stoma from injury.
    B. Change the appliance every day to prevent leakage and decrease peristomal skin discomfort.
    C. Empty the pouch when it is one-third to half full.
    D. Monitor the color of the stoma and assess for bleeding. Teach the patient to use silver nitrate sticks to stop bleeding.

43. M.H., A 59-year-old patient with advanced metastatic breast cancer, is at home and receiving palliative care. She has severe bone pain and is taking scheduled and PRN opioids. Her daughter, a primary caregiver, states that M.H. has begun to experience some constipation. Which statement from M.H.'s daughter shows the need for further instruction about preventing constipation?
    A. "Mom needs to drink at least 8 glasses of fluid every day."
    B. "Mom needs more fiber in her diet, such as whole-grain breads, legumes, and fresh fruits and vegetables."
    C. "Some light exercise such as walking may help to keep my Mom regular."
    D. "Magnesium citrate used daily will help to prevent constipation."

44. Small bowel obstructions typically occur as a result of
    A. nonsurgical adhesions.
    B. volvulus.
    C. diverticulitis.
    D. gastrointestinal bleeding.

45. Which of these clients is at greatest risk for acute infectious diarrhea?
    A. A 36-year-old client with human immunodeficiency virus (HIV) who has just completed a 6-week course of antibiotics
    B. A 66-year-old client with acute myelogenous leukemia (AML), currently in remission, who is traveling in the northeastern United States
    C. An 8-year-old child, previously treated for rhabdomyosarcoma, in whom there has been no evidence of disease for the past 3 years
    D. A 70-year-old client with prostate cancer who is receiving intramuscular leuprolide (Lupron) monthly

46. Which of these laxatives chemically stimulates smooth muscles of the bowel and increases contractions?
    A. Senna
    B. Methylcellulose
    C. Docusate
    D. Sodium phosphate

47. According to the NCI grading criteria, a patient experiencing more than seven stools per day or who has a need for parenteral support for dehydration is classified as
    A. grade 1.
    B. grade 2.
    C. grade 3.
    D. grade 4.
    E. grade 5.

48. Which of the following is a secondary mechanism for slowing of intestinal mobility?
    A. Lack of privacy for defecation
    B. Decreased physical activity
    C. Spinal cord compression
    D. Anticonvulsant medications

49. In secretory diarrhea, the intestinal mucosa secretes excessive amounts of fluid and electrolytes. What can cause secretory diarrhea?
    A. Enteral tube feedings
    B. Graft-versus-host disease
    C. Inflammatory bowel disease
    D. Bacteria such as *Escherichia coli* and *Clostridium difficile*

50. L.I. is a 39-year-old client with ovarian cancer. She has completed a number of months of chemotherapy and has undergone a laparoscopic surgery, which revealed no evidence of malignancy. She presents to the clinic for the first postoperative visit with a complaint of constipation. Which of the following statements indicates that she understands a possible cause of her constipation?
    A. "Surgery can cause constipation because of the anesthesia and handling of the intestines."
    B. "My cancer must have returned and caused my bowels to close off."
    C. "I've not been very active since my surgery so that I can save my energy to be able to have a bowel movement."
    D. "I haven't eaten much lately; maybe that's why I haven't had a bowel movement."

29 Alterations in Genitourinary Function

1. Which type of incontinence is defined as the involuntary loss of urine associated with an abrupt and strong desire to void?
   - A. Stress
   - B. Urge
   - C. Reflex
   - D. Functional
   - E. Total

2. Which of the following is not an example of a urinary storage problem?
   - A. Intrinsic sphincter dysfunction
   - B. Reduced bladder wall compliance
   - C. Urethral or prostatic obstruction
   - D. Unintentional bladder contraction during filling

3. D.O. is a 72-year-old man diagnosed with prostate cancer who recently underwent a radical prostatectomy. After surgery, he has experienced incontinence and asks the nurse why. Which statement would the nurse not want to include in the answer to his question?
   - A. As you age, there is evidence that one of the sphincters controlling urine flow can weaken and nerves can degenerate, causing incontinence.
   - B. Tissue injury around the sphincter may have been caused by lack of blood flow to that area during surgery.
   - C. Your urologist is new and not very experienced in doing these procedures. He probably injured your pudendal nerve.
   - D. Sometimes stress and urge incontinence occurs because your bladder muscles are weak; I can teach you some exercises that may help strengthen your muscles.

4. Which of the following is not considered a comorbid condition associated with urinary incontinence that may be elicited when conducting a patient history?
   - A. Endocrine conditions, such as hyperglycemia and diabetes insipidus, that can lead to diuresis
   - B. Estrogen depletion during menopause may induce urethral epithelium thinning
   - C. Increased bladder or rectal contractions in clients with lesions in the brain cortex as a result of a cerebrovascular accident, multiple sclerosis, or Parkinson disease
   - D. Immobility commonly associated with chronic degenerative disease

5. What medications are associated with urinary incontinence?
   - A. Antiemetic agents, nonopioids, and antihistamines
   - B. Nonopioids
   - C. Laxatives
   - D. Diuretics
   - E. Certain chemotherapeutic agents such as vinca alkaloids and doxorubicin

6. L.P. is a 61-year-old woman with urinary incontinence after ovarian cancer debulking surgery. She is very discouraged because she has to wear protective urinary drainage pads constantly, especially when she exercises, and wants to know what she can do to regain her urinary function. When asked about her oral intake, she eats a regular diet, drinks 2 cups of coffee in the morning, has 2 or 3 glasses of wine with dinner, enjoys herbal tea in the evening, and drinks plenty of fluids throughout the day. What instructions will the nurse not include because it would have little effect on L.P.'s incontinence?
   - A. Limit alcohol intake.
   - B. Limit caffeine intake.
   - C. Limit fluid intake several hours before bedtime.
   - D. Recommend she stop exercising until the incontinence subsides.

7. H.C., a 78-year-old woman with metastatic breast cancer to bone, presents with hypercalcemia. She is admitted to the oncology unit with symptoms of polyuria, nausea, clouded sensorium, increased pain, weakness, fatigue, and immobility. She is receiving continuous IV hydration at 250 mL/hr, adequate replacement of potassium and magnesium, IV Zometa, hydromorphone 0.2 mg on demand by PCA, and ondansetron 4 mg IV PRN for nausea and vomiting. She is a fall risk and has difficulty getting out of bed for toileting because of increased pain and weakness. Frequent urinary incontinence is a problem. What nursing intervention should be incorporated into her plan of care? ⚠
   - A. Insert an indwelling urinary catheter for comfort.
   - B. Use absorbent incontinence pads.
   - C. Don't set a voiding routine because that could put stress on the patient and deter voiding.
   - D. Apply lotion after each incontinent episode.
   - E. Clean the perineal and perianal areas after each voiding or bowel movement with soft washcloth and chlorhexidine, rinse thoroughly, and pat dry.

8. Which of the following patients would be suitable candidates for neobladder surgery? A patient
   A. with a history of benign prostatic hypertrophy (BPH).
   B. with inflammatory bowel disease.
   C. who has received radiation therapy.
   D. with urethral cancer.

9. Which of the following is a true statement about urinary diversions?
   A. Voiding is accomplished by concurrent relaxation of the urinary sphincter and a Valsalva maneuver in patients with a neobladder.
   B. An ileal conduit does not require an external collection device.
   C. Patients with a continent diversion require intermittent catheterization (every 3 hours) through the stoma to drain urine from the reservoir.
   D. Patients with an ileal conduit have a low risk for urinary tract infections.
   E. Patients with an ileal conduit have a high risk for urinary tract infections.

10. Mr. Y, a 64-year-old man with a new diagnosis of bladder cancer, is 5 days post ileal conduit surgery. He is going home in a few days with an external collection device for urine. He is planning to start chemotherapy in 7 to 10 days when healed. The nurse starts discharge teaching and reviews care for his urinary diversion with Mr. Y and his wife. Which of the following instructions are appropriate to review?
   A. Cut the pouch opening of your appliance so that the barrier clears the stoma by ½ inch. Protect your exposed skin with barrier paste as needed.
   B. Change the appliance every morning to prevent odor buildup and leakage.
   C. Examine your stoma and skin around it for redness, bleeding, irritation, and stoma issues with each appliance change.
   D. Empty the pouch when full and before chemotherapy treatment.

11. Treatment-related renal dysfunction can occur in all the following except
   A. administration of 5-fluororacil (5-FU).
   B. administration of gemcitabine.
   C. radiation to renal structures that can lead to long-lasting fibrosis.
   D. renal obstruction caused by tumor lysis syndrome.

12. Which of the following cancers does not cause hypercalcemia of malignancy (HCM)?
   A. Squamous cell cancer of the lung
   B. Renal cell cancer
   C. Multiple myeloma
   D. Pancreatic cancer

13. Which of the following laboratory data indicate renal impairment?
   A. ↑Serum Cr, normal BUN, ↓uric acid
   B. ↑Uric acid, ↑calcium, ↓potassium, ↓magnesium
   C. A positive urine culture and sensitivity
   D. ↓Uric acid, ↓creatinine, ↑potassium, ↑albumin

14. What interventions (both pharmacologic and nonpharmacologic) must be considered to maintain adequate fluid volume and electrolytes during and immediately after chemotherapy administration? ⚠
   A. Monitor urine output. If output is less than 60 mL/hr, this may indicate renal impairment.
   B. Ensure aggressive hydration before cisplatin administration. When a patient is adequately hydrated, additional fluids are not necessary during and after administration.
   C. If a patient is receiving diuretics, maintain a greater intake than output unless contraindicated.
   D. Administer oral sodium bicarbonate to maintain acid urine.

15. After extensive surgery for metastatic bladder cancer, a patient returns to the outpatient clinic for a follow-up appointment and to begin chemotherapy treatment. He is newly married and expresses sexual health concerns. What is the nurse's response?
   A. Encourage him to verbalize his feelings about having a urinary diversion device to his doctor; it is uncomfortable for the nurse to talk with him about these issues.
   B. Acknowledge that it is normal to have these feelings and concerns. Stress that it is important to relax; things will get better over time.
   C. Actively listen to his concerns, assist him to incorporate changes into his activities of daily living, discuss his interpersonal relationships, and ask if he would like to be referred to a sexual health counselor.
   D. Tell the patient that the infusion area is so busy right now that the nurse does not have time to talk with him about his concerns. Refer him to an ostomy support group where he can get the needed support.

16. Which of the following is true about the tests used to evaluate urinary incontinence?
   A. An electromyogram is used to identify the site of obstruction.
   B. A cystoscopy is used to determine presence and amount of post void residual urine.
   C. Bladder scanning is used to evaluate micturition and bladder filling.
   D. A culture and sensitivity test is used to assess for hematuria, bacteriuria, and glucosuria.

17. J.V. is a 68-year-old man with prostate cancer. He has had a radical prostatectomy for stage II disease. He comes to the surgical oncology clinic for his 1-month follow-up and reports to the nurse that he has experienced urinary incontinence several times a day for the past week. Which statement made by J.V. indicates he understands his urinary symptoms?

A. "Urinary incontinence commonly occurs after removal of the prostate, so I will probably always be incontinent."

B. "The incontinence should have stopped by now, so I need to have an indwelling catheter, just like I did after my surgery."

C. "Urinary incontinence may continue for several months but should improve with a scheduled voiding program and pelvic muscle exercises."

D. "I need to take antibiotics. My incontinence is probably caused by a bladder infection."

18. Which of the following chemotherapy agents requires aggressive hydration before, during, and after therapy to prevent renal toxicity?

A. Daunorubicin (Cerubidine)

B. 5-FU

C. Cisplatin (Platinol)

D. Flutamide (Eulexin)

19. A patient has breast cancer with bone metastases. Which condition commonly occurs with her disease and can cause the kidneys to lose the ability to concentrate urine?

A. Hyperkalemia

B. Hypocalcemia

C. Hyponatremia

D. Hypercalcemia

20. A new patient with metastatic breast cancer was admitted to the oncology unit for management of treatment-induced congestive heart failure. On admission, she was given 40 mg of furosemide (Lasix). Because she is elderly, frail, and in a strange environment, the nurse is concerned about urinary incontinence. A nursing care plan would include

A. providing adult briefs for the patient so she will not have to worry about incontinence.

B. inserting an indwelling urinary catheter to avoid incontinence.

C. placing a commode at the bedside and instructing the patient in its use.

D. no special measures.

21. Which of the following is a risk factor that can lead to renal dysfunction?

A. Radiation therapy to the renal structures

B. Diuretic use

C. Hypocalcemia of malignancy

D. Renal hyperperfusion

30 Alterations in Musculoskeletal, Integumentary, and Neurologic Functions

1. P.E. is a 74-year-old breast cancer survivor and avid gardener. Over the past few months she has noticed increasing shoulder discomfort and back and neck pain. When conducting a physical examination to access P.E.'s alteration in musculoskeletal functioning, which of the following would most likely not be part of the assessment?
   A. Examine joint structure and alignment.
   B. Assess deep tendon reflexes of the biceps, brachioradial, triceps, Achilles, and patellar.
   C. Evaluate the patient's mobility and sensory function.
   D. Teach patient to inspect affected areas for cuts, burns, and bruises.

2. Which of the following is the most appropriate nursing action in a cancer patient at risk for fungal infection?
   A. Apply povidone-iodine (Betadine) to moist areas.
   B. Dry the skin folds of the patient thoroughly.
   C. Bathe the patient daily.
   D. Keep the patient's room cool.

3. A 67-year-old patient was treated for a nasopharyngeal carcinoma a few years ago with chemotherapy and was considered to have a complete clinical response. He has recently been found to have perineural tumor spread (PNS) along the fifth to seventh cranial nerves. Which symptoms would indicate a change in his neurologic status?
   A. Reduced ability to feel pain and changes in temperature in the feet or hands
   B. A consistently small pupil and a drooping of the upper eyelid
   C. Pain and paresthesia
   D. Pain in or behind his ear, drooling, and increased sensitivity to sound

4. A patient with impaired skin integrity is receiving an antineoplastic medication that causes myelosuppression. The nurse should assess the patient for which of the following? ⚠
   A. Diarrhea
   B. Infection
   C. Constipation
   D. Dysrhythmia

5. M.W., a 74-year-old patient with a history of prostate cancer, presents at the emergency department (ED) with numbness and tingling of the legs. What is the most appropriate nursing action?
   A. Immobilize the body and instruct the patient not to flex his head.
   B. Reassure the patient that the change in sensation is temporary.
   C. Turn him every 2 hours and check his skin.
   D. Initiate a complete neurologic examination.

6. After further evaluation, M.W. (from the previous question) has a diagnosis of spinal cord compression caused by metastatic disease. What nursing actions are necessary to maintain skin integrity?
   A. Perform range of motion (ROM) exercises to the extremities.
   B. Set up regular bowel and bladder programs.
   C. Logroll every 2 hours and inspect the skin.
   D. Monitor for edema of the extremities.

7. A patient begins chemotherapy treatment and, within 1 hour after infusion has begun, presents with itching and redness of the skin. This skin reaction is typically the result of which drug class or mechanism?
   A. Platinum derivatives (cisplatin, carboplatin)
   B. Epidermal growth factor receptor (EGFR) inhibitors (cetuximab, gefitinib)
   C. Rituximab
   D. None of the above

8. With a diagnosis of ataxia, the patient should be assessed for
   A. skin integrity issues.
   B. ambulation and mobility status.
   C. heart rate and respiratory rate.
   D. dehydration, electrolyte imbalance, and renal compromise.

9. Which of these symptoms is most associated with a grade 3 diagnosis of skin rash mediated by EGFR inhibition?
   A. Pruritus
   B. Severe generalized erythroderma or macular or papular eruption
   C. Acneiform rash
   D. Generalized exfoliative, ulcerative, or blistering skin toxicity

10. Which activity is most related to tertiary prevention in a patient with impaired physical mobility?
    A. Educating
    B. Promoting
    C. Immunizing
    D. Rehabilitating

11. Which of the following is not a psychoeducational intervention used in patients with anxiety and depression?
    A. Counseling and psychotherapy
    B. Cognitive distraction
    C. Requesting a sitter if the patient is considered unsafe
    D. Behavioral therapy

12. A patient has a nursing diagnosis of impaired physical mobility related to calcium loss resulting from extended bed rest. What is an important function of calcium?
    A. Keeping the stomach acidic
    B. Muscle contraction
    C. Preventing blood clotting
    D. Production of insulin

13. A 26-year-old patient has been diagnosed with gastric cancer at the esophageal gastric junction. He is receiving second-line chemotherapy with paclitaxel and ramucirumab. The nurse notices the palms of his hands are reddened with spotty areas that seem to contain small welts. He states that it does not hurt, but it itches to some extent and feels hot. The nurse suspects this is
    A. erythema multiforme.
    B. candidiasis.
    C. erythema nodosum.
    D. rosacea.

14. H.B. is an 87-year-old breast cancer patient with delirium. In planning her care, you would
    A. remove calendars from the patient's environment because they increase confusion.
    B. allow family photos only if the patient can identify the people in the photos.
    C. encourage the patient to consistently use assistive devices such as eyeglasses and hearing aids.
    D. maximize the patient's exposure to environmental sounds, such as alarms, to remind her that she is in a hospital and not at home.

15. Which of the following is a nursing intervention to protect skin integrity?
    A. Moisturizing and lubricating skin
    B. Teaching about the use of sterile technique for invasive procedures such as insertion of tubes
    C. Use of medications to manage rash
    D. Instructing on gentle skin cleansing with mild pH-balanced skin cleanser

16. Which assessment finding would support the nursing diagnosis of impaired physical mobility?
    A. Curvature of the spine
    B. Muscle atrophy in the lower extremities
    C. Generalized decreased upper muscle mass
    D. Bilateral hypertrophy of paired muscle groups

17. Which of the following nursing interventions should be used to support and communicate with a patient who is cognitively impaired and receiving chemotherapy?
    A. Call the patient by a term of endearment when addressing him or her.
    B. Identify the patient using the identification band.
    C. Identify yourself and give a simple explanation to the patient.
    D. Avoid touching the patient to decrease the risk of anxiety.

18. A patient is on strict bed rest. Which of these interventions would be most commonly used in increasing a patient's physical functioning?
    A. Placing the bed in low position and the two side rails at the head of bed (HOB) to use
    B. Changing the patient's position every hours
    C. Discussing risk factors for impaired mobility with both the patient and the family
    D. Placing the call light within reach when the patient is left alone

31 Alterations in Respiratory Function

1. Abnormal accumulation of air within the pleural space is known as
   A. an empyema.
   B. a pneumothorax.
   C. parenchymal disease.
   D. a pleural effusion.

2. A patient is scheduled for surgery after being diagnosed with non–small cell lung cancer. He says that the doctor called the surgery a pneumonectomy. Which statement from him indicates he has a basic understanding of the type of surgery?
   A. I was always afraid of lung cancer like my father had, but I am glad they only have to take part of the lining off my lung at this time.
   B. I knew this was a risk for me because I couldn't stop smoking, but am hopeful removing a segment of my lung will remove all the cancer.
   C. I guess I should be thankful my lungs have multiple sections so that when they remove part of one, I will still be able to function.
   D. I never knew that a person could learn to do OK after having a whole lung removed.

3. Which client has the highest number of risk factors for alterations in ventilation? A client with
   A. tuberculosis receiving treatment with isoniazid (INH) and vitamin B6 for 6 months, who is a smoker, had a cholecystectomy 3 months ago, and has a productive cough with yellow sputum.
   B. a non–small cell lung cancer diagnosis, a history of left upper lobe lung removal, chronic obstructive pulmonary disease (COPD), and atherosclerotic heart disease.
   C. ovarian cancer with total hysterectomy 3 weeks ago, type 2 diabetes mellitus for 5 years with abnormal HgB A1C levels, history of latex allergies, and history of asthma.
   D. cardiac stents placed 3 months ago, prostate cancer diagnosed 2 months ago, currently receiving radiation therapy for his prostate cancer, and a history of abdominal aortic aneurysm (AAA) repair 12 years ago.

4. Which of the following would the nurse anticipate for the client who has just been given the diagnosis of empyema?
   A. Radiation therapy to the lung field(s) involved
   B. Systemic antibiotics to treat the infection
   C. Subcutaneous epinephrine 1:100 solution
   D. Semi-Fowler position and oxygen at 30% face mask

5. The nurse is preparing a teaching plan for the family of an elderly client with lung cancer who currently lives alone. What would be the priority for client safety and optimal outcomes? ⚠
   A. Activity prioritization and energy conservation strategies
   B. Medication management and availability of emergency care
   C. Signs and symptoms to report to the local health care provider
   D. Enhanced understanding of the impact on cognitive function

6. J.J. has been receiving radiation therapy and bleomycin (Blenoxane) chemotherapy for treating his cancer. He is at risk for which type of pulmonary toxicity?
   A. Hemothorax
   B. Pulmonary empyema
   C. Pneumonitis
   D. Pleural effusion

7. D.T. is being treated with glucocorticoids for her radiation-induced pneumonitis. Her symptoms have begun to improve by 50%. The physician writes an order to "stop the glucocorticoids; she is doing much better." The nurse knows that ⚠
   A. the glucocorticoids can and should be discontinued as prescribed.
   B. she should auscultate the client's lungs and review her blood count first.
   C. she will also need to request a prescription for a cough suppressant.
   D. abrupt discontinuation of glucocorticoids can flare up the pneumonitis.

8. N.K. is receiving his first dose of gemcitabine (Gemzar) chemotherapy as treatment for pancreatic cancer. During treatment, the client begins to have significant dyspnea, a fever of 100.5° F (38.05° C), and a nonproductive cough. What would the nurse prioritize as the initial nursing intervention?
   A. Get the code cart and prepare for emergency intubation.
   B. Stop the chemotherapy immediately but maintain the venous access.
   C. Obtain STAT chest radiography to check for ground-glass opacities.
   D. Administer oxygen at 2 L by nasal cannula and give epinephrine 1:1000.

9. T.K. has just been given the diagnosis of pulmonary toxicity as a result of radiation therapy and chemotherapy. What would the nurse expect to see?
   A. Hyperoxygenation and hypercapnia
   B. Metabolic acidosis with an increased pH
   C. Hypoxia and hypocapnia
   D. Hypoxia and hypercapnia

10. The nurse is providing care for a client receiving targeted therapy, cetuximab, and concomitant radiation therapy. What pulmonary abnormalities would she need to watch for?
    A. Radiation pneumonitis and isolated acute chest pain
    B. Acute pneumonitis and hypersensitivity reaction
    C. Hemoptysis and acute radiation pneumonitis
    D. Bronchiolitis and increased lung diffusion capacity

11. Which of the following classes of pharmacologic agents is used to decrease local inflammation in the client with dyspnea?
    A. Bronchodilators
    B. Glucocorticoids
    C. Antibiotics
    D. Diuretics

12. M.T. developed dyspnea after being up and showering. The nurse wants to determine the severity of his hypoxia. What is the best intervention to accomplish this? Obtain a STAT
    A. lung diffusion capacity.
    B. pulse oximetry.
    C. chest radiography.
    D. sputum culture.

13. Which of the following body positions would be recommended to the client experiencing dyspnea?
    A. Lie flat and on the right side.
    B. Lie in semi-Fowler position at a 45-degree angle.
    C. Sit upright with his legs crossed and hands over the head.
    D. Sit upright and lean forward with both elbows on a table.

14. Which of the following is a complementary therapy that can help decrease the sense of dyspnea and enhance psychosocial well-being?
    A. Grape seed extract
    B. Prayer and meditation
    C. Intravenous morphine sulfate
    D. Use of an incentive spirometer

15. The greatest challenge in working with clients experiencing dyspnea is?
    A. Similar to pain, dyspnea is a subjective experience.
    B. Abnormal assessment findings may be lacking.
    C. Dyspnea may be present with many different conditions.
    D. Clients often do not know how to describe it.

16. B.D. has just had a thoracentesis for treatment of a pleural effusion that was transudative in nature. The nurse knows that he may present with decreased oncotic pressure in the microvasculature as a result of
    A. hypoproteinemia.
    B. heart failure.
    C. atelectasis.
    D. acute pain.

17. K.J.T. comes in for her 1-month postoperative visit for breast cancer, and on physical examination she has tachypnea, dullness to percussion in the right lower lobe (RLL) of the lung, absent breath sounds in the RLL, egophony on the right side of the chest, and a slight fever. This client most likely has
    A. lung metastasis
    B. severe anemia.
    C. pulmonary fibrosis.
    D. a pleural effusion.

18. When caring for a client who has just been identified as having a pleural effusion, it is important to know that
    A. symptoms are typically related to speed of fluid accumulation rather than the amount of fluid present.
    B. transudative fluid is probably related to local factors, such as metastatic tumor or infections causing an effusion.
    C. exudative fluids are related to systemic factors such as congestive heart failure (CHF) and nephrotic syndrome causing an effusion.
    D. the patient will probably need video-assisted thoracoscopic surgery (VATS) for talc pleurodesis.

19. A patient's family member has just been given information about abnormal accumulation of air within the pleural space. She asks, "Doesn't air belong in the lungs?" The nurse would explain that
    A. the air is accumulating in the pleural space, the space between the lung tissue and the chest wall. This is called a pneumothorax.
    B. the client most likely has metastatic spread of the cancer at this time.
    C. the radiation therapy and the bleomycin cause this type of problem.
    D. the patient will need to have surgery to remedy this problem.

32 Alterations in Cardiovascular Function

1. Lymphedema secondary to cancer treatment is
   A. an obstruction of the lymphatic system that causes lymph fluid overload in the interstitial space.
   B. accumulation of fluids in the interstitial space, occurring most frequently with breast cancer.
   C. lower limb swelling that occurs secondary to the accumulation of fluid in the peritoneal cavity.
   D. the presence of edema in an extremity that includes the presence of pain and erythema.

2. Nursing actions for treatment and prevention of problems related to lymphedema include
   A. sterile technique before administration of chemotherapy in the limb.
   B. using an electronic or automated rather than a manual blood pressure cuff.
   C. massage therapy and vigorous weight lifting of the affected limb.
   D. regular measurement of extremities and elevation of the affected extremity.

3. If a client with breast cancer has not developed lymphedema in the first 3 years after surgery, she
   A. will probably not develop problems in the arm.
   B. must be instructed that the potential for its development remains a concern.
   C. probably had sentinel node mapping at the time of her initial surgery.
   D. benefited from breast conservation and radiation therapy.

4. A client presents with increased pigmentation; prominent superficial venous patterning; and thickening, pitting, and erythema of the skin on her arm. This is probably
   A. lymphedema.
   B. deep venous thrombosis.
   C. interstitial edema.
   D. arterial emboli.

5. Risk factors associated with the development of lymphedema include
   A. history of deep vein thrombosis (DVT).
   B. infection in the extremity with surgical alterations.
   C. low-dose radiation therapy.
   D. immobility of extremity.

6. A client calls stating her arm has become tight and red after a long plane trip. The most appropriate advice to give her is: ⚠
   A. keep the arm elevated and see her provider in a week—this is probably just because her extremity was dependent during the flight.
   B. don't worry—this is a normal response to trav, and it will most likely improve in a couple of day
   C. to promptly make arrangements to see her provide the same day for probable antibiotics for cellulitis.
   D. refer her to physical therapy to start manual lymph drainage and the application of a pressure dressing.

7. An appropriate outcome for a client with lymphedema includes the client
   A. verbalizing an acceptable level of pain control.
   B. reporting weight gain of more than 2 lb per day.
   C. reporting absence of dyspnea.
   D. exhibiting normal vital signs.

8. Which statement by a family member of a client with breast cancer would indicate adequate comprehension of the teaching regarding her treatment?
   A. "I am glad my wife had a sentinel node mapping so that we don't have to worry about swelling like her mother had."
   B. "My wife's surgery was 6 months ago. She doesn't still need to worry about the use of her affected extremity."
   C. "I'm glad the new medications for breast cancers have decreased the risk of lymphedema."
   D. "We want to plan a plane trip for us to go see our newest grandchild; what do we have to do for her arm?"

9. A decrease in which of the following leads to edema?
   A. Capillary pressure
   B. Capillary permeability
   C. Plasma oncotic pressure
   D. Hydrostatic pressure

10. Which of the following may be associated with edema in clients with cancer?
    A. Hyperthyroidism and sepsis
    B. Hyperproteinemia and poor nutrition
    C. Hyperalbuminemia and nephrotic syndrome
    D. Angiogenesis inhibiting chemotherapy agents

11. Nursing assessment of potential risk factors for edema would include identification of what?
    A. Deep venous thrombosis and hypotension
    B. Hypertension and history of edema
    C. Pain or stiffness in an extremity
    D. Paroxysmal nocturnal dyspnea

12. Findings related to edema of cancer include
    A. the presence of S2 heart sound.
    B. decreased serum albumin and protein.
    C. increased peripheral pulses.
    D. decreased blood pressure and heart rate.

13. Which of the following is a safety-related concern for individuals with edema? ⚠
    A. Sepsis from an infected central line
    B. Skin breakdown on the extremity
    C. Fluid retention after prolonged standing
    D. Need for bedrest to promote diuresis

14. Which statement is true regarding pericardial effusions?
    A. They are often caused by spread of the cancer, or metastatic disease involvement in the cardiac space.
    B. Radiation therapy to the heart increases the risk pericardial infections secondary to immune suppression.
    C. They occur in individuals who have received cardiotoxic agents that decrease capillary permeability.
    D. Common causes include hemorrhagic tamponade from a severe direct injury to the anterior chest.

15. All of the following are findings associated with pericardial effusions except
    A. weakness and a productive persistent cough, especially with physical activity.
    B. chest radiography showing cardiac enlargement and a wide mediastinum.
    C. tachycardia, jugular vein distention, and decreased peripheral pulses.
    D. echocardiography findings of the presence of fluid.

16. Risk factors associated with malignant pericardial effusion include
    A. low fraction size of radiation therapy daily but covering a majority of the heart.
    B. diabetes mellitus and a history of bacterial endocarditis.
    C. history of deep venous thrombosis in a client with lung cancer.
    D. existing cardiac disease and systemic lupus erythematosus.

17. High-dose cyclophosphamide (Cytoxan) is associated with which cardiac toxicity?
    A. Asymptomatic bradycardia with nonspecific electrocardiogram changes
    B. Coronary artery spasm causing positional chest pain on exertion
    C. Cardiomyopathy leading to significant activity intolerance
    D. Myocardial necrosis caused by endothelial damage

18. As a nurse caring for a client with malignant pericardial effusion, which intervention should be implemented?
    A. Keep the head of bed flat and elevate feet.
    B. Administer diuretics to mobilize excess fluid.
    C. Increase the level of physical activity.
    D. Administer no intervention if the patient is asymptomatic.

19. Which of the following interventions is not recommended for patient education when relieving symptoms and improving quality of life in patients with malignant pericardial effusion?
    A. Relaxation techniques
    B. Energy conservation strategies
    C. Sleep with the head of the bed elevated
    D. Oxygen therapy

20. Potential cardiovascular toxicities in a client receiving treatment for cancer include
    A. alteration in the electrical conduction within the heart.
    B. increased risk of myocardial infarction caused by treatment-induced hypertension.
    C. bilateral lower limb edema caused by deep venous thrombosis.
    D. asymptomatic bradycardia caused by radiation therapy to the chest.

21. Early heart failure and left ventricular dysfunction (LDV) are likely to be related to which of the following chemotherapy agents?
    A. Daunorubicin combined with tamoxifen
    B. Methotrexate
    C. Doxorubicin combined with paclitaxel or docetaxel
    D. High-dose 5-fluorouracil (5-FU)

22. Cardiac toxicities that begin 24 hours after chemotherapy administration are
    A. chronic.
    B. permanent.
    C. acute.
    D. irreversible.

23. Factors that are associated with increased risk of cardiotoxicity from chemotherapy include
    A. standard dose cyclophosphamide over multiple days, advanced age, and history of smoking.
    B. history of smoking, bony metastasis, and history of lung cancer with pericardial effusion.
    C. high-dose cyclophosphamide, radiation therapy to the chest, and history of lung cancer.
    D. high doses of potentially cardiotoxic chemotherapeutic agents administered over relatively short periods of time.

24. Prevention of doxorubicin (Adriamycin)-related cardiomyopathy includes
    A. exercise and low-dose dexamethasone.
    B. smoking cessation and oxygen therapy
    C. exercise and use of dexrazoxane (Zinecard).
    D. lipid-lowering drugs and low-fat diet.

25. When the ejection fraction is less than 45%, the nurse should expect ⚠
    A. an increase in the dexrazoxane (Zinecard) dose.
    B. a decrease in the dose of cardiotoxic chemotherapeutic agents.
    C. close monitoring of client with serial electrocardiograms.
    D. an increase in intravenous fluids.

26. Which statement correctly identifies the classifications of chemotherapy agents and their potential effects?
    A. Protease inhibitors and tyrosine kinase inhibitors can cause early heart failure and left ventricular dysfunction.
    B. Antimetabolites have the potential to cause coronary artery spasm, resulting in cardiac-related sudden death.
    C. Anthracyclines given with taxanes have the potential to cause coronary artery spasm, resulting in cardiac-related sudden death.
    D. Monoclonal antibodies can cause cardiac toxicities by impeding immune system response to infection.

27. A client is admitted with congestive heart failure. Records indicate a history of breast cancer treated with chemotherapy and radiation therapy. The most likely late effect of this treatment is
    A. pulmonary fibrosis from radiation therapy.
    B. pleural effusion causing dyspnea on exertion.
    C. cardiomyopathy caused by anthracycline therapy.
    D. coronary artery disease and hypertension.

28. Which is considered a risk factor for a thrombotic event?
    A. Thrombocytopenia.
    B. Anemia.
    C. Disseminated intravascular coagulation (DIC)
    D. Neutropenia.

29. Family members of a client contact the nurse to report the client is very anxious, complaining of chest pain and breathing rapidly with shallow breaths. This presentation would be typical of
    A. arterial embolus.
    B. venous occlusion.
    C. pulmonary embolus.
    D. paroxysmal nocturnal dyspnea.

30. The presence of which of the following would point to a venous occlusion in an extremity rather than an arterial embolus?
    A. A dull ache, tight feeling, or pain in the calf
    B. Severe pain in the involved extremity
    C. Coolness and pallor of the affected extremity
    D. Absent or decreased pulse in the extremity

31. Which of the following would assist the nurse planning care for a client with DVT?
    A. A diagnostic spiral CT
    B. Knowledge that tamoxifen use places women at increased risk for problems
    C. Education regarding risk factors such as family history of cancer with no coagulopathy abnormalities
    D. Knowledge that monoclonal antibodies increase the potential risk for problems

32. Which is an appropriate outcome for the client with DVT? The client
    A. reports cool extremities.
    B. maintains intact skin.
    C. has increased blood pressure.
    D. reports increased fatigue.

33 Alterations in Nutritional Status

1. A patient is concerned about metabolic changes caused by cancer. The nurse explains the impact of malignancy on the metabolism of
   A. vitamins and minerals.
   B. pharmaceutical products.
   C. protein and carbohydrates.
   D. mono- and polyunsaturated fats.

2. What are possible complications associated with prolonged anorexia?
   A. Bone atrophy
   B. Hyperalbuminemia
   C. Compromised humoral and cellular immune function
   D. Increased white blood cells

3. What syndrome occurs when a patient's protein and calorie requirements are not met, his or her condition progressively worsens, and muscle wasting ensues?
   A. Cachexia
   B. Anorexia
   C. Secondary cachexia
   D. Failure to thrive

4. Which medications may stimulate appetite?
   A. Dexamethasone and opioids
   B. Megestrol acetate and dexamethasone
   C. Muscle relaxants and methylphenidate
   D. Opioids and metoclopramide

5. Although patients and their families often believe that total parenteral nutrition (TPN) is superior to oral or enteral nutrition, the most important reason for using the GI tract is that it
   A. is less expensive than TPN.
   B. makes nutrients available faster.
   C. prevents atrophy of the GI mucosa.
   D. promotes adequate vascular fluid volume.

6. J.K. is 2 weeks post gastric resection for stomach cancer. She has lost 20 lb since her surgery. What is the most likely cause of her significant weight loss?
   A. NPO status before and after surgery
   B. Postprandial dumping syndrome
   C. Cancer cachexia
   D. Depression associated with her diagnosis

7. Which of the following cancer types are associated with cachexia?
   A. Lung and pancreatic cancers
   B. Breast and ovarian cancers
   C. Leukemias and lymphomas
   D. Malignant melanoma and gastric cancer

8. What would not be considered a physiological factor associated with cancer-related anorexia?
   A. Metabolic disturbances such as hypercalcemia
   B. Treatment-induced side effects from chemotherapy
   C. Anxiety and depression
   D. A proinflammatory cytokine environment created by the tumor

9. When a nurse reviews the nutrition-related laboratory data for the patient with cancer and compromised nutritional status, he/she expects to review
   A. erythrocyte sedimentation rate (ESR).
   B. serum creatinine and bicarbonate.
   C. prothrombin and activated partial thromboplastin time (APTT).
   D. serum albumin and transferrin.

10. A patient has received aggressive chemotherapy for Hodgkin lymphoma and has been nauseated and vomiting for the past 2 days at home despite anti-emetic use. His wife calls the clinic and is concerned about his inability to keep anything down. Which of the following is not a symptom indicative of dehydration?
    A. Scant urine
    B. Poor skin turgor
    C. Decreased energy
    D. Dry mucous membranes

11. Primary cachexia is
    A. associated with decreased metabolic rate.
    B. mediated by proinflammatory cytokines including tumor necrosis factor (TNF).
    C. associated with increased gluconeogenesis.
    D. present in 50% of cancer patients at death.

12. The patient with evidence of malnutrition is likely to experience which of the following?
    A. Beneficial weight loss
    B. Shortened hospital stays
    C. Prolonged wound healing
    D. Increased tumor response to treatment

13. L.R. has recently been diagnosed with pancreatic cancer and has severe weight loss and decreased appetite. What teaching points might the nurse make to L.R. and his family to increase caloric intake?
    A. Increase the kilocalorie (kcal) protein content of foods by adding instant breakfast powders to puddings and other foods.
    B. Discourage access to favorite foods as the patient may get "turned off" from them if eaten too frequently.
    C. Try hot, spicy foods to improve taste and intake.
    D. Encourage liquids at mealtime and at bedtime; they may decrease nausea and stimulate appetite.

14. Which of these would not be considered a nutritional anthropometric measurement that would be assessed before and during therapy?
    A. Height and weight
    B. Body mass index (BMI)
    C. Midarm circumference
    D. Skin turgor

15. Which metabolic changes occur with malignant tumor development?
    A. Tumors use aerobic glycolysis.
    B. Tumors have a decreased rate of gluconeogenesis.
    C. Tumors have a decreased uptake of amino acids.
    D. Tumors have altered protein metabolism; muscle tissue is mobilized to meet increased metabolic demands.

16. What would not be considered a reason why cancer patients experience weight gain?
    A. Inactivity
    B. Effusions
    C. Steroids in treatment regimen
    D. Metabolic effects of the tumor

17. A patient has been recently diagnosed with B-cell lymphoma. She informs the nurse that she has lost her appetite and food actually tastes strange and unpleasant. What is her condition called?
    A. Hypogeusesthesia
    B. Dysgeusia
    C. Ageusia
    D. Cachexia

18. Which nursing intervention should be instituted to prevent nasogastric tube complications? ⚠
    A. Check placement of tube by aspirating gastric contents before each use.
    B. Change feeding bag and tube three times per week to avoid contamination.
    C. Keep the head of the bed elevated 30 degrees during and for 15 minutes after infusion.
    D. Inject water and listen for gurgling sounds with stethoscope over stomach before use.

19. Which taste alteration do patients undergoing chemotherapy typically experience?
    A. Constant or intermittent metallic taste
    B. Increased threshold for bitter taste
    C. Aversion to tea
    D. Decreased threshold for salty food

20. Which of the following precautions should be taken when administering TPN? ⚠
    A. Do not leave TPN solution unrefrigerated for longer than 4 hours prior to administration.
    B. Observe for signs of hyperkalemia.
    C. If sudden cessation of TPN occurs, infuse 50% dextrose in water solution peripherally at same rate of TPN.
    D. Verify blood return before connecting TPN IV tubing to central line catheter and check for blood return every 2 hours while infusing.

21. What laboratory value is most commonly used to measure malnutrition and nutritional risk?
    A. Cholesterol
    B. Albumin
    C. Red blood cell count
    D. White blood cell count

22. A patient has chemotherapy-related severe taste alterations. What can the nurse suggest to improve taste bud sensitivity?
    A. Decrease fluid intake with meals.
    B. Use spices and flavorings to enhance taste.
    C. Decrease smells associated with food preparation.
    D. Use amifostine (Ethyol) to prevent tissue damage and subsequent taste loss.

23. Which of the following changes in patient condition would merit nutritional intervention?
    A. Weight loss of greater than 2% of body weight
    B. Dehydration and inability to eat or drink
    C. Mouth soreness or sensitivity
    D. Queasiness

24. Taste alterations can lead to or indicate which more serious conditions?
    A. Anorexia
    B. Positive nitrogen balance
    C. Dysphagia
    D. Disease progression

25. A patient is receiving enteral feedings per nasogastric tube. The nurse monitors for complications by assessing for ⚠
    A. euthyroidism.
    B. aspiration and diarrhea.
    C. dehydration and dyspnea.
    D. hypoglycemia and edema.

26. Enteral therapy has been offered to H.M., a patient who has been diagnosed with lung cancer. H.M. is being treated with chemotherapy, has severe weight loss of greater than 5% body weight, and has malabsorption syndrome. A percutaneous endoscopic gastrostomy (PEG) has been placed, and the choice of formula needs to be determined. Which of the following is an appropriate tube-feeding formula for this patient?
    A. A polymeric formula containing nitrogen, carbohydrate, fat, and fiber
    B. A formula containing low carbohydrate-to-fat ratio to minimize carbon dioxide production
    C. A predigested formula containing nitrogen, proteins as free amino acids, carbohydrates, and triglycerides
    D. A renal failure formula containing modified protein, electrolytes, and volume

27. Which of the following is appropriate for managing taste alterations?
    A. Use commercial mouthwashes such as Scope® or Listerine® to eliminate the bacteria that cause bad taste.
    B. Suggest that the client try meat served hot.
    C. Have the client suck on sugar-free lemon drops or other smooth, flat, tart candies to stimulate saliva.
    D. Suggest doing oral care once a week.

28. Cancer-associated nutritional problems, rather than treatment-related nutritional problems, are best reversed by
    A. extensive nutrition counseling.
    B. self-care actions.
    C. medications.
    D. successful treatment of the tumor.

29. At what stage does nutritional intervention have the best chance to alter client outcomes?
    A. Early, before treatment begins
    B. Later, when the malignancy is aggressive
    C. During treatment
    D. After treatment has ended

34 Comfort

1. Healthcare professionals demonstrate acceptance of the International Association for the Study of Pain (IASP) definition of pain by
   A. carefully reviewing the client's medical record for test results supporting the cause of the reported pain.
   B. acknowledging the most important component of care planning is hearing the client's description and perception of pain.
   C. involving the client's family in planning for pain management strategies they think will work.
   D. working collaboratively as a team using pharmacologic and nonpharmacologic interventions.

2. A safety concern for individuals with peripheral neuropathy is ⚠
   A. pain caused by blankets on the feet at night.
   B. inability to keep feet warm.
   C. risk of falls because of poor position sense of lower extremities.
   D. the impact of the peripheral neuropathy on quality of life.

3. Managing pain in clients with cancer is complex because they can have
   A. pain related to chronic injuries.
   B. pain medications that interact with chemotherapy.
   C. multiple types of pain from their disease.
   D. a tendency to become addicted to pain meds.

4. A patient indicates he has pain that shoots down his right leg sometimes and at other times there is just a burning sensation. This is probably
   A. centrally mediated neuropathic pain.
   B. peripheral neuropathic pain from the treatments.
   C. caused by autonomic dysregulation and maintained by sympathetic nerves.
   D. from nociceptor activation secondary to changes in the hip joint.

5. Pain assessment can determine the presence of nociceptive pain, such as
   A. sympathetically maintained pain that was caused by autonomic dysregulation.
   B. abdominal visceral pain that arises from a targeted local area of intense pressure.
   C. somatic pain from bone, joint, or connective tissue, typically described as localized, sharp, throbbing, or pressure.
   D. pain that radiates down the arm and is described as burning and aching in a background of numbness in the fingers.

6. The process of nociception includes
   A. transduction—as the noxious stimuli is recognized, neurotransmitters and excitatory substances that inhibit nociceptive transmission are released in the spinal cord.
   B. transmission—neurotransmitters that were released at the time of injury include prostaglandins, bradykinin, serotonin, substance P, and histamine, which initiate an inflammatory response.
   C. perception—the cerebral cortex processing the experience of pain and responding to the noxious stimuli to reduce pain perception via descending modulating mechanisms.
   D. modulation—neurons in the brainstem descend to the dorsal horn and release neuromediators (norepinephrine and serotonin), which promote the transmission of the pain impulses at the dorsal horn.

7. The most common source of pain related to cancer is
   A. bone metastases.
   B. liver metastases.
   C. pancreatic involvement.
   D. nerve compression or injury.

8. A patient has completed four rounds of chemotherapy and is complaining of burning, numbness, and tingling of his or her hands and feet. Agents with the highest incidence of this side effect are
   A. platinum compounds, vinca alkaloids, antimetabolites, and interferon.
   B. bortezomib, trastuzumab, vincristine, and paclitaxel.
   C. platinum compounds, gemcitabine, and thalidomide.
   D. thalidomide, bortezomib, taxanes, and platinum compounds.

9. After experiencing nausea and vomiting for 48 hours, a client is unable to take the scheduled opioids for cancer pain and begins to withdraw. The withdrawal is attributable to
   A. physical dependence.
   B. drug tolerance.
   C. addiction.
   D. equianalgesia.

10. When assessing pediatric patients for pain the nurse should
    A. ask the parent about the child's level of pain.
    B. use the "0 to 10" scale to assess pain intensity for children age 7 years and older.
    C. encourage children 7 to 10 years of age to use the pain faces to describe pain.
    D. use a pain scale that is appropriate to the developmental level of the child.

11. S.J. was recently given the diagnosis of multiple myeloma and is undergoing her first cycle of chemotherapy. Although her pain is rated as 2 on a scale of 0 to 10 when she is at rest and not moving, the pain increases to 8 with any type of movement or activity. She is taking 30 mg of controlled-release oxycodone every 12 hours and 5 to 10 mg of immediate-release oxycodone every 4 hours as needed. The nurse's best recommendation for the management plan would be to
    A. add a nonsteroidal antiinflammatory medication for the bone pain.
    B. increase the dose and frequency of the breakthrough opioid medication and administer before anticipated activity.
    C. encourage S.J. to use a bedside table to keep items near her to prevent movement.
    D. encourage her that the pain will decrease once the chemotherapy begins to work.

12. H.Q. has a history of rheumatoid arthritis and has been taking pentazocine (Talwin) for the last 2 years. She was recently diagnosed with metastatic breast cancer and has been experiencing low back pain, rated at an 8, related to bone metastases. She is given a fentanyl (Duragesic) patch. What should be considered with this client?
    A. The pentazocine and Duragesic will work synergistically to provide more optimal pain relief.
    B. H.Q. will have an exacerbation of side effects related to the two opioids she is taking.
    C. The pentazocine, an agonist–antagonist, should be discontinued because the Duragesic will not work effectively in combination with an agonist–antagonist.
    D. An alternative agent to pentazocine, such as nalbuphine (Nubain), should be substituted for the arthritic pain.

13. Bisphosphonates such as pamidronate (Aredia) and zoledronic acid (Zometa) are a component of the supportive care management of clients experiencing pain associated with
    A. visceral metastases.
    B. neuropathic pain.
    C. osteolytic bone metastases.
    D. headache associated with increased intracranial pressure.

14. One type of autonomic nervous system block used to prevent or relieve pain from pancreatic cancer is the
    A. peripheral nervous system block.
    B. celiac plexus block.
    C. dorsal rhizotomy.
    D. commissural myelotomy.

15. A client who has been receiving thalidomide as cancer treatment reports burning pain and an inability to tolerate the covers on his feet at night. Which class of analgesic adjuvants is helpful for this pain?
    A. Analeptics
    B. Tricyclic antidepressants
    C. Serotonin-specific reuptake inhibitor antidepressants
    D. Benzodiazepines

16. A client with cancer has a pain score of 2 on a 0 to 10 scale but reports "always being sleepy." An appropriate intervention would be to recommend the addition of
    A. amitriptyline (Elavil).
    B. phenytoin (Dilantin).
    C. methylphenidate (Ritalin).
    D. a nonsteroidal antiinflammatory drug.

17. Mediators of pruritus include
    A. prostaglandins E6 and H3 released from mast cells.
    B. substance P synthesized in C fibers and epinephrine.
    C. TSH, opioids along the afferent pathway, and serotonin.
    D. physical stimuli (pressure, electricity, and temperature).

18. Which classification of antineoplastic agents increases the risk of pruritus?
    A. EGFR inhibitors and erythromycin
    B. Taxanes and platinum compounds
    C. Monoclonal antibodies and mTOR inhibitors
    D. Mycosis fungoides and renal disease

19. Clinical findings related to pruritus would typically include all the following except
    A. occurrence usually increases at night.
    B. patient describing constant, intermittent, and transient burning and numbness.
    C. elevated creatinine and hypoglycemia.
    D. elevated blood urea nitrogen (BUN) and abnormal liver function test results.

20. Pharmacologic interventions for pruritus include
    A. Oradol, ketamine, and dexamethasone.
    B. diazepam, gabapentin, and clonidine.
    C. modafinil, alprazolam, and corticosteroids.
    D. cimetidine, naloxone, and capsaicin.

21. Which statement is true about the physiology of pruritus?
    A. It is closely linked to the physiology of pain.
    B. Delta fibers are the neurons responsible for itch.
    C. The initiating stimulus occurs external to the body.
    D. Serotonin is the neurotransmitter responsible for the transmission of pruritus.

22. Risk factors for pruritus include
    A. history of alcohol abuse, lymphoma, and dehydration.
    B. age older than 70 years, iron deficiency, and polycythemia vera.
    C. male gender, melanoma, and diabetes.
    D. hematologic malignancies, dehydration, and age younger than 60 years.

23. C.O. returned from colon resection surgery 2 hours ago. Client-controlled analgesia morphine was initiated in the postanesthesia recovery unit, and he is now complaining of pruritus. What is the best intervention in this situation?
    A. Administer an opioid antagonist to block the pruritic influence.
    B. Administer diphenhydramine, an H1-receptor antagonist.
    C. Change the opioid to meperidine.
    D. Place a fan in the room to control the pruritus.

24. On assessment of a client with pancreatic cancer, the nurse notices scratch marks and scabs on her trunk and upper extremities. The client reports that she has been itching in the evenings before bedtime, and the itching is "driving her crazy." In addition to managing the underlying cause, an appropriate nursing intervention to would be to ⚠
    A. encourage the family member to scratch the affected area to prevent skin irritation.
    B. encourage a warm bath in the evening when the pruritus is most likely to occur and relaxing activities for distraction.
    C. encourage to drink a glass of wine each evening before bedtime for relaxation.
    D. encourage the client and family to understand the safety risk of developing a significant infection from organisms located on the skin.

25. Cancer related symptoms that frequently cluster with fatigue include
    A. pain, nausea, and vomiting.
    B. sleep disturbances and diarrhea.
    C. depression, pain, and sleep disturbances.
    D. hyperthyroidism and pain.

26. Fatigue
    A. can persist as a chronic condition for up to 10 years after treatment.
    B. occurs in 40% to 50% of individuals receiving cancer treatment.
    C. is more common in individuals who have been otherwise healthy.
    D. is treatment related and seldom persists into survivorship after treatment.

27. In which treatments has fatigue become a dose-limiting side effect?
    A. Drugs that cross the blood–brain barrier
    B. Immunotherapy or biotherapy
    C. Hormone therapy
    D. Radiation therapy

28. Red blood cell growth factors used in the management of anemia include
    A. erythropoietin (rHuEPO) (Epogen, Procrit) and oprelvekin (Neumega).
    B. darbepoetin alfa (Aranesp) and erythropoietin.
    C. oprelvekin and pegfilgrastim (Neulasta).
    D. erythropoietin and sargramostim (Leukine).

29. A patient with lymphoma is undergoing chemotherapy, has completed 2 of 6 cycles of therapy, and is reporting a fatigue level 8 on a 0 to 10 scale. What suggestions would help her with her fatigue?
    A. Maintain a vegetarian diet to increase the vitamin stores in her body.
    B. Sleep during the day when fatigued and get up only as needed.
    C. Engage in some activity as tolerated during the day to maintain energy stores.
    D. Continue the regular schedule that was used before the illness.

30. According to National Comprehensive Cancer Network (NCCN) guidelines, fatigue assessment should include all the following except
    A. onset, patterns, alleviating factors, and impact it has on overall functioning.
    B. pattern of hemoglobin and platelet count related to intensity of fatigue.
    C. family perception of the impact the fatigue has on the client's quality of life.
    D. depression scales and the client's self-report as the gold standard.

31. Many individuals with cancer have not mentioned their sleep problems because they
    A. assumed sleep problems were caused by treatment.
    B. thought that the physician would give them medicine that would make them feel groggy during the day.
    C. did not believe it was impacting their quality of life.
    D. have always had a problem falling asleep or staying asleep.

32. For adults, sleep
    A. consists of 2 to 4 cycles of rapid eye movement (REM) and non–rapid eye movement (NREM) sleep.
    B. involves three distinct stages from the lightest to deepest level of a sleep cycle and then starting over again.
    C. is regulated by melatonin and circadian rhythm, which are regulated by the body's clock genes.
    D. remains constant throughout the adult life unless altered by diseases such as cancer.

33. Melatonin is a hormone released by the pineal gland that
    A. mediates night and day rhythms.
    B. increases with age.
    C. increases during the daylight hours.
    D. increases with menopause.

34. Nonpharmacologic interventions for sleep include
    A. going to bed at a scheduled time whether sleepy or not.
    B. arising at the same time each morning.
    C. exercising 1 hour before retiring for bed.
    D. staying in bed (upon awakening at night) until sleep resumes.

35. What is a safety concern for individuals with significant sleep deprivation? ⚠
    A. Sleep is important for thermoregulation and immune function.
    B. Regular use of sleep medications is likely to result in addiction.
    C. Patients should be cautioned about driving or operating dangerous equipment.
    D. Patients will not be able to tolerate their cancer treatment.

36. Which of the following characteristics or lifestyle factors may interfere with sleep?
    A. Male gender
    B. Younger age
    C. Regular physical activity
    D. Alcohol intake

37. Physical signs of sleep deprivation include
    A. dark circles under the eyes, nystagmus, and incorrect word use.
    B. dark circles under the eyes, overpronunciation of words, and a loud voice.
    C. stuttering, nystagmus, and loss of balance.
    D. slurred speech, a loud voice, and an impaired gait.

35 Cultural, Spiritual, and Religious Diversity

1. Which concept is most difficult to clearly define?
   A. Culture
   B. Religion
   C. Spirituality
   D. Diversity

2. Which of these statements about race and/or ethnicity is correct?
   A. Asian American and Pacific Islanders are examples of ethnic groups composed of more than one racial group.
   B. Race is socially defined based on phenotype (appearance) rather than the genetics of the individuals in the group.
   C. Cubans are an example of a racial group of individuals that includes multiple ethnic groups.
   D. Ethnicity encompasses a group's world view, religion, language, and social structure.

3. What role does poverty as a culture play in healthcare?
   A. With the same treatment, poverty has little impact on outcome.
   B. Poverty crosses racial and ethnic groups and has an impact on health status.
   C. Its influence on access to healthcare can be remedied with free screenings.
   D. It increases a person's willingness to accept sliding scale services offered.

4. G.K. is a patient from a culture different than others on the unit. When the nurse enters her room, she maintains a downward gaze and avoids eye contact. This is most likely an indication that
   A. G.K. is not comfortable with culture diversity in healthcare providers.
   B. G.K.'s culture may view direct eye contact as disrespectful.
   C. G.K. is dealing with depression related to her cancer diagnosis.
   D. G.K. wants the nurse to avoid close physical contact.

5. A coworker claims he has a high level of cultural competence. What concern might be indicated?
   A. If he does not have a high level of professional education, others will not be inclined to believe him.
   B. To be very cautious if he is from a different culture than your own.
   C. None, try to make arrangements for him to participate in the cultural diversity taskforce being established.
   D. Knowing we often overestimate our knowledge about persons from other cultures, try to emphasize that everyone benefits from more education on cultural differences.

6. Although African American women have a lower incidence of breast cancer, they are less likely to survive 5 years than are white women. This difference in outcome is likely caused by all factors except
   A. late stage at detection.
   B. more aggressive tumor types.
   C. presences of multiple chronic conditions.
   D. decreased adherence to treatment.

7. A 72-year-old American Indian woman with advanced cancer is unresponsive. She has a small discolored pouch around her neck. While bathing her, the most appropriate action for the nurse is to
   A. discard the pouch; it is a source of infection.
   B. remove it and place it in the drawer with any personal belongings.
   C. leave it on and talk with the family when they come.
   D. remove it and talk with the family when they come.

8. A wife has been at her husband's bedside continually since his admission 3 days ago. She is clearly tired. Considering their Japanese American background, the most appropriate nursing action is to
   A. insist that the wife go home at night.
   B. talk with the client; have him tell his wife to go home at night.
   C. do nothing. It is the wife's duty to be at the bedside at all times.
   D. talk with the family about other family members who might help stay with the client.

9. Given the increase in cultural diversity in our society and the diverse populations receiving care at the institution, the hospital is establishing a cultural competence committee. During the initial planning session, which of the following is an appropriate first step?
   A. Developing family-focused interventions
   B. Conducting an assessment of one's own cultural beliefs and values
   C. Emphasizing that good health comes from good luck despite cultural heritage
   D. Conducting focus groups with diverse communities

10. Cultural competence is an ongoing process. A healthcare provider may demonstrate a genuine passion to be open and flexible with others, referred to as a cultural
    A. desire.
    B. knowledge.
    C. skill.
    D. encounter.

11. As an outreach worker with an American Indian community, the nurse notes a sudden decrease in mammography participation even after several diagnoses of breast cancer. After many unsuccessful attempts to increase mammography participation, what is the most appropriate strategy to pursue?
    A. Continue to explore beliefs and practices with outside consultants.
    B. Extend mammography screening hours.
    C. Prepare more culturally appropriate materials.
    D. Consult with respected American Indian leaders for assistance and suggestions.

12. When planning programs targeting culturally diverse populations, which of the following would likely not facilitate success?
    A. Creating and sustaining partnerships with community leaders
    B. Recognizing intracultural variability
    C. Incorporating traditional values, beliefs, and traditions
    D. Developing a proposal with the nurses in the clinic

13. Culture can have an impact on all the following except
    A. responses to the cancer diagnosis.
    B. participation in clinical trials.
    C. coping with advanced stage disease.
    D. the organized system of faith and worship.

14. Spirituality and religion are not mutually exclusive and cannot be used interchangeably. Which statement about these two concepts is accurate?
    A. Religion describes organized systems of faith that follow regulated group practices.
    B. Spirituality applies to persons who practice the tenets of organized religions.
    C. A fatalistic view is seldom seen in an individual with strong spiritual or religious beliefs.
    D. The role of spirituality and religiosity will stay consistent across the stages of cancer.

15. An individual who was regarded as highly spiritual comes into the outpatient setting, and he appears downcast and rejected. The nurse
    A. knows this may be an indication of spiritual distress.
    B. would encourage him to speak with a member of the clergy.
    C. offers to contact the spiritual leader listed on his medical record.
    D. asks the patient if he has been able to participate in religious services.

16. A core action to provide support to individuals with diverse religious beliefs and sense of spirituality would be to
    A. participate in educational opportunities to learn more about other belief systems.
    B. attend religious services of the primary groups receiving care at the institution.
    C. conduct a personal assessment of personal beliefs, values, and practices.
    D. seek the input of other healthcare professionals in the practice.

17. Which of these practices would not be considered an evidence-based alternative practice that supports or enhances spiritual well-being?
    A. Prayer
    B. Expressive therapies
    C. Herbal drinks
    D. Mindfulness meditation

36 Altered Body Image

1. A patient returns for her third round of chemotherapy for ER-negative breast cancer and indicates she just doesn't feel like going out with her family anymore; she feels like everyone stares at her everywhere they go. How would the nurse respond?
   A. Provide reassurance that she has been tolerating the treatment really well and that she is on the road to being cancer free.
   B. Query her for more details; she was able to have conservative surgery and will be eligible for reconstruction later.
   C. Discuss the changes she has experienced and acknowledge that the hair loss can be challenging because it is so visible to others, but it is temporary.
   D. Provide her with a referral to Look Good Feel Better and encourage her husband to be supportive.

2. A patient is scheduled to receive radiation therapy for cancer that will include a portion of the head, and he is concerned about hair loss. The radiation oncologist acknowledges that this can be a concern and tells him that it is feasible to adequately treat his cancer and minimize hair loss by treating with a maximum dose of
   A. 10 to 15 gray units (Gy).
   B. 20 to 25 Gy.
   C. 30 to 35 Gy.
   D. 40 to 45 Gy.

3. A patient is scheduled to start a chemotherapy regimen that includes two agents that will place her at risk for alopecia. She states she is very worried about hair loss. She has heard about scalp cooling and would like to try it. What knowledge would guide the nurse's response?
   A. The efficacy of scalp cooling to prevent alopecia depends on the chemotherapy agents, dosages, duration, and the client's liver function.
   B. The emphasis should be focused on optimal treatment results, not appearance. Hair loss is temporary and should not be a concern.
   C. Shaving the head is a common practice that makes hair loss more acceptable.
   D. The availability of alternatives (wigs, designer turbans) for head covering should completely counterbalance the client's concerns about hair loss.

4. How would the nurse address safety for a client who thinks hair loss will mean "just less time getting ready in the morning"? ⚠
   A. Focus on the true impact for the client psychologically—is she merely in denial and not coping?
   B. Determine the risk of the client developing self-destructive behaviors when the hair loss actually occurs.
   C. Provide education regarding risk related to potentially severe sunburns and significant heat loss during cold weather.
   D. Emphasize the multiple resources that are available as hair loss often makes others incomfortable.

5. Persons with body image disturbance may need assistance in dealing with their feelings. The primary goal of the nurse is to assist the client to identify the ⚠
   A. logical basis for behavior.
   B. adverse effects of feelings on behavior.
   C. moral implications of behavior.
   D. psychological basis for behavior.

6. Which of the following client outcome behaviors represents the highest level of adaptation to body image changes?
   A. Discusses plans to return to previous work role
   B. Discusses changes in body structure and function
   C. Serves as a volunteer in a client-to-client visitation program
   D. Lists emergency resources to deal with self-destructive behavior

7. Evidence supports which approach to potential body image disturbances?
   A. Address cultural similarities because the response across diverse cultures is usually very similar.
   B. If a client does not express concerns related to body image, she or he probably does not want to discuss it.
   C. The impacts of the changes are usually short term or at least remain fairly stable over time for a given client.
   D. A lower quality of life can contribute to problems with body image changes over time throughout treatment.

8. The impact of cancer treatment on body image can sometimes create a misconception among health professionals regarding what outcomes are concerning to patients. In contrast to health professionals' concerns, patients with head and neck cancer were more concerned about
   A. anatomical defects.
   B. body image changes.
   C. speech and exercise tolerance.
   D. response by family members.

9. What body image concerns should be discussed when considering hormone therapy instead of the surgical removal of an organ associated with sexuality (e.g., testicles, breast)?
   A. Negative body image can occur secondary to the weight gain associated with hormone therapy.
   B. Weight management is less difficult with hormone therapy than in patients who have had surgery to remove organs related to sexuality.
   C. Surgical loss of sex organs causes more stress than hormone therapy and its related side effects.
   D. Hormone-related changes and side effects are easier to avoid with proper treatment.

10. Nurses can assist clients in the acceptance of a changed body image. Which of the following nursing interventions is the most supportive?
   A. Stressing a time frame to grieve and then quickly moving on
   B. Facilitating conversations between client and long-lost family
   C. Educating family immediately regarding body image changes
   D. Allowing ventilation of negative emotions, especially anger and guilt

11. A nursing intervention that may increase the severity of a body image disturbance is to
   A. use active listening skills and facilitate discussion of concerns.
   B. educate the client and family about body image changes after surgery.
   C. stress the temporary nature of some side effects and limits in function.
   D. allow the client to return to work after head and neck surgery before talking about the reactions of coworkers.

12. There are many complementary health approaches that are potentially beneficial as adjuvant therapies for actual or potential body image disturbances. Which option is not considered a complementary health approach?
   A. Support from family and friends
   B. Art therapy
   C. Strength training and physical exercise
   D. Mindfulness focus
   E. Reconstructive surgery

37 Coping Mechanisms and Skills

1. Which percentage of clients with cancer experience some level of distress related to their diagnosis or treatment?
   A. 33%
   B. 50%
   C. 66%
   D. 100%

2. A client asked, "Why did this happen to me? I never smoked, and no one in my family has had lung cancer." This demonstrates what type of coping?
   A. Problem focused
   B. Emotion focused
   C. Meaning focused
   D. Behavioral focused

3. Multiple types of distress may be observed in those with a cancer diagnosis and those dealing with symptoms and treatment effects. Which of these words would not be used to describe distress related to cancer diagnosis?
   A. Psychological
   B. Social
   C. Avoidance
   D. Spiritual

4. The family of A.D., who is 6 months post cancer treatment, contacts the clinic and reports that he is demonstrating significant behavior changes including absences from work and increased alcohol intake. He is using these behaviors to help him deal with what appear to be panic attacks. A.D. is probably experiencing
   A. the realization that his cancer is cured and a desire to celebrate.
   B. a long-term effect of the chemotherapy he received.
   C. a normal phase of recovery from the stress of the cancer.
   D. posttraumatic stress disorder (PTSD) from his cancer experience.

5. What is the major safety-related concern for individuals experiencing cancer-related distress? ⚠
   A. Ineffective coping that can lead to suicidal ideation and threats or attempts to take one's life
   B. The frequent mistakes resulting from similar names of drugs for treatment of cancer-related anxiety
   C. The potential for drug-to-drug interaction between medicines used for treating distress and the cancer therapy regimen
   D. The potential for family members to self-medicate with the client's medications

6. Which of the following would be considered a coping response for clients with cancer and their family members?
   A. Gender and family influences
   B. A conscious or unconscious attempt to deny the disease
   C. Cultural factors, including healing practices and beliefs
   D. Physiologic effects of the disease and the chemotherapy treatment

7. J.P. will be seen in the clinic today for treatment of pancreatic cancer. His family members called yesterday to report periods of increased activity and an expressed sense of urgency to do things before it is too late followed by near exhaustion and withdrawal and complaints of chest pain and shortness of breath. This is consistent with
   A. PTSD.
   B. severe manic-depressive disorder.
   C. signs of cancer-related anxiety.
   D. a normal response to poor prognosis.

8. Depression at the time of a cancer diagnosis can be caused by all except
   A. endocrine abnormalities and metabolic changes.
   B. pancreatic and head and neck cancer.
   C. long waiting times in the clinic.
   D. poorly controlled symptoms, including pain.

9. Metabolic changes and endocrine abnormalities that are potential medical causes of cancer-related depression include
   A. hypocalcemia and anemia.
   B. sodium or potassium imbalance.
   C. increased hormone levels.
   D. vitamin D deficiency and fever.

10. Denial can be a primary coping mechanism in a client with cancer. It is
    A. considered dysfunctional and should be addressed.
    B. a conscious attempt to deny the knowledge of the diagnosis.
    C. a significant concern when it leads to denial of the relevance of symptoms.
    D. likely to delay healthcare team response to symptoms.

11. What score on the NCCN Distress Thermometer should lead to further action by the healthcare professional?
    A. 85
    B. 50
    C. 8
    D. 2

12. Caregiver role strain often accompanies cancer-related distress. What would be an appropriate initial expected outcome to address this?
    A. The caregiver identifies resources available to help and verbalizes mastery of the care situation.
    B. The client exhibits enhanced social interaction skills and involvement in activities.
    C. Family caregivers demonstrate signs of emotional distress and anxiety.
    D. Caregiver identifies mastery of new coping skills and relaxation techniques.

13. What should be included in an appropriate distress-related intervention plan for individuals with cancer and their caregivers?
    A. Active listening and avoiding confrontation to prevent increased stress
    B. Having them establish stretch goals that promote positive growth through this experience
    C. Avoiding discussions regarding either sexuality or spirituality as causes of distress
    D. Collaborating with the client and caregiver(s) to identify strengths and available resources

14. Self-care should be encouraged for individuals experiencing cancer-related distress. Knowledge of which of the following factors should not be considered in self-care plans?
    A. Multi-focused education programs, including preparatory education, cognitive restructuring, and building on current coping skills, have all shown merit.
    B. Individual preferences play a role in the effectiveness of complementary or alternative approaches.
    C. Identification of strengths and the recognition and management of sources of stressors will improve outcomes.
    D. Pharmacologic interventions are the critical cornerstone to the effectiveness of most alternative approaches.

15. The evidence-based NCCN Distress Management Guidelines support
    A. universal intervention plans to allow the collection of data to advance practice.
    B. screening based on the professional judgment of the primary provider.
    C. limiting the number of different disciplines involved to streamline care and avoid distress.
    D. screening all clients at the initial visit and then as indicated with disease status changes.

16. What would be considered an indicator of depression?
    A. Greater dysfunction related to cancer
    B. Evidence of persistent irrational beliefs regarding diagnosis
    C. Significant change in appetite and sleep patterns
    D. A weak social support system and solitary work environment

17. Selective antidepressants include
    A. tricyclic antidepressants: venlafaxine (Effexor) and nortriptyline (Pamelor).
    B. selective serotonin reuptake inhibitors (SSRIs): paroxetine (Paxil) and sertraline (Zoloft).
    C. monoamine oxidase inhibitors: bupropion (Wellbutrin) and trazodone (Desyrel).
    D. atypical antidepressants: mirtazapine (Remeron) and amitriptyline (Elavil).

38 Psychosocial Disturbances and Alterations

1. What is the best description of emotional distress related to cancer?
   A. A normative response to the life-threatening nature of cancer that frequently does not require intervention
   B. A combination of social, spiritual, physical, financial, and psychiatric stressors that strains coping abilities
   C. A normative response, different from clinical depression, posttraumatic stress disorder (PTSD), or anxiety disorder
   D. Psychiatric distress and existential concerns common in clients with cancer and their family members

2. A nurse wants to prioritize a nursing intervention for a client identified as at risk for emotional distress. Which one of the following risk factors are nurses more likely to be able to influence?
   A. Disruption of age-specific developmental-like tasks
   B. Lack of prognostic certainty regarding the cancer
   C. Knowledge of cancer diagnosis, treatment, and expected outcomes
   D. Previous life experiences and learned coping ability

3. Which of the following is supported by the National Comprehensive Cancer Network Guidelines for distress?
   A. Developmental stage, phase of disease, past coping skills, and available resources determine psychological needs.
   B. Most clients seen in the outpatient setting will not require screening; they will self-identify.
   C. Identifying and treating psychological issues is usually a simple straight-forward process for the experienced clinician.
   D. Because emotional distress is a normal response, referral to mental health specialists is not usually indicated.

4. In caring for a client with a diagnosis of ineffective individual coping, which intervention will require the most participation on the part of the client?
   A. Evaluation of the effectiveness of current coping strategies with the client
   B. Instruction in relaxation, imagery, and other holistic stress reduction techniques
   C. Providing referrals as needed to the psychiatric liaison nurse, psychologist, or social worker
   D. Strengthening the client's social support system

5. A.R. is a 76-year-old retired banker who has done well for 2 years after pelvic exoneration. Recently she experienced a recurrence. She now has multiple draining fistulae and has been told that she is not a candidate for further treatment. Her son said that her response has been complete withdrawal. She has changed from a meticulous dresser and housekeeper to neglecting both. She refuses to eat and blames herself for not going for regular Pap smears. She refuses help from her son, saying he is "wasting his time; I deserve to die." Her responses reflect developmental, situational, and disease-related characteristics most suggestive of
   A. fear of death.
   B. low self-esteem.
   C. neurotic anxiety.
   D. role abandonment.

6. C.D. had become disinterested in attending to her own care caused by a wound-related fistula with uncontrolled fecal drainage. During this hospitalization, control of the drainage has improved, and C.D. is showing more interest in learning how to manage the drainage. During this phase, the most therapeutic nursing approach to facilitate adaptive behavior would be to
   A. initiate a referral for rehabilitative counseling.
   B. make no demands on C.D. for her own care.
   C. positively reinforce C.D.'s approaches to self-care.
   D. ask her family to assume responsibility for C.D.'s care.

7. Emotional distress can be seen as a sense of hopelessness, symptoms of PTSD, and ineffective role performance. Which nursing intervention would be indicated for a client demonstrating a sense of hopelessness?
   A. Assist the individual in identifying perceived threats and provide accurate information on actual risks.
   B. Assist the individual in listing priorities within his or her personal, professional, and social responsibilities.
   C. Offer to provide a referral to supportive and expressive group therapy and a rehabilitation specialist.
   D. Assist the client to explore his or her personal value system and sense of purpose and meaning in life.

8. A.L. is admitted to an oncology unit, and assessment reveals flushed skin, sweating, jerky hand movements, and asking questions repeatedly. The most probable nursing diagnosis would be which of the following?
   A. Anxiety
   B. Fear
   C. Delirium
   D. Phobias

9. Awareness of disease, treatment, and interpersonal-related risk factors for anxiety in clients with cancer can facilitate early recognition of symptoms and intervention. Which of the following are abnormal metabolic states that can increase the risk for anxiety?
   A. Hyperthyroidism, hormone-secreting tumors, and hypoglycemia
   B. Hormone-secreting tumors, hypercapnia, delirium, and hyperglycemia
   C. Paraneoplastic syndromes, hyperglycemia, and electrolyte imbalance
   D. Electrolyte imbalance, hypoglycemia, hypothyroidism, and delirium

10. Medications are an important component of treatment for anxiety, but they can also serve as a risk factor for anxiety in individuals with cancer. Which of the following medications actually fall into both categories?
    A. Azaperones and antihistamines
    B. Antihistamines and neuroleptics
    C. Bronchodilators and antidepressants
    D. Neuroleptics and anxiolytics

11. Spiritual belief systems can be an important factor in anxiety reactions for clients with cancer. Which of the following would be prioritized as important for an individual recently informed of metastatic spread of his or her cancer?
    A. Provide for privacy and time alone to meditate.
    B. Inquire about the client's fears related to death.
    C. Contact a clergy person to visit the client.
    D. Determine the desire to participate in spiritual rituals.

12. L.B. had a minimally emetogenic chemotherapy protocol 5 days ago. He has contacted the infusion center with complaints of persistent nausea, vomiting, and diarrhea. These symptoms and signs of apparent distress indicate which of the following as a psychosocial distress reaction?
    A. Psychotic stress disorder
    B. Bipolar disorder
    C. PTSD
    D. Anxiety disorder

13. J.L. returns to the oncology outpatient clinic for his 1-year follow-up appointment. He states that he is having problems with sleeping, flashbacks of his initial treatment, and difficulty concentrating. The nurse refers him for psychiatric evaluation, suspecting that he is experiencing
    A. bipolar disorder.
    B. generalized anxiety stress disorder.
    C. PTSD
    D. psychotic disorder.

14. S.S. is admitted to the hospital for the evaluation of metastatic disease related to her diagnosis of breast cancer. Her family is concerned about recent changes in her behavior such as crying, lack of interest in her appearance, and changes in sleeping and eating. In considering a referral for evaluation of depression in this client, it is most important to assess the
    A. effect of behavior on family members.
    B. meaning of the illness to the client.
    C. meaning of appearance to client and family.
    D. mental status as an indicator of delirium.

15. The nurse's assessment of treatment-related risk factors for depression in individuals with cancer should include the
    A. chemotherapeutic agents being given.
    B. sleeping and eating patterns.
    C. symptom control, particularly pain.
    D. type of cancer.

16. Which of the following risk factors for development of depressive symptoms is most amenable to direct nursing interventions?
    A. Family developmental and situational crises
    B. Inadequate social support
    C. Inadequate symptom control
    D. Client history of suicidal thoughts

17. Clinical assessment findings most descriptive of a depressed state include
    A. facial pallor, tense posturing, vocal tremors, and diaphoresis.
    B. fatigue, psychomotor agitation, and change in appetite.
    C. inappropriate affect, sweaty hands, and tremors.
    D. labile emotions, hyperactivity, sighing respirations, and overtalkativeness.

18. Which of the following responses by the nurse would be most therapeutic in helping the client deal with the somatic complaints often associated with depression?
    A. Advising the client to minimize these symptoms, thus conserving energy to fight the disease.
    B. Explaining that the symptoms being experienced are not "real" and therefore need no treatment.
    C. Listening nonjudgmentally and trying diversional techniques as a possible method of alleviation.
    D. Validating that symptoms do or do not have a physiologic basis and planning interventions.

19. R.B. has been diagnosed as major depressive disorder based on the DSM-V. What would be a priority to address as a nursing intervention in the client with cancer? ⚠
    A. Interference with social roles
    B. Lack of compliance with medical treatment
    C. Severe psychological regression with loss of function
    D. Suicidal ideation or attempt

20. H.G. returns to the oncology clinic for treatment of recurrent lymphoma after bone marrow transplant. He verbalizes that it is hard to believe that there is a purpose to his experience, tearfully stating, "I'm really angry and I don't trust anything anymore." The most probable nursing diagnosis would be
    A. anxiety.
    B. ineffective coping.
    C. self-esteem disturbance.
    D. spiritual distress.

21. From past contact with A.G., nurses know him to be a deeply spiritual person, attending church and using prayer to manage the demands of his illness and treatment. Today he angrily refuses when a nurse volunteers to call his pastor for him. The best response to this would be:
    A. "Getting angry with God isn't going to help."
    B. Determine if he would like to talk about the current feelings that seem to be present.
    C. "Sounds like some privacy might be helpful. I'll be back soon."
    D. Attempting to get him to reconsider his decision.

22. C.J., a 48-year-old businessman, has recently been given the diagnosis of lung cancer. His family states that since his diagnosis, he has refused to participate in decision making about his treatment, is ignoring postbiopsy instructions, and has become more withdrawn. The most accurate nursing diagnosis would be
    A. anxiety.
    B. ineffective coping.
    C. powerlessness.
    D. spiritual distress.

23. An individual's response to the loss of personal control during cancer treatment depends primarily on which of the following?
    A. Duration of time since diagnosis
    B. Individual patterns of coping
    C. Personal meaning of the loss
    D. Response of family and friends

24. What response would be appropriate to a client stating, "I don't feel like I have any control over what is happening to me"?
    A. "Ask the doctor about your care, and he will answer your questions."
    B. "Ask your wife to let you regularly do more things for yourself."
    C. "Let's spend some time talking a little more about your feelings."
    D. "Let's develop a routine schedule for your care so you will know what to expect."

25. What would the nurse prioritize as the most basic nursing intervention designed to facilitate C.J.'s sense of personal control?
    A. Asking family to make decisions regarding burdensome areas of care
    B. Discussing with him his feelings regarding personal control
    C. Encouraging identification of areas over which control can be maintained
    D. Providing successful management of current cancer related symptoms

26. Before discharge, what is the most important nursing intervention for facilitation of a sense of control for both C.J. and his family?
    A. Make a referral to an appropriate home care agency for regular visits.
    B. Organize a health team meeting to work on a detailed plan for his care.
    C. Provide specific instructions for family members regarding what to monitor.
    D. Seek the client's and family's opinions and suggestions about his care at home.

27. A sense of loss of control can have a tremendous impact on the client with cancer. Which of the following behaviors would indicate a need for immediate professional assistance?
    A. Inability to perform activities of daily living
    B. Noncompliance with treatment regimen
    C. Refusal to discuss personal feelings
    D. Verbalization of self-harm intentions

28. A client with cancer has indicated that she feels sad, almost like when a parent died in the past, and asks why. What would be an appropriate response?
    A. "You are probably reliving that loss; how long ago did that happen?"
    B. "Your cancer has an excellent prognosis. Are you concerned about dying? I can contact the social worker."
    C. "Maybe you are depressed. Would you like to try some medications that could be helpful for depression?"
    D. "People can experience feelings of grief from more than just the loss of a valued person, including loss of abilities."

29. In addition to the developmental and situational factors that most people experience with a loss, individuals with cancer may also experience
    A. changes in body structure or function.
    B. changes in employment, including retirement.
    C. multiple losses and unanticipated losses.
    D. symbolic losses, including independence.

30. A daughter from a distant state is currently visiting her father who has advanced stage lung cancer. Nurses know from previous conversations with the client that the daughter has been estranged from her father for more than 10 years. She seeks information regarding the likelihood that his drinking and smoking caused the cancer. What would be the primary concern at this time?
    A. This daughter will be at risk for complicated grief because of the apparent ambivalent relationship with her father.
    B. Be certain to keep the client's pain control at an optimal level so she does not see him suffer because that is his wish.
    C. Primarily for the client with cancer; the daughter has made choices and will have time to resolve her feelings in the future.
    D. Help her to understand that blaming her father for causing his cancer by life choices is not beneficial.

31. In discussing the process of grief with clients or family members, what is the main, most basic point to emphasize?
    A. One's grief response will be influenced by past experiences with loss and grief.
    B. Each family member will grieve in his or her own fashion.
    C. Somatic symptoms of grief often occur and should be addressed.
    D. Specific stages of grief exist; be prepared for changes over time.

32. Resolution of the grief process may be facilitated by which of the following interventions?
    A. Encouraging discussion of the feelings related to the loss
    B. Discouraging expression of negative feelings, such as anger
    C. Providing sedation and diversion as suggested by others
    D. Restricting visitors other than immediate family members

33. Which of the following client responses is most representative of a dysfunctional grief response?
    A. A 76-year-old man who cared for his wife during the terminal phases of colon cancer reports frequent vivid dreams about his wife and himself.
    B. A mother who cries continuously and keeps saying, "No, he can't die," as she tends to her 21-year-old son who is dying of leukemia.
    C. A 35-year-old woman who, at 6 weeks after a mastectomy, avoids hugs and physical contact with family and friends and has not allowed her husband to look at the surgical site.
    D. A 35-year-old widower prides himself on keeping all of his wife's possessions and visiting her grave daily for the 5 years since her death while neglecting his other responsibilities.

34. The family of a client who died 8 weeks ago is coming to visit the cancer center staff. Which of the following grief responses would cause the nurse the greatest concern?
    A. Crying, angry outbursts, and accusations
    B. Preoccupation with deceased person
    C. Somatic symptoms like the deceased
    D. Withdrawal or social isolation

39 Sexuality

1. What statement is not accurate regarding sexuality during cancer care?
   A. With appropriate intervention, 70% of clients with cancer can have their sexual function return to baseline rather than decreasing over time.
   B. Decreasing sexual function can increase the risk of emotional morbidity with a cancer diagnosis and treatment.
   C. The majority of clients across all cancer types reported that client–provider conversations on sexual issues were important.
   D. Sexuality issues are seldom significant if they had not been a problem for the client and partner before treatment.

2. When nurses do not include discussions about sexuality as an integral part of treatment, it can communicate that
   A. sexuality is a legitimate topic, but it should be discussed with a physician.
   B. changes in sexual function is a "cost" of successful treatment.
   C. standards of care do not allow nurses to discuss this aspect of care.
   D. education about sexuality will occur before treatment begins, but not during this appointment.

3. What are sexuality-related safety concerns for a 36-year-old woman receiving chemotherapy? ⚠
   A. The client is probably already infertile because of the cancer.
   B. There is a significant risk of pain with intercourse.
   C. Vaginal mucositis will place the individual at increased risk for infection during intercourse.
   D. Pregnancy is not desirable at this time because of the negative effects of the chemotherapy on the new fetus.

4. An individual receiving hormonal therapy for cancer expresses intense sexuality-related concerns. What should be discussed with him?
   A. Hormone therapy has fewer sexuality-related concerns than other antineoplastic agents.
   B. The majority of effects are reversible once treatment has been completed.
   C. Hormone therapy can have multiple short- and long-term effects in both women and men.
   D. The cancer treatment will cause fatigue, which will have a large effect on sexuality.

5. Because radiation therapy (RT) is usually a local or regional therapy, the sexuality-related side effects are often regarded less significant because
   A. many professionals lack adequate knowledge of the side effects of RT.
   B. RT is more common for prostate cancer, and many of these clients are already older than 70 years of age.
   C. unless RT for females includes the ovaries, there are few long-term side effects.
   D. prostate brachytherapy only causes erectile dysfunction in less than 30% of the recipients.

6. Which statement is true about the side effects of chemotherapy agents and is an important basis for discussions regarding sexuality?
   A. Antimetabolites and targeted therapies have the greatest impact on sexual dysfunction because of their systemic effects.
   B. Unless the individual has vaginal- or ovarian-related effects, the impact on sexuality remains limited.
   C. Combining antimetabolites or antitumor antibiotics with alkylating agents increases the effect on sexuality.
   D. The risk of infection during bone marrow suppression from systemic chemotherapy outweighs sexuality concerns.

7. J.S., a 38-year-old woman, is considering a mastectomy or a lumpectomy for a new diagnosis of breast cancer. She is discussing her plans with the nurse. Which statement would not indicate a need for a sexuality-related discussion of the treatment options?
   A. "A lumpectomy eliminates my concern about the impact of loss of my breast, so I don't have to worry about my partner's reaction."
   B. "At least with lumpectomy, I won't have to be concerned about all the sensation changes with a mastectomy."
   C. "My husband and I are more concerned about disease outcomes than potential effects on sexuality."
   D. "I can have an implant after my mastectomy and then will not have to worry about disease or my appearance."

8. An unexpected impact of surgical changes on sexuality with prostatectomy is
   A. the need for hormone replacement therapy.
   B. shrinkage of the testicles and resulting body image changes.
   C. the potential for retrograde ejaculation, which may affect sensation for the client's partner.
   D. sleep disturbances and thus the incidence of fatigue.

9. The spouse of an individual undergoing surgical resection for head and neck cancer expresses concern about her loss of emotional attraction to her husband. What would NOT be included in potential approaches for addressing causative factors?
   A. The concept of providing nutrition as a demonstration of caring
   B. Discussing the role for communication during lovemaking
   C. Sensations of respirations from the stoma on his neck
   D. The occurrence of drooling during close physical contact

10. The PLISSIT (permission, limited information, specific suggestions, intensive therapy) model for sexuality counseling
    A. is so complex that the generalist nurse should not use it and should refer clients to nurses with an advanced degree.
    B. requires only limited knowledge about sexuality or how sexuality is affected by a diagnosis of cancer or the treatment for cancer.
    C. is a useful model for levels of nursing interventions based on the nurse's comfort and knowledge about the subject.
    D. is used primarily for clients with cancer who have long-standing or severe problems with sexuality.

11. The first level of assessment P (permission) in the PLISSIT model conveys the message that
    A. any sexual activity is appropriate behavior.
    B. discussing sexual issues is appropriate.
    C. they must remain sexually active.
    D. sexual discussions should be referred to other sources.

12. Which statement is true about exposure to radiation and its effect on fertility?
    A. The age of males at the time of exposure affects risk of sterility.
    B. Dosage levels that cause sterility are similar in males and females.
    C. About 95% of women older than 40 years of age will be sterile with 20 Gy over 5 to 6 weeks.
    D. Pelvic radiation in men at greater than 6 Gy causes temporary sterility.

13. Models for sexual assessment include
    A. arousal, timing the discussion, and partner response.
    B. alarm, better, and pleasure.
    C. attitudes, symptoms, and reproduction.
    D. bringing up the topic and being sensitive.

14. The type and dose of chemotherapy are determining factors for infertility as a result of cancer treatment; therefore, it is important for nurses to be aware that
    A. only 40% of men and women who receive mechlorethamine, Oncovin (vincristine), procarbazine, prednisone (MOPP) combination therapy have fertility effects.
    B. 60% of men treated with Adriamycin (doxorubicin), bleomycin, vinblastine, dacarbazine (ABVD) combination therapy experience fertility issues.
    C. more than 50% of individuals do not recall having a fertility risk discussion when diagnosed.
    D. when chemotherapy has caused infertility, couples no longer have to worry about birth control.

15. Cancer during pregnancy requires careful consideration of
    A. anesthesia risk during surgery and the need for high-risk obstetric care.
    B. the risk to the fetus and the couple's beliefs and values.
    C. the inability to have diagnostic procedures and receive chemotherapy
    D. the importance of treating early to avoid problems late in the pregnancy.

16. Which use of the PLISSIT model should guide planning and implementation of interventions regarding sexuality?
    A. Providing information regarding different options to consider and giving your input on what you think is the best option
    B. Discussing how treatment can affect feelings about themselves and how these impact identified gender roles
    C. Suggesting the need for referral to a counselor because of the complexity of the issues involved
    D. Providing the client and family member with resources to provide for enhanced erotic stimulation

17. A 28-year-old client who was just diagnosed with cancer asks if this means she will not be able to have children of her own. She adds, "Will I even live that long?" The nurse's responses would be guided by
    A. awareness of the need to address preservation of fertility from a preventive model.
    B. stressing the improvements in survival with cancer treatment and the need to focus on cure.
    C. understanding that at her current age, there will be multiple options available in the future.
    D. providing the reassurance that when she survives the treatment, adoption will always be an option.

18. A 36-year-old woman is undergoing chemotherapy for ovarian cancer. It is important for her to know that
    A. she may be affected by premature menopausal changes.
    B. her libido will be increased.
    C. intercourse will be impossible because of pain.
    D. side effects of chemotherapy will not interfere with sexual activity.

19. Education and anticipatory guidance to prevent sexual dysfunction should include
    A. assuming the client knows basic sexuality information.
    B. encouraging the couple to avoid discussing fears or concerns with each other.
    C. dispelling myths and misconceptions.
    D. using models or drawings to explain how sexuality can be affected.

20. A client and his partner have some concerns after his abdominoperineal resection. Which concerns are the most realistic and appropriate to discuss with him?
    A. The variety of ways to achieve sexual pleasure
    B. Erectile dysfunction caused by the surgery
    C. Ability to ejaculate with intercourse
    D. Effect of surgery on his masculinity

21. A client is scheduled to have a mastectomy for breast cancer. Which of the following questions would be most appropriate for the nurse to ask when discussing the potential impact of surgery on sexuality?
    A. "Do you have any concerns about how the loss of your breast may affect how others see you?"
    B. "Some women have concerns about how the surgery will affect their sexual life. Do you have any concerns?"
    C. "Do you have any problems with your sexual life at this time?"
    D. "Some women don't see themselves as feminine after the surgery. How about you?"

22. A client is receiving RT to the pelvis. She states that she has not had intercourse for several weeks, although she desires sexual intimacy. What suggestions would be most appropriate for the nurse to make to this client ?
    A. "Let your partner know you are interested in having sex."
    B. "Limit the amount of time you and your partner initially spend on intercourse."
    C. "Ask your partner why he hasn't wanted to have sex."
    D. "Concentrate on pleasing your partner during intercourse."

23. A client has returned to the clinic for a follow-up visit after her colostomy for a bowel obstruction. She and her partner are asking questions about resuming sexual activity. The nurse's suggestions might include
    A. to avoid anal intercourse.
    B. how to secure the ostomy bag for sexual activity.
    C. to place a folded towel over the ostomy site.
    D. avoid face-to-face sexual positions.

24. A total abdominal hysterectomy, including the ovaries, in a 40-year-old woman will cause
    A. fear of sexual intimacy.
    B. vaginal changes.
    C. total loss of sexual desire.
    D. destruction of self-concept as a woman.

25. A client is receiving a continuous cisplatin infusion for treatment of testicular cancer. Upon entering his room, the nurse discovers he and his partner engaged in sexual activity. The best response would be to
    A. report it to his physician.
    B. instruct the client and his partner to use condoms.
    C. explain that oral sex is a safe method of sexual satisfaction.
    D. reprimand them for unacceptable behavior in a hospital.

40 Metabolic Emergencies

1. Disseminated intravascular coagulation (DIC) features increased intravascular coagulation in which coagulation factors and platelets are consumed. This process may be more gradual in patients with cancer. During cancer treatment, the risk of DIC
   A. increases.
   B. decreases.
   C. initially increases and then normalizes.
   D. is not an issue.

2. DIC represents an imbalance of normal coagulation. Which of the following statements best summarizes the characteristics of this condition?
   A. Failure of the fibrinolytic system
   B. Blocked internal pathway of clotting
   C. Excessive amounts of clotting factors
   D. Accelerated coagulation and the formation of excessive thrombin

3. The nurse should be aware that which of the following is considered a contributing factor for the development of hypercalcemia?
   A. Male sex
   B. Young age
   C. Immobility
   D. Fluid overload

4. M. is a 55-year-old woman with lymphoma. She has received high-dose Rituxan and is experiencing tumor lysis syndrome (TLS). What symptoms would the nurse expect to see?
   A. Muscular weakness, cardiac arrhythmias, and acute renal failure
   B. Bell's palsy, hypertension, anorexia, nausea, and vomiting
   C. Rigors, diaphoresis, confusion, and azotemia
   D. Kussmaul breathing, blurred vision, confusion, and delirium

5. J.M. is a young man with acute promyelocytic leukemia (APL) undergoing induction therapy. On day 4 of chemotherapy, he develops a fever of 101.5° F (38.6° C). The nurse notices new petechiae, pallor, ecchymosis, and some shortness of breath. He is complaining of pain in his ear. A diagnosis of DIC has been made. What would the nurse expect his laboratory values to show?
   A. Anemia, elevated serum iron, and low platelet count
   B. Increased prothrombin and BUN, and decreased fibrinogen
   C. Decreased activated partial thromboplastin time (APTT) and increased platelet count
   D. Increased protein C level, decreased BUN, and schistocytes on peripheral smear

6. J.M., the patient with DIC from the previous question, is being given antibiotic therapy. Which other strategies will be used next to treat his DIC?
   A. Vasopressors
   B. Fibrinolytic therapy
   C. Mechanical ventilation
   D. Heparin therapy

7. A patient's risk for anaphylaxis increases when medications are
   A. given at low dose.
   B. given intravenously.
   C. given as a single dose.
   D. synthetically prepared.

8. L.C. is a 62-year-old man with lung cancer who has metastatic disease to the right hip. He is admitted to the hospital with serum calcium of 16 mg/dL. His wife explains that he has been "acting very funny" and has not been eating or drinking like usual for the past 3 days. The patient reports that he is quite nauseated. The nurse suspects he has?
   A. Williams syndrome
   B. Local osteolytic hypercalcemia of malignancy (LOH)
   C. Renal sarcoidosis
   D. Increased intracranial pressure

9. Which is a hallmark sign on assessment of a patient for DIC?
   A. Bradycardia
   B. Mottled extremities
   C. Decreased bowel sounds
   D. Elevated specific gravity

10. What is the most commonly seen oncologic emergency?
    A. Hypercalcemia
    B. TLS
    C. Syndrome of inappropriate antidiuretic hormone secretion (SIADH)
    D. DIC

11. Platelet transfusion are used in the treatment of DIC to
    A. promote volume expansion.
    B. inhibit thrombin formation.
    C. increase RBCs and clotting factors.
    D. decrease hemorrhage and convert prothrombin to thrombin.

12. During the administration of L-asparaginase (Elspar), a patient complains of "feeling funny" and being short of breath. The nurse hears wheezes in bilateral lung fields. Suspecting hypersensitivity, what is the most appropriate immediate nursing intervention? ⚠
    A. Call a code.
    B. Stop the infusion.
    C. Intubate the patient.
    D. Initiate cardiopulmonary resuscitation.

13. How would a nurse *assess* the pulmonary status for a patient with DIC? ⚠
    A. Obtain sputum for cytology.
    B. Auscultate for wheezes, crackles, and stridor.
    C. Provide adequate hydration.
    D. Measure for intake and output.

14. G.H. is a 71-year-old woman with a diagnosis of breast cancer. She was admitted to the hospital this afternoon with mental status changes. In reviewing the laboratory reports, the nurse notes that G.H.'s serum calcium is 14 mg/dL, her potassium is 3.0 mEq/L, and her phosphorus is 7 mg/dL. What metabolic emergency should the nurse be most concerned about based on these laboratory values?
    A. Hypercalcemia
    B. TLS
    C. DIC
    D. SIADH

15. Hypercalcemia is often described as mild, moderate, or severe, usually based on clinical lab results. Which of the following symptoms are usually seen in patients diagnosed with "moderate hypercalcemia?
    A. Anorexia, nausea and vomiting, restlessness, generalized weakness, and frequent urination
    B. Ileus, seizures, coma, ataxia or pathological fractures, renal failure, and abnormal EKG
    C. Constipation, bloating, increasing abdominal pain, weakness, and dehydration
    D. Dysuria, flank pain, hematuria, paralysis, weakness, and spasms of the feet and hands

16. P.A., who is 72 years old, has a new diagnosis of multiple myeloma. Prior to his diagnosis, he lost 27 lb. He had a port-a-cath placed and received cyclophosphamide, lenalidomide, and dexamethasone for induction treatment a few days ago. P.A. is acutely at risk for
    A. TLS.
    B. DIC.
    C. systemic inflammatory response syndrome (SIRS), sepsis, and septic shock.
    D. hypersensitivity reactions.

17. Treatment of hypercalcemia may include all of these therapies except
    A. vasopressors.
    B. calcitonin.
    C. diuretic medications.
    D. bisphosphonates.

18. In monitoring the patient's vital signs and laboratory results, the nurse should realize which of these clinical signs and symptoms indicate SIRS? ⚠
    A. Temperature greater than 100.4° F (38° C) or less than 96.8° F (36° C)
    B. Heart rate between 50 and 60 beats/min
    C. Respiratory rate greater than 40 breaths/min
    D. Anemia with hemoglobin less than 8.0 and hematocrit less than 26

19. Signs and symptoms of anaphylaxis include ⚠
    A. fatigue.
    B. urticaria.
    C. pain around an intravenous insertion site.
    D. itching around an intravenous insertion site.

20. A 26-year-old disoriented and irritable young man with Hodgkin disease and diabetes is admitted to the hospital. His temperature is 100° F (37° C), pulse is 110 beats/min, blood pressure is 90/40 mm Hg, respiratory rate is 30 breaths/min, WBC count is 500/mm³, and platelets are 150,000/mm³. Urine output is normal and positive for glucose (blood sugar, 190 mg/dL). Which condition would the nurse suspect in this patient? ⚠
    A. DIC
    B. Septic shock
    C. Hypocalcemia
    D. Diabetic shock

21. A patient with ovarian carcinoma has agreed to participate in a clinical trial involving a new agent with anaphylactic potential. What precautions should the nurse take the first time the drug is given? ⚠
    A. Premedicate the patient with diazepam.
    B. Reject the patient as a candidate for the study.
    C. Take vital signs before the agent is administered and every 4 hours thereafter.
    D. Administer the agent only in an environment where emergency medications and equipment are available.

C.F. is a 62-year-old woman who has previous history of stage III kidney disease related to long-term use of medications for rheumatoid arthritis. She presented with lower abdominal discomfort, and a computed tomography (CT) of the abdomen and pelvis showed extensive ascites, thickened omentum, and large pelvic mass. After a complete hysterectomy and tumor bulking, the final diagnosis was poorly differentiated papillary serous carcinoma originating from the ovaries. She was treated initially with 5 cycles of paclitaxel and carboplatin. When her CA-125 levels increased, she was switched to topotecan. C.F. is at risk for TLS because of which of the following?
    A. Cancer with large bulky tumor mass
    B. Chronic renal insufficiency
    C. Radiation therapy
    D. Many

23. Which of the following patients is most at risk for developing SIADH?
    A. A patient with colon cancer undergoing a colon resection
    B. A patient with small cell lung cancer receiving weekly paclitaxel (Taxol) and carboplatin (Paraplatin)
    C. A patient with acute myelogenous leukemia receiving induction therapy with cytarabine (Cytosar) and idarubicin (Idamycin)
    D. A patient with breast cancer who is admitted to the hospital for pneumonia and is taking morphine for pain control

24. A patient with a diagnosis of non–small cell lung cancer is admitted to the hospital with altered mental status and vomiting. His serum sodium is 118 mEq/L, urine sodium is 30 mEq/L, and potassium is 3.0 mEq/L. What is the appropriate immediate nursing intervention with this patient? ⚠
    A. Medicate the patient for pain.
    B. Implement seizure precautions.
    C. Encourage the patient to do frequent mouth care.
    D. Encourage the patient to increase his fluid intake.

25. Emergency treatment of SIADH may be required if ⚠
    A. serum sodium is 125 mEq/L.
    B. serum sodium is 135 mEq/L.
    C. cardiopulmonary changes are present.
    D. significant neurologic changes are present.

41 Structural Emergencies

1. A patient has leukemia with a new diagnosis of lepto-meningeal metastases. The nurse should understand that the patient has metastatic disease located in which location?
   A. Lymph nodes
   B. Spleen
   C. Cerebrospinal fluid
   D. Liver

2. The patient with leptomeningeal metastases has been, according to her daughter, mentally "off" for several weeks. The nurse should assess the patient for the presence of what additional symptoms?
   A. Bradycardia, respiratory distress, and hypertension
   B. Constipation, increased appetite, and esophageal spasm
   C. Euphoria, labile emotions, and manic episodes
   D. Reduced urination and painful urination

3. Increased Intracranial Pressure (ICP) can be diagnosed and monitored via a catheter placed in intraventricular, intraparenchymal, subarachnoid, or epidural site. The goal of this technique is to achieve ⚠
   A. a negative Romberg test result.
   B. intracranial pressure less than 20 mm Hg.
   C. intracranial pressure between 20 and 40 mm Hg.
   D. a cerebral perfusion pressure (CPP) between 30 and 45 mm Hg.

4. Early detection of spinal cord compression (SCC) is essential for prompt intervention and preventing loss of function. The most common presenting symptom of SCC in patients with cancer is ⚠
   A. motor weakness and motor loss.
   B. sensory loss.
   C. neck and back pain.
   D. bowel or bladder incontinence.

5. A patient with elevated ICP is admitted to the hospital. The oncology nurse should expect which treatment to be initiated most rapidly? ⚠
   A. Corticosteroids
   B. Radiation therapy
   C. Emergent surgery
   D. Hyperventilation

6. What measures should the nurse include in the care of a patient with increased ICP? ⚠
   A. Maintaining the patient in a supine position without elevation of the head of the bed
   B. Administration of stool softeners and laxatives to prevent constipation
   C. Encourage the patient to perform isometric exercises and the Valsalva maneuver
   D. Active range of motion exercises with 5-lb weights

7. What is the most common cause of spinal cord compression (SCC) in patients with cancer?
   A. Syndrome of inappropriate diuretic hormone secretion (SIADH)
   B. Herpes zoster infection
   C. Carcinomatous meningitis
   D. Metastatic tumor invasion

8. C.N. is 76 years old and has lymphoma. He has a new onset of tingling and numbness in his lower extremities and back pain, usually more noticeable at night. He had surgery about 10 years ago for a herniated disc. The nurse understands that the patient should be assessed for a new diagnosis of SCC rather than for pain from the herniated disc based on which factors?
   A. Pain caused by SCC worsens in the supine recumbent position and may be relieved in the sitting position; the opposite is true for a herniated disc.
   B. Pain caused by SCC worsens in the sitting position and may be relieved in the supine recumbent position; the opposite is true for a herniated disc.
   C. Pain caused by SCC causes severe frontal and occipital headache upon waking in the morning.
   D. Pain caused by a SCC, not by a herniated disc, is always localized to one area of the spinal column.

9. What should the nurse include in the physical examination of C.N., the patient in Question 8?
   A. Lumbar palpation and percussion
   B. Vertebral palpitation and percussion
   C. Digital rectal examination to rule out rectal bleeding
   D. Auscultation of the chest to detect new or existing murmurs

10. What is the most common cause of cardiac tamponade?
    A. Pericarditis caused by chemotherapy such as doxorubicin
    B. Radiation therapy–induced pericarditis
    C. Malignant disease that causes pericardial effusion
    D. Diseases such as rheumatoid arthritis or systemic lupus erythematosus

11. To obtain a definitive diagnosis of SCC, the nurse should expect to complete the appropriate forms for which imaging procedure?
    A. Magnetic Resonance Imaging (MRI) myelography.
    B. Plain spine radiography.
    C. Bone scan.
    D. Myelography.

12. What is the least important prognostic factor for functional outcome in patients with SCC?
    A. Neurologic status before the initiation of therapy
    B. The ability to "walk in" to the health facility at diagnosis and to "walk out" upon discharge
    C. Ambulatory status at the time of diagnosis
    D. Weight loss

13. In providing teaching to new nurses on the oncology unit, the nurse should explain that superior vena cava syndrome (SCVS) occurs when
    A. excess fluid collects in the pericardial space.
    B. excess fluid collects in the pleural cavity.
    C. extrinsic compression causes an obstruction of the superior vena cava.
    D. excess fluid accumulates and causes intrinsic pressure within the vessel.

14. A diagnosis of SCC requires prompt attention. The oncology nurse educator should teach nurse orientees that which method is the accepted initial medical treatment for SCC? ⚠
    A. Surgery
    B. Radiation therapy
    C. Corticosteroids
    D. Chemotherapy

15. The oncology nurse should explain that which conditions are most commonly associated with the development of SVCS?
    A. Non-Hodgkin lymphoma
    B. Advanced thyroid cancer
    C. Radiation therapy–induced pneumonitis
    D. Mediastinal fibrosis caused by histoplasmosis

16. What are diagnostic techniques used to determine SVCS?
    A. Electrocardiography and echocardiography
    B. MRI and CT with contrast
    C. Chest radiography and barium swallow
    D. Cervical spine and myelography

17. What are possible early signs of SVCS? ⚠
    A. Muffled heart rate of 100 beats/min, abdominal distention, and fever
    B. Hypertension, bradycardia, widening of pulse pressure, and abnormal respirations
    C. Jugular vein distention and edema of the face, periorbital area, back, neck upper thorax, breasts, and upper extremities
    D. Hypotension and Cheyne-Stoke respirations

18. In patients with lung cancer, what is the principal cause of increased ICP?
    A. Metabolic complications from the syndrome of inappropriate antidiuretic hormone secretion (SIADH)
    B. Side effects of chemotherapy and radiation therapy
    C. A space-occupying metastatic mass within the brain
    D. Cerebrovascular accident or transient ischemic attack

19. What are medical treatments for patients with early clinical signs of SVCS?
    A. Instillation of tissue plasminogen activator (TPA) in a patent central catheter
    B. Chemotherapy after diagnosis of lymphoma or small cell lung cancer is made
    C. Anticoagulation with heparin for all patients who have superior vena cava syndrome
    D. Immediate chemotherapy before histologic diagnosis is obtained in patients with unknown cause of SVCS

20. Immediate medical treatment of ICP includes administration of ⚠
    A. calcium channel blockers and β-blockers.
    B. a vascular smooth muscle relaxer, such as nitroglycerin.
    C. an osmotic diuretic such as Mannitol and a corticosteroid.
    D. a cardiac glycoside.

21. What instructions should the oncology nurse provide to a patient with newly diagnosed SVCS?
    A. Report inability to complete usual activities.
    B. Rest or sleep in the supine position in bed.
    C. Call the physician if temperature reaches 102° F (38° C).
    D. Take blood pressure measurements in either arm every 4 hours.

22. The nurse should monitor a patient receiving treatment for SVCS for which treatment-related side effects?
    A. Hypoglycemia with corticosteroids
    B. Hypertension caused by diuretics
    C. Pancytopenia from chemotherapy or radiation therapy
    D. Generalized rash caused by systemic antibiotics

42 Survivorship

1. In relation to cancer survivorship, the term *survivor* refers to what population?
   A. Anyone who is given the diagnosis of more than one cancer
   B. Someone who recurs with the original primary disease
   C. A family member who also has a cancer diagnosis
   D. Anyone with a cancer diagnosis or a member of a social network of the individual with cancer

2. A client finished breast cancer treatment 5 years ago. She reports to her practitioner with complaints of arm swelling and pain and states, "I thought I was done with my breast cancer; is this related?" The nurse knows that
   A. her symptoms are unrelated because her initial treatment involved only sentinel node biopsy and lumpectomy.
   B. because of the amount of time that has elapsed since her surgery and limited radiation, these symptoms are unrelated.
   C. this is likely a late effect of her sentinel node resection, lumpectomy, and the radiation therapy.
   D. because she made it to the 5-year progression-free window, she will be considered disease free and a survivor.

3. Survivorship issues are important for any nurse in the cancer care spectrum because
   A. with the advances in treatment, cancer survivors today have a high likelihood of being free of disease-related concerns.
   B. the minority of cancer survivors are individuals who are 65 years of age or older; this number will continue to increase.
   C. the majority of cancer survivors have survived 5 years or more since the original diagnosis of their cancer.
   D. survivorship has equal representation from each cancer site population.

4. How are long-term, short-term, and late side effects of cancer treatment differentiated?
   A. Long-term side effects are those that begin as a complication of treatment and persist throughout treatment but do not persist after treatment is completed.
   B. Late effects are those that begin after treatment is completed, may have been subclinical at the end of treatment, and may manifest years later.
   C. Short-term recurring side effects often become long-term side effects but do not become late effects.
   D. Long-term and late effects are primarily related to the treatment the individual received for cancer.

5. Evidence shows that long-term and late effects of cancer
   A. include the increased risk of cardiovascular problems as the individual ages, including valvular heart disease and electrical or conductive changes.
   B. will pass. Any psychological and cognitive impairment concerns, if they persist, should prompt a referral for counseling.
   C. include spiritual impact, but will not affect the survivor's thoughts of illness, transcendence, and finding inner strength to continue.
   D. are not a factor that influences treatment or insurance issues for survivors who have passed the 5-year mark.

6. A 32-year-old female client was diagnosed at the age of 17 years. She received mantle radiation for Hodgkin disease (HD). Now she wonders why a baseline mammogram was ordered for her. The nurse explains that
   A. this is a mistake. She is too young for a baseline mammogram, and her breasts would be too dense for a definitive procedure.
   B. she should have had a baseline mammogram before treatment began and needs to be monitored closely.
   C. the radiation would prevent any cancer from developing in her nodes.
   D. guidelines suggest a mammogram at approximately age 25 years, or 8 years after initial therapy, because of an increased risk of breast cancer after mantle radiation.

7. Which statement best describes the current state of long-term follow-up care for adult cancer survivors in the United States?
   A. All long-term survivors are seen in specialty follow-up clinics for the rest of their lives.
   B. Although pediatric survivors undergo follow-up for indefinite periods of time in long-term survivor specialty clinics, adult cancer survivors rarely have access to this type of oncology follow-up.
   C. Adult survivors are eligible to be seen in follow-up clinics after being free of disease for 5 years.
   D. Primary care physicians are best prepared to identify oncology-related follow-up problems.

8. A cancer survivorship care plan (CSCP) should include all the following except
   A. verbal discussion with client and family members regarding the long-term and late effects of treatment.
   B. recommended follow-up surveillance and recommended health promotion behaviors and health maintenance.
   C. a list of healthcare team providers with their contact information and role on the team.
   D. a treatment summary, including the cancer site, type and stage of cancer, date of diagnosis, and any treatment(s) received.

9. Which of the following statements accurately describes a psychosocial effect of long-term survival?
   A. Most cancer survivors have severe and permanent psychological adjustment problems.
   B. After therapy is completed, there is rarely, if ever, any need for continued psychosocial support.
   C. The fear of recurrence may persist for many years after completion of therapy and range anywhere between a mild or chronic anxiety to disabling fear.
   D. The family remains overprotective and reactive to any new indication of illness such as colds, flu, etc., not allowing reintegration into societal roles.

10. What major barriers persist in the provision of survivorship care?
    A. An aging population with inadequate number of providers with expertise in care of elderly
    B. A lack of knowledge regarding the late and long-term effects that should be addressed
    C. Resistance on the part of clients to return to the institution where they received their care
    D. Increased number of comorbidities in the individuals being diagnosed with cancer

11. A client is having a difficult time going to her breast cancer support group. Although she is doing well and is free of disease 2 years after completing treatment, she feels sad and despondent when she sees others suffer or die of the same illness she had. She asks herself why she is alive and doing well when so many others are not. This is
    A. posttraumatic stress disorder (PTSD).
    B. acute reactive syndrome.
    C. bipolar disorder.
    D. survivor's guilt.

12. Survivorship care focusing on prevention and detection would include all the following factors except
    A. encouraging healthy behaviors such as physical activity and tobacco cessation.
    B. promoting sun protection and regular screening based on established guidelines.
    C. assessing for occurrence of late effects related to cancer diagnosis and treatment.
    D. intervening with a psychological referral for PTSD.

43 Palliative and End-of-Life Care

1. A client has been admitted for pain control because of bone metastases from advanced prostate cancer. He is still seeking aggressive treatment. Which of the following types of care is indicated?
   A. Acute care
   B. Palliative care
   C. Rehabilitative care
   D. Hospice care

2. Family of individuals in palliative care can expect
   A. that symptoms will be addressed as they occur throughout the treatment.
   B. an emphasis on the physical comfort of the client receiving the care.
   C. to be included in the planning of care along with their loved one.
   D. entry into a clinical trial to manage pain and extend life.

3. Palliative care should be included for all situations below except
   A. advanced disease with a prognosis of less than 1 year.
   B. significant social or psychosocial distress.
   C. Karnofsky performance status that is less than 50%.
   D. families that are not being realistic about the prognosis and are unable to assist with care.

4. Palliative care is becoming more widely accepted, as evidenced by
   A. its availability in multiple venues and levels of care facilities and home care.
   B. certification programs for nurses through Oncology Nursing Society and physicians with plans for future expansion.
   C. family member acceptance of the program referrals.
   D. healthcare providers developing a skill set in management of multiple symptoms.

5. Evidence supporting the positive impact of palliative care on cancer client outcomes includes
   A. the ability to provide more aggressive care until the final phase of the disease.
   B. clients in palliative care programs are dying sooner with better symptom control.
   C. increased desire of family members to allow the disease to run its course.
   D. improved quality of life and less aggressive end-of-life care.

6. When clients with multiple symptoms are admitted to palliative care, the important first step is
   A. assessing the client's symptoms.
   B. assessing how the family is coping.
   C. talking with the family about hospice plans.
   D. developing a therapeutic relationship with client and family.

7. Hospice care can be defined as all the following statements except
   A. based on the understanding that dying is part of life.
   B. a regulated insurance benefit that includes a Medicare benefit.
   C. separate and distinct from palliative care.
   D. supports meticulous management of symptoms to promote quality of living.

8. A challenge with providing hospice is
   A. clients living beyond the expected 6 months.
   B. not being able to provide life-prolonging therapies.
   C. physicians tending to be overly optimistic when estimating life expectancy.
   D. accepting the unique way families live out their cultures.

9. Definitions related to grief include
    A. anticipatory grief—the experience of emotions related to the absence of an object, position, ability, or attribute.
    B. disenfranchised grief—the experience of psychological, social, and somatic responses before the death of a loved one.
    C. complicated grief—the outward expression of emotions related to the death of a loved one that continues for 4 months.
    D. prolonged grief—persistent and severe yearning for the deceased beyond 6 to 12 months after the loss.

10. The dual process model of coping with bereavement
    A. is a theoretic approach to integrate the two processes in grief, loss and restoration.
    B. discusses restoration as the individual concentrates on working through some aspect of the loss.
    C. focuses on the work of experiencing the pain of the loss so that it becomes real.
    D. counsels families to resolve relationship conflicts before death of client.

11. Certification programs are currently available to assure programs meet predetermined standards, including
    A. acute hospital-based palliative care programs.
    B. ambulatory palliative care as part of a cancer center.
    C. community-based nonhospice palliative care.
    D. nursing home–based services for progressive chronic diseases.

12. What is an appropriate nursing care role for individuals where hospice or palliative care services are not available?
    A. Explain to clients and families they must waive traditional curative care to qualify for supportive services.
    B. Assist clients and families to complete necessary documentation to articulate wishes for end-of-life care.
    C. Collaborate with social work and other support services to establish a coordinated plan with available support services.
    D. Assume responsibility to contact agencies such as American Cancer Society for hospice support.

13. Interdisciplinary care is an essential component of comprehensive palliative care and requires
    A. collaboration to create a client- or family-directed plan of care.
    B. each discipline to clearly articulate the aspect of care for which they will be responsible.
    C. all professional team members to be certified by their individual professional organization.
    D. all disciplines to assess the client and family to formulate an individualized plan of care.

14. The initial priority in end-of-life care is
    A. identifying the meaning of quality of life for the client and family.
    B. identifying interventions for optimal pain control for the client.
    C. continuing interventions identified initially as the disease progresses.
    D. addressing the underlying cause rather than treating the outward symptoms.

15. The family members of an individual express concern about malnutrition and starvation. An appropriate response would be to
    A. offer to meet with the physician with them to discuss a feeding tube.
    B. assist the family to understand cancer cachexia in advanced stage disease.
    C. encourage them to review the client's living will and end-of-life preferences.
    D. initiate a calorie count to determine caloric intake over 24 hours.

16. What are some hydration-related interventions to improve a client's comfort?
    A. Providing frequent oral care (avoiding drying rinses)
    B. Discontinuing interventions such as complex chemotherapy regimens
    C. Addressing hydration needs with intravenous or enteral fluids
    D. Encouraging the family to provide fluids hourly

17. During a home visit to a hospice client with advanced stage disease, the family mentions their loved one seems to cough frequently with oral intake. Safety concerns include: ⚠
    A. maintaining adequate hydration for client comfort.
    B. encouraging the family to offer favorite foods and avoid fluids.
    C. discussing positioning of the client to avoid aspiration.
    D. discussing placement of an enteral feeding tube for fluids.

18. Potential causes of excess fluid loss include all the following except
    A. nausea and vomiting.
    B. diarrhea and diuresis.
    C. diaphoresis with fever.
    D. excessive pulmonary secretions.

19. Anticholinergic medications may be indicated to treat
    A. hormone-induced diuresis.
    B. diaphoresis at the end of life.
    C. opioid toxicity at the end of life.
    D. excessive secretions.

20. The need for supplemental fluids may outweigh the benefit of natural dehydration when the client is
    A. sedated with complaints of headache, dizziness, and somnolence.
    B. coughing and appears to choke on thick secretions.
    C. on morphine and demonstrates signs and symptoms of myoclonus, hyperalgesia, and allodynia.
    D. sleeping more, and family are expressing concern about fluid intake.

21. A client is demonstrating ineffective breathing; an assessment will explore potential causes, including all of the following except
    A. disease process.
    B. generalized weakness.
    C. renal failure.
    D. dying process.

22. Which position would be most likely to lessen the work of breathing?
    A. Lying on the side when the head of bed is elevated.
    B. Elevate the head of the bed at 45 degrees and the feet at approximately 30 degrees.
    C. Have the client sit in a chair at the side of the bed.
    D. Elevate the head of the bed with the client leaning forward over the bedside table supported with pillows.

23. If pneumonia is determined to be a likely cause of dyspnea, use of antibiotics should be
    A. routinely indicated unless it is likely to trigger an ethics consult.
    B. based on the client's perceived quality of life.
    C. determined by underlying disease processes.
    D. initiated if family dreads listening to the "death rattle."

24. The palliative care team has concluded that a pleural effusion is contributing to dyspnea. The decision to tap the effusion will be guided by
    A. whether it is new or recurring.
    B. the client's life expectancy.
    C. likelihood the effusion will recur.
    D. likelihood that the underlying disease will respond to chemotherapy.

25. Which factors should guide care planning regarding oxygen therapy at the end of life?
    A. A mask would be the preferred mode of delivery.
    B. Many clients need oxygen at the end of life, even when they have not needed it previously.
    C. Clients who have needed oxygen previously will no longer need it at the end of life.
    D. A fan blowing on the face may be adequate if the individual did not need oxygen previously.

26. Which symptomatic treatments of dyspnea are effective?
    A. Providing a hot sensation to the face such as a hot compress on the cheeks
    B. Using benzodiazepines at same dose as recommended for moderate levels of anxiety
    C. Avoiding long-acting opioids; all others are equally effective for treating end-of-life dyspnea
    D. Providing reassurance, presence, and sup   rt to lessen the anxiety associated with dyspne

27. What are some interventions for noisy respira   is?
    A. Help the family to understand the significa   of the "death rattle."
    B. Position with the head of the bed elevat   or lying on the side for drainage.
    C. Try to avoid mouth care to decrease secreti   .
    D. Suction deeply to provide a longer lasting be   fit.

28. Assessment findings indicate that the client is   n-onstrating decreased cardiac output and poor t   e perfusion. The nurses realize that
    A. the process starts centrally, moves toward   e periphery, and involves the skin.
    B. the body temperature may decrease. Prepar   o add extra blankets and heating devices.
    C. mottling is an indication of progression. Reinfe   e to the family this is an indicator of immir   t death.
    D. continue regularly monitoring vital signs to co   municate availability to the family members.

29. Morning assessment of an elderly client in yc   hospice program indicates delirium. The nurs   response would be to:
    A. consider evaluation of exposure to toxins a   evaluate for additional evidence of neurocogniti   changes.
    B. determine the need to administer sedative med   cation at night to prevent sleep deprivation.
    C. recognize that hypoactive delirium in older adult   can be related to dehydration and metabolic ab   normalities.
    D. anticipate the current hypoactive state may change   quickly to a hyperactive delirium from withdrawa   of medications.

30. Pharmacologic management of delirium includes
    A. use of a benzodiazepine titrated to effect.
    B. use of haloperidol, but if the client has Parkinson disease, then use quetiapine.
    C. discontinue the use of opioids; they are most likely contributing to the problem.
    D. treating metabolic abnormalities; the delirium can be reversed.

31. What factors can contribute to end-of-life delirium and should be eliminated or treated?
    A. Constipation, pain, infections, dehydration, and hypoxia
    B. Fever, age, cognitive status, and malnutrition
    C. Hypercalcemia
    D. Overstimulation, noise, unnecessary lighting, and constant interruptions

32. Diagnostic criteria for delirium includes
    A. increasing evidence of a comatose state.
    B. disturbance in attention and awareness.
    C. disturbance that develops slowly over multiple days or weeks with little fluctuation.
    D. disturbances explained by preexisting neurocognitive disorder.

33. Possible causes of delirium may include
    A. antibiotics.
    B. antiemetics.
    C. bowel obstruction.
    D. urinary tract infection.

44 Evidence-Based Practice and Standards of Oncology Nursing

1. As the nurse is discussing nursing care related to a central venous catheter (CVC) with a new clinician, he states that his former clinic used alcohol–povidone–iodine, not chlorhexidine, preparations for the skin around the CVC. Chlorhexidine preparations increase the risk of infection, he was told. The nurse is aware of the evidence-based practice (EBP) standards for CVC care and knows that ⚠
   A. either product is probably acceptable as long as care includes using antibacterial ointment at the exit site.
   B. there is limited documented research comparing the two agents for skin preparations of a CVC.
   C. the risks and benefits of a CVC should be carefully weighed.
   D. multiple antiseptics have been studied; povidone–iodine is the best option.

2. An individual nurse can use the standards of care to
   A. ensure patient participation in health promotion and health prevention.
   B. provide a basis for organizational policies, procedures, and protocols.
   C. identify gaps in his or her knowledge base regarding cancer care.
   D. provide educational content to a client about his or her treatment protocol.

3. The Oncology Nursing Society (ONS) Standards of Practice emphasize the importance of all the following except
   A. intra- and inter-professional collaboration and collegiality.
   B. ethical practice and ensuring universal quality cancer care.
   C. recognition of racial and ethnic diversity and the need for diversity awareness.
   D. nurses guiding evidence-based quality cancer care.

4. The standards of care can provide the advanced practice nurse and generalist nurse in oncology a nursing proc   s framework, which ensures that
   A. da   collection is systematic, characterized by div   ity awareness, and limited to a brief episode of c
   B. outco   s flow from collaborative diagnoses and are ind   dualized to the patient's needs.
   C. the plan   f care is implemented in concordance with the n   se's identified priorities for the patient.
   D. nursing an   collaborative diagnoses are derived from data re   cted to the patient's potential health problems.

5. What do the standa   s of care provide to society at large?
   A. Identification of th   4 most likely problem areas common to patients   th cancer
   B. A guide for ensuring e   ence-based quality cancer nursing care
   C. An indication that onc   gy nursing is able to define and govern the q   ity of cancer nursing practice
   D. An indication of key nursi   actions, which include assessment, diagnosis,   nning, implementation, and evaluation

6. A nurse has just started practicing at a   w facility and notes that the organizational protoc   for care of intravascular catheters references the g   deline from the Centers for Disease Control and Prevention (CDC). This indicates that the facility
   A. may not be invested in the establishment o   vidence-based practice that is sensitive to unique   eds of patients.
   B. should adopt a preestablished aggregate l   l of performance, which can be used to dete   ine quality of care.
   C. uses established standards to develop curricu   r content for orientation of the new generalist nurs
   D. uses established evidence-based guidelines for the development of practice-setting specific plans of care for a high-incidence problem area.

7. An institution is planning a quality-improvement initiative using the framework of the Standards of Professional Performance for Quality of Practice. What instructions would you not include in the framework?
   A. Use the measurement criteria provided as a statement to guide acceptable practice.
   B. Define a minimum acceptable level of performance and actions that will result from an unacceptable performance level.
   C. Collect and analyze data to monitor effectiveness of care and to identify areas to improve.
   D. Implement recommendations from the project and then focus on other areas for improvements.

8. What statement addresses the relevance of the standards for nursing management and leadership?
   A. Their strength in evidence-based practice and research restrict the relevance for staff nurses.
   B. They provide a problem-solving approach for addressing clinical concerns at the specific institution.
   C. The systematic approach recommended emphasizes using the best evidence to make decisions about concern.
   D. They can provide a framework to evaluate resource utilization and to justify additional resources for quality care.

9. The primary goal of EBP in oncology nursing is to
   A. guide the selection of interventions that are likely to facilitate priority nursing outcomes.
   B. integrate a problem-solving approach for clinical practice related to the nurse's personal clinical expertise.
   C. guide nursing interventions that are demonstrated to enhance the quality and outcomes of care.
   D. provide an approach to respond to patient preferences and facilitate cost-effective care.

10. The standards address the professional mandate for EBP through
    A. the use of EBP to guide performance improvement for quality outcomes.
    B. the inclusion of EBP in each of the six standards of care.
    C. the extensive detail of the Professional Performance EBP standards.
    D. the integration of nursing practice, research, and education into each standard.

11. Oncology nurses contribute to the scientific base of cancer nursing practice, education, management, quality improvement, and research through multiple avenues, including all of the following except
    A. identifying clinical dilemmas and problems appropriate for rigorous study.
    B. integrating relevant research into practice to improve outcomes.
    C. reading published literature in area of expertise.
    D. collecting data.

12. According to the nursing education standard, graduates of generic nursing programs should be able to
    A. care for multiple patients who are receiving cancer treatment and their family members.
    B. develop a proposal for a nursing research study and submit the proposal for funding.
    C. address the concerns of patients and family members regarding nonpayment of services.
    D. develop and evaluate an evidence-based plan of care for a patient receiving cancer treatment.

13. Examples of nonresearched evidence to guide EBP include
    A. clinical questions, quality improvement data, and risk data.
    B. benchmarking data, principles of pathophysiology, and legal data.
    C. cost-effectiveness analysis, international, national, and personal standards of care.
    D. retrospective chart review data and qualitative patient interview data.

14. According to the standards, involvement in EBP
    A. is an expectation for nurses prepared at all levels.
    B. requires participation in nursing research.
    C. is a necessary component to evaluate clinical quality.
    D. increases the benefit of pay-for-performance programs.

15. EBP provides for safety by ⚠
    A. focusing efforts on performance improvement.
    B. orienting nurses to risks, including look-alike medications.
    C. requiring the reporting of incidents involving patients.
    D. integrating evidence with clinical expertise and patient values.

16. Factors contributing to the need for EBP include
    A. the Institute of Medicine mandate that all health-care decisions will be evidence based by 2020.
    B. the need for comprehensive, outcomes-driven healthcare.
    C. healthcare costs are more likely to soar without EBP.
    D. cost-effective analysis requires EBP.
    E. using research evidence to collect and analyze data.

17. What are some potential research roles of the oncology nurse generalist that can facilitate EBP?
    A. Identification of problems by observing patients and focusing on quality improvement
    B. Directing the evaluation of existing nursing research study data analysis
    C. Participating in research activities under the guidance of qualified researchers
    D. Providing nursing care to clients on a medical/surgical acute care unit

18. A nursing peer shares an abstract from a published research study and asks if this can be used to support the development of a new practice protocol. What would be an appropriate response?
    A. Give him professional evaluation of the research abstract and recommendation for action.
    B. State that the decision cannot be made on the abstract alone; all parts of the study must be critiqued.
    C. Because this is a high-incidence area for us, let us try to implement the recommendations presented.
    D. Ask to hear if he thinks the findings will be of value to the patients with cancer and why.

19. A research study reports statistically significant results, what additional information would be important to know?
    A. Are the results clinically significant, and can they be generalized?
    B. Is the physician leading the care of these clients supportive of nursing research?
    C. Who can determine if the clients in the clinic will be receptive to recommendations?
    D. Is this something clinic staff would be interested in addressing for clients?

20. The 14 high-incidence problem areas in oncology nursing, cited in the Statement on the Scope and Standards of Oncology Nursing Practice, are
    A. key areas in which oncology nurses assess, plan, and intervene.
    B. the problems with the highest incidence rates in cancer care.
    C. problems that most often affect the client in the acute care setting.
    D. clinical indicators that are measurable dimensions of the quality of client care.

21. The standard of care on outcome identification states that the oncology nurse identifies expected outcomes individualized to the client. Which of the following measurement criteria supports this standard? The oncology nurse
    A. communicates the client's responses with the healthcare team.
    B. ensures that expected outcomes provide direction for continuity of care.
    C. incorporates preventive, therapeutic, rehabilitative, palliative, and comforting nursing actions into the plan of care.
    D. reviews and revises the nursing diagnoses, expected outcomes, and plan of care based on the findings of the evaluation.

22. Using evidence to influence clinical practice is a multistep process. After clarifying the problem of interest, the next step in the process is
    A. conducting a literature review of relevant research.
    B. getting "buy-in" from colleagues and administration.
    C. identifying the information needed to solve the problem.
    D. developing a clinical protocol to address the problem.

23. A phase IV treatment clinical trial is designed to evaluate
    A. drug toxicities.
    B. which tumor will be responsive to a drug.
    C. new areas of use after Food and Drug Administration (FDA) approval.
    D. activity of a new combination in relation to the standard of treatment.

45 Education Process

1. Which statements accurately describe learning theories that can be useful for guiding clinical teaching strategies?
   A. Learning is based on observable behaviors, which are reinforced to increase the strength of the behavior as presented in motivational learning theory.
   B. There is an internal process requiring attention, thought, and reasoning for information to be retrieved and applied, as presented in cognitive learning theory.
   C. Human behavior is activated and directed by internal cues or drive or environmental cues as put forward by behavior learning theory.
   D. Each individual is unique, and all individuals have a desire to learn and grow in a positive manner as supported by adult learning theory.

2. Which questions should be addressed before developing an educational program for a client?
   A. What the client knows and wants to know, cultural and religious beliefs and practices that might impact the process for the client, and the content the nurse knows to be important
   B. What the client knows and wants to know, physical and cognitive impairments that might impact learning, preferred learning style, and the budget available
   C. What the client knows and wants to know, the language used by the client (speaking and reading), and the educational background of the client
   D. What the client knows and wants to know, the preferred learning style, the nurse's understanding of the topic, and the time the nurse has available for the teaching

3. What factors should serve as a priority to guide initial client education in order to avert a potential threat to patient safety? ⚠
   A. The similarity between the nurse's SMART goals and the client's ability to learn
   B. The components of the teaching content that would be important to cover initially
   C. Cultural practices that guide the consumption of food and supplements
   D. The client's family history with cancer and cancer treatment

4. It is important for educational programs to include SMART goals because they
   A. are the best way to organize the educational content.
   B. encourage the nurse to individualize the content.
   C. let clients know what to expect from the program.
   D. facilitate the evaluation of a program based on meaningful outcomes.

5. After participation in the chemotherapy teaching class, the client will be able to address management of common side effects. What is this sentence an example of?
   A. A teaching goal that is well-written based on SMART criteria for education
   B. An objective that lacks clear articulation of the degree of performance expected. ABCD objective rule
   C. Evaluation criteria for a chemotherapy class targeting a group of clients
   D. A guide for evaluation of the evaluation of a client's learning

6. In the process of planning an education program for patients, the nurse identifies teaching practices in the literature, establishes standards of care and relevant hospital procedures, and consults with experts. This facilitates
   A. development of a teaching program with excellent visuals.
   B. establishment of a process for assessment of cultural concerns.
   C. development of an evidence-based teaching program.
   D. awareness of limitations related to staffing resources and budget.

7. What are major potential barriers to evaluation of an educational program?
   A. Goals and objectives of the program were not articulated prior to the teaching.
   B. Evaluation required documentation of learning outcomes.
   C. Recipients of the content found it to be irrelevant to them.
   D. The nurse involved in the evaluation did not provide the content.

8. A 48-year-old woman is discharged after a lumpectomy for a newly diagnosed malignant breast tumor. What subjects would be her priority learning needs?
   A. Postmastectomy wound care
   B. Breast self-examination
   C. Breast cancer and its treatment
   D. Follow-up mammography

9. The purpose of the educational component of nursing practice is to help people acquire the knowledge they need in order to
   A. comply with the physician's orders.
   B. learn what health professionals believe they need to know.
   C. understand the particular diagnosis.
   D. participate in their treatment decisions and self-care.

10. A nurse prepares an educational plan for a client who is about to receive chemotherapy. The client verbalizes a desire to continue working during the treatment. Which of the following statements represents an important learning principle in addressing the client's needs?
    A. Learning should be subject centered, not client centered.
    B. The learner's needs should receive priority.
    C. Learning is often negated by life experiences.
    D. Learning occurs when the teaching plan is completed.

11. Participation in cancer-related public education is an important nursing activity because
    A. these programs have an impact on cancer prevention, incidence, morbidity, and mortality.
    B. programs enhance the professional image of cancer nursing.
    C. the participants' fear of cancer will be modified.
    D. the competence of the nurse as a cancer-client educator will improve.

12. D.J. is hospitalized for shortness of breath. A mass is seen on chest radiograph, and a biopsy reveals non–small cell lung cancer (NSCLC). She and her husband have smoked 2 packs of cigarettes per day for the past 20 years. Her mother died of lung cancer when D.J. was 15 years old. How would the nurse begin the educational process with this client?
    A. Teach her about the pathophysiology of lung cancer.
    B. Educate D.J. and her husband regarding the causes of lung cancer.
    C. Enroll D.J. and her husband in a smoking cessation program.
    D. Ask D.J. what she knows about lung cancer and about her past experiences with cancer.

13. When planning public education programs, what factors should the nurse take into consideration?
    A. Problems identified by the nurse; behaviors related to the health problem, development, and implementation of a program; and evaluation of the program
    B. Problems of concern to the community, specific behaviors related to the health problem, development and implementation of a program, and evaluation of the program
    C. Problems of concern to the community, general behaviors that might address the health problem, and presentation of a program
    D. Problems identified by the nurse, general behaviors that might address the health problem, presentation of a program, and evaluation of the program

14. A nurse responsible for staff education at her facility starts with an awareness of what nurses must know and understand to provide safe care. This nurse is
    A. using her intuition and critical thinking as part of the assessment of staff learning needs.
    B. likely to not address the needs of the nurses starting on the unit.
    C. bypassing the step of self-assessment by the nurses on the unit.
    D. not accounting for performance analysis to guide the plan.

15. Healthy People 2020 is an example of an initiative with the Department of Health and Human Services (DHHS) to improve health and
    A. address health literacy.
    B. the effectiveness of interventions.
    C. optimize scope of practice
    D. reduce health disparities.

16. Diffusion of innovations, a theory of technological innovation, identifies which stages of change?
    A. Innovators, early adopters, early majority, late majority, and laggers
    B. Knowledge, persuasion, decision, implementation, and confirmation
    C. Assessment, design, implementation, and evaluation
    D. Awareness, interest, trial, decision, and adoption

17. "Citizens are at risk for social isolation because of lack of public transportation" is an example of
    A. an intervention for an identified health need.
    B. a community health diagnosis based on data.
    C. illness prevalence data to guide an intervention.
    D. using community resources, advocates and agencies to foster change.

46 Legal Issues

1. What are characteristics of quality nursing documentation?
   A. Patient centered and written to reflect the subjective opinion of the direct care nurse
   B. Contains the work of the multidisciplinary team, including education
   C. Reflects variances in the patient's condition, including changes in response or nursing intervention
   D. Provided in structured format with specific labels and written as the events occurred

2. The nurse is preparing a presentation regarding the regulation of nursing practice to help peers understand key components. How are nursing regulations defined?
   A. The state boards of nursing define nursing roles, titles, and scopes of practice.
   B. Educational program standards are defined by the Nursing Council of State Boards of Nursing.
   C. Nurse Practice Acts define the scopes of practice and requirements for licensure.
   D. State boards of nursing develop the NCLEX-RN exam for new graduates.

3. What are key patient's rights changes resulting from the Affordable Care Act (ACA) in 2012? The ACA
   A. protects consumer privacy, restricts annual dollar limits on coverage, and protects consumer choice of doctors.
   B. ensures coverage to Americans with preexisting conditions and ends lifetime limits on coverage.
   C. ensures a clean and safe healthcare environment and helps consumers get the most from their premium dollars.
   D. ends arbitrary withdrawals of insurance coverage and provides help when leaving the hospital.

4. There are several standards of practice and position statements for oncology nursing. Which statement accurately describes one of these standards of practice?
   A. Lifelong learning for professional oncology nurses, which focuses on the importance of ongoing formal and informal education
   B. Oncology certification for nurses that supports specialized education for nurses who administer chemotherapy and biotherapy
   C. Cancer pain management, which addresses the essential nature of palliative care as part of cancer programs
   D. Survivorship in cancer care, which is a joint position statement with the American Society of Clinical Oncology (ASCO), mandating care for survivors

5. What primary source of law serves as the basis for most malpractice litigation?
   A. Statutes
   B. Legislation
   C. Common law
   D. Administrative law

6. Which one of these situations would not be considered an oncology nursing professional practice issue with legal implications?
   A. Off-label drug or device use and risk evaluation mitigation strategies
   B. Mandatory reporting of elder abuse, communicable diseases, and death
   C. Professional certification to provide for quality cancer care
   D. Adverse drug events and chemotherapy medication errors

7. State-specific definitions of nursing practice are found through
   A. licensure.
   B. credentialing.
   C. nurse practice acts.
   D. required continuing education.

8. A nurse applies evidence-based practice and participates in symptom management administering opiates to a client dying from metastatic lung cancer. The client's family blames the nurse, believing the opiates contributed to client weakness, and threaten legal action. The nurse feels secure with her clinical decision making because she
   A. practices under protocol.
   B. is familiar with the current literature.
   C. is a member of her state nursing organization.
   D. follows the nurse practice acts and professional standards of care.

9. A cognitively impaired client who is unable to participate in his or her medical decision making can rely on receiving appropriate medical care by having a(n)
   A. legal will updated since recent diagnosis.
   B. insurance policy with adequate coverage.
   C. durable power of attorney and advance directive.
   D. known and documented organ and tissue donation preferences.

10. A registered nurse calls in a new prescription for her client without a physician order. She states that she did so because she knew what the physician would order and that he would back her up. This is an example of ⚠
    A. team duty.
    B. malpractice.
    C. negligence.
    D. breach of duty.

11. Professional documents used in legal decision making to establish minimal standards of care include state-specific nurse practice acts and
    A. statutes.
    B. licensure requirements.
    C. professional standards of care.
    D. state-determined competencies required for practice.

12. An advance directive
    A. is a living will.
    B. creates a do not resuscitate order.
    C. appoints an agent whom the client trusts to make medical decisions.
    D. informs healthcare providers (in writing) of medical management requests.

13. What are some strategies for minimizing risk of malpractice or disciplinary action?
    A. Verify job description fits within the federally defined scope of practice.
    B. Participate in professional speakers bureaus in cancer care.
    C. Keep a list of community service activities such as support groups and teaching life support.
    D. Establish close relationships with patients and families through their cancer treatment process.

47 Ethical Issues

1. Morals differ from ethics in that
   A. morals involve personal values or rules.
   B. ethics are based on upbringing, conscience, cultural, and religious beliefs.
   C. ethics serve as a guide to moral choice and behavior.
   D. morals involve the intentional practice of analyzing choices.

2. The American Nurses Association (ANA) Code of Ethics for Nurses includes provisions with interpretative statements that include all of the following except
   A. serve to establish or maintain healthcare policies.
   B. guide duty to self.
   C. provide a framework for ethical nursing practice.
   D. interpret collaboration to meet health needs.

3. Utilitarianism theory of ethics
   A. ensures that anticipated treatment benefits outweigh any anticipated harms and offer only potentially therapeutic interventions.
   B. starts with the assumption that what makes an action better or worse is some intrinsic property of the action itself.
   C. supports that the end never justifies the means; the right question to ask is, "What are the likely consequences?"
   D. holds that actions are right in proportion as they tend to promote happiness and wrong as they tend to produce the reverse of happiness.

4. Deontologic theories
   A. are based on a calculation of duties rather than on consequences.
   B. begin with the assumption that what makes an action better or worse is the tendency to promote happiness.
   C. support that the end justifies the means, if proposed actions are in accordance with the morality of the person taking the action.
   D. judge actions by the consequence of what will happen if the action is or is not performed at this time.

5. A nurse hears a group of coworkers in the break room saying that a client does not deserve good quality care because of his poor past behavior. This is an example of a violation of which core ethical principle?
   A. Justice
   B. Veracity
   C. Maleficence
   D. Beneficence

6. Which ethical principle applies when a nurse is deciding whether to complete an incident report regarding a failure to administer a medication to a client?
   A. Autonomy
   B. Nonmaleficence
   C. Veracity
   D. Justice

7. A nurse educator uses paradigm situations for comparison and analysis of nursing actions in particular cases to approach ethical decision making. This demonstrates
   A. a focus on relationships involved.
   B. casuistry
   C. narrative-based ethics.
   D. virtue-based case approach.

8. When a nurse focuses on the client's relationships and their effect on ethical care, his emphasis will be on all the following except
   A. sympathy.
   B. compassion.
   C. fidelity.
   D. justice.

9. A clinical unit has decided to focus on a quality improvement project that would place emphasis on learning the client's story. This approach
   A. views the illness as a story and emphasizes showing empathy and compassion.
   B. can assist the nurse in time allocation based on the story the client and family share.
   C. emphasizes the goal of living a good life by the development of good character with an emphasis on education.
   D. will most likely require more nursing time than currently allotted for the client admission process.

10. Ethics committees
    A. articulate the core competencies for healthcare ethics consultation.
    B. serve three functions: case consultation, policy development, and education.
    C. provide a mechanism to address ethical issues but are not required by The Joint Commission.
    D. increase nurses' sensitivity and require the nurse to hear the details of a case before taking action.

11. Which statement regarding communication with clients is true?
    A. Sending clear messages is the critical component of communication.
    B. Approximately 60% of communication is of a nonverbal nature.
    C. Clients require direct professional guidance to make appropriate decisions.
    D. The ethical principle of veracity should guide all communication with clients.

12. Communicating bad news using the approach proposed by Buckman involves all of the following except
    A. honestly describing any news that will potentially, drastically, and negatively alter a client's view of his or her future.
    B. a multistep process that starts with finding out how much the client knows and wants to know.
    C. nurses being advocates, showing sensitivity and support for the client and family receiving bad news.
    D. listening attentively to what is being said and not said.

13. Nurses' responsibilities regarding confidentiality and privacy operationalize the ethical principle of
    A. protected health information.
    B. nonmaleficence.
    C. autonomy.
    D. veracity.

14. A staff member is overheard revealing details about an incarcerated client. What is the responsibility of a professional nurse colleague in this situation?
    A. Ask if the client is accompanied by the appropriate number of law officials.
    B. Remain busy; this happens commonly and is not a problem when stated within the confines of healthcare staff workspace.
    C. Inquire about the source of the information.
    D. Discuss this with the staff member as a violation of protected health information.

15. Kleinman's explanatory model of illness is used to guide the assessment of the client's cultural perspective. The next step would be to
    A. provide education materials in the client's language.
    B. ask the family members to serve as the interpreter for the client.
    C. determine how closely the practices align with others from that culture.
    D. obtain informed consent to document the information in the medical record.

16. From an ethical and legal perspective, informed consent
    A. is open to interpretation by all parties to the situation.
    B. can be interpreted according to the objective standard for a particular client.
    C. is consistent across all clients for a given situation.
    D. sees an individual's decision-making capacity as an absolute.

17. A nurse working with clients undergoing a treatment must be aware of her or his role related to presence, including
    A. being aware of her or his own value system, beliefs, and biases that may influence decision making and informed consent.
    B. being present when the informed consent is obtained so that he or she can be certain what the client was told.
    C. advocating for the client in relation to the client's value system and current level of anxiety or ambivalence.
    D. discussing the potential benefits of the clinical trial for a specific individual with the family.

18. A newly hired nurse on the clinical unit expresses concern about a client's involvement in a clinical trial. What would be the appropriate response?
    A. Because the unit is a research unit, the nurse must learn to support client involvement in research as a priority.
    B. Even though the clinical focus of the unit is research, the first obligation is to care for the client.
    C. Perhaps the client or family just did not understand the informed consent process; attempt to repeat the information.
    D. Assure the nurse that because the client signed the informed consent, there is little reason to be concerned.

19. What would not be considered a challenge with clinical research?
    A. The client may or may not receive benefit from participation in the study.
    B. The client may agree because she believes she is out of treatment options.
    C. The nurse must be comfortable answering questions about the study.
    D. After the informed consent has been signed, the client must follow through with finishing the study.

20. The family of a client who has advanced stage cancer and is experiencing significant pain is concerned about the physician's recommendation to consider a transition to palliative care. The nurse needs to clarify that
    A. palliative care will mean that curative care will no longer be administered.
    B. good symptom management is the focus of palliative care, but curative goals do not have to be abandoned.
    C. the secondary goal of palliative care will be that the client experiences a good death.
    D. palliative care should be delivered in a hospice setting.

21. According to the Patient Self-Determination Act (PSDA),
    A. all clients in healthcare institutions must complete advance directives for healthcare.
    B. healthcare providers must be certain all clients have received information about their right to participate in healthcare decisions.
    C. medical power of attorney allows clients to indicate when they no longer wish to make decisions for themselves.
    D. advance directives must be honored for clients receiving healthcare in a facility across state lines.

22. When addressing questions regarding do not attempt resuscitation (DNAR) orders and physician orders for life-sustaining treatment (POLST), nurses must clarify that
    A. DNARs are one type of advance directive.
    B. a DNAR must be directed by the client only.
    C. all therapies should be guided by the client's values, goals, and preferences.
    D. the need for renewal of the orders is based on state laws.

23. Clients and family should be encouraged to participate in discussions about care preferences early in the course of care. This can decrease problems related to
    A. the articulation of advance directives.
    B. quality of care and patient safety.
    C. informed consent for treatment.
    D. preferences for care providers.

24. A decision by a healthcare team to initiate legal action to administer blood transfusions to a pediatric client
    A. can be based on the wishes of an older child who does not desire to have blood transfusions.
    B. is not necessary when parents are morally bound by cultural expectation.
    C. can be resolved by taking the decision to an ethics committee.
    D. is based on the professional responsibility to protect the welfare of a child as a member of a broader community.

25. A client with an advance directive requesting no heroics is brought to the emergency department (ED) after a car accident. The ED physician determines that the client's condition is a reversible event and institutes treatment. This is an example of
    A. allowing professional values to dictate care decisions.
    B. violating a do not attempt resuscitation request.
    C. beneficence.
    D. nonmaleficence.

48 Professional Issues

1. A patient was admitted to receive her first round of chemotherapy. During the night, she had diarrhea and tried to go to the bathroom herself. She was found on the floor after falling and hitting her head. This incident demonstrates a(n): ▲
   A. failure of communication.
   B. failure of prevention.
   C. error in treatment.
   D. failure to act on results of monitoring.

2. Strategies for increased safety within the health system recommended by the Institute of Medicine (IOM) include all the following except ▲
   A. improved identification of errors through a mandatory reporting system.
   B. raising performance standards and expectations to decrease errors.
   C. implementing safety systems where safety is an explicit organizational goal.
   D. mandatory continuing education and professional education.

3. The IOM paper "Charting a New Course for a System in Crisis" did not identify which action to deliver high-quality, safe patient care?
   A. Including older adult patients and those with multiple comorbidities in cancer clinical trials
   B. Including patient outcome data in quality monitoring plans to guide future care of clients
   C. Providing free services to clients and family members without the resources to receive adequate care
   D. Developing a healthcare information technology (IT) system to meet meaningful use criteria

4. The oncology nurse plays a vital role in multidisciplinary collaboration and coordination of care, such as
   A. obtaining specialty certification through the Oncology Nursing Society (ONS).
   B. involving individuals with comorbidities in nursing research studies.
   C. providing clients and families with health related literacy information.
   D. working with others to use available community-based hospice services.

5. The key priority in planning for quality improvement involves
   A. asking, "Are we identifying nurse-sensitive patient outcomes?"
   B. considering if involved team members can collaborate efficiently for the task.
   C. setting aims for the project that are time specific and measureable.
   D. questioning if the project will result in adequate cost savings.

6. PDSA (plan, do, study, act) is used to
   A. prepare for certification.
   B. perform clinically meaningful research.
   C. propose a review of a clinical pathway.
   D. plan and direct a special assignment.

7. Clinical implementation of the ONS's statement on multidisciplinary collaboration would involve
   A. determining the health literacy of the client and family to prepare multidisciplinary teaching materials.
   B. implementing the standard care plan from a former institution that improved client outcomes.
   C. working with team members and the client and family to determine cultural factors that guide their care expectations.
   D. preparing for the integration of client and family education materials into the current electronic information system.

8. What would not be considered a barrier to multidisciplinary collaboration?
   A. Administrative directives regarding the need to provide oversight
   B. Varied skill levels of individuals involved
   C. Identification of resource options available for client community
   D. A tendency to identify more closely with another discipline

9. A nurse oversees an infusion center and is concerned about an incident involving protocol variation. Collaboration across roles would include
   A. encouraging staff nurses on the unit to identify the causative factor and the best solution.
   B. working with educators, administration, and clinicians on orientation of new nurses on the unit.
   C. hiring an experienced nurse consultant to direct the quality improvement project to address the issue.
   D. identifying a nurse researcher with expertise and interest in problem areas to assist with review of literature to guide performance improvement.

10. An employee has just taken a new position for a certified oncology nurse at an acute care facility. The nurse is attempting to engage the nurses on the medical surgical unit in the care of clients with cancer. Which intervention is likely to be the most useful in obtaining the cooperation of staff nurses with these clients' care?
    A. Conduct an education program about the importance of symptom management of clients receiving chemotherapy.
    B. Require staff nurses to complete an evaluation form on the care provided to their oncology clients.
    C. Collaborate with the nursing staff to develop critical pathways and reach individual discharge goals.
    D. Provide a 24-hour pager number so that the staff can reach the certified nurse when clinical decisions are needed.

11. Nurses on the oncology unit notice during an audit of the nursing admission assessment forms that nurses are consistently leaving blank or putting "N/A" on the sexuality portion of the tool. They further evaluate that the nurses are reluctant to ask clients questions to assess for sexuality concerns. The auditing nurses would best correct this deficiency by
    A. suggesting deletion of the sexuality category from the admission form.
    B. designing a sexuality continuing education program to enhance the nurses' knowledge.
    C. developing a poster of the admission form highlighting the sexuality portion.
    D. recommending the use of Annon's PLISSIT model for sexuality assessment.

12. Client navigation
    A. was originally proposed by the IOM report focusing on patient safety.
    B. resulted in reduced healthcare access barriers and increased screening of underserved populations.
    C. is included in the National Comprehensive Cancer Network recommendations for care.
    D. is included as an ONS cancer program guideline for optimal patient outcomes.

13. Which statement accurately describes specific nurse navigator competencies?
    A. Professional role—living out healthy living practices
    B. Education—pursuing continuing education and certification
    C. Care coordinator—identifying barriers to care and potential referral resources
    D. Communication—contributing content regarding role to professional literature

14. A nurse who conveys a client's needs and concerns to the client's physician is practicing which type of advocacy?
    A. Consumer advocacy
    B. Paternalistic advocacy
    C. Simplistic advocacy
    D. Consumer-centric advocacy

15. After a nurse clarifies a procedure for a client, the client decides he does not want to have it. The nurse supports the client by informing the physician of the client's decision. What type of advocacy is this?
    A. Simplistic advocacy
    B. Consumer-centric advocacy
    C. Paternalistic advocacy
    D. Consumer advocacy

16. What are some risks and problems associated with advocacy?
    A. Published evidence may not be available to nurses in the clinical setting.
    B. Independent action may be restricted.
    C. Nurses are not qualified to deal with difficult controversial issues.
    D. Ethical consultation services may not be perceived as available.

17. A goal has been established by the Institute of Medicine to ensure that 80% of nurses have bachelor's degrees by 2020, which
    A. would provide the majority of nurses with the scientific basis for providing services to clients in an evolving healthcare system.
    B. provides further regulation of nursing education by the healthcare system.
    C. is an indirect attempt to eliminate the associate degree education programs in many regions.
    D. will be supported because more nurses with bachelor's degrees will mean less need for advanced practice nurses.

18. Professional certification
    A. requires employers to provide incentives to pursue certification and to openly acknowledge certified nurses on staff.
    B. establishes standards of performance in cancer care that will serve to improve client outcomes.
    C. upgrades nursing services provided by the institution in which the certified nurse practices.
    D. provides the public with assurance that the certified nurse has the knowledge and qualifications to practice in the role.

Answer Key

1. **Answer:** B

Rationale: The cancer mortality rate is the number of deaths attributed to cancer in a defined population during a 1-year period. Mortality rate is helpful in understanding the significance of a public health problem, but it must be interpreted alongside incidence rates in order to provide beneficial information. For example, some cancers have a high incidence (i.e., skin cancer) but a low mortality rate. Other cancers have a relatively low incidence but a high mortality rate (pancreatic cancer). A is incorrect because cancer is the second leading cause of death; heart disease is the leading cause of death in the United States. C is incorrect because one in every four deaths is caused by cancer. D is incorrect because among men, the five leading causes of cancer-related death in the United States are lung, prostate, colorectal, pancreas, and liver and intrahepatic bile duct. B is the only correct statement.

2. **Answer:** A

Rationale: Combined estrogen and progesterone hormone replacement therapy in postmenopausal women has been shown to increase the breast cancer risk. Certain fertility drugs, such as Pergonal, may actually increase the ovarian cancer risk. White women are more likely to develop breast cancer. D is also not a lifestyle-related risk. A is implicated in increasing the breast cancer risk in women. Selective estrogen receptor modulators reduce the risk of developing breast cancer.

3. **Answer:** B

Rationale: B is the correct statement according to the global cancer statistics compiled by the International Agency for Research on Cancer and Cancer Research in the United Kingdom. Lung continues to be the number one cancer in the world because of increased tobacco use. Breast and prostate cancer incidences have increased in more developed regions of the world.

4. **Answer:** A

Rationale: Incidence is the number of new cancers of a specific type that occur in a defined population during a 1-year period. Incidence rates are published annually and help nurses understand how many individuals a cancer affects each year. A is correct because the worldwide cancer incidence has increased due to an aging population; increased tobacco use; and exposure to reproductive, dietary, and hormonal risk factors. For all cancers combined, trends in cancer incidence rates in the United States steadily declined.

5. **Answer:** C

Rationale: Infection with hepatitis B virus has been directly linked with but not proven as a single cause of primary cancer of the liver. Mammography and colonoscopy are not associated with cancer development; they are screening tools for breast and colorectal cancer. Alcohol consumption is a risk factor for multiple cancers, including cancer of the mouth, pharynx, larynx, esophagus, liver, colorectum, pancreas, and breast. In particular, alcohol consumption has a synergistic effect with tobacco. A diet high in fat and low in fiber, fruits, and vegetables is associated with several cancers, including colorectal, breast, prostate, and endometrial cancer.

6. **Answer:** D

Rationale: A total of 59% of cancer survivors are older than 65 years of age. A is incorrect because among all cancer survivors, 54.3% were female and 45.7% were male. B is incorrect because 64% of cancer survivors have survived 5 years or more. C is incorrect because most common cancer sites in the survivor population are breast (22%) and prostate (20%) followed by colorectal (9%) and gynecologic (8%) cancers.

7. **Answer:** C

Rationale: The U.S. Public Health Service 5As model is Ask, Assess, Advise, Assist, and Arrange for follow-up. Smoking cessation programs aim to support patients in their endeavors to quit, not scare them. Offering medications to assist individuals to stop smoking, including culturally tailored educational materials, may have the greatest impact. D is incorrect. Electronic cigarettes or "e-cigarettes" are battery-operated devices in which the inhaled vapor is produced from cartridges that contain nicotine, flavor, and other chemicals. E-cigarette use may lead nonsmokers, especially children, to smoking. They should not be considered therapeutic or an aid for smoking cessation.

8. **Answer:** D

Rationale: Cancer health disparities are adverse differences in incidence, prevalence, mortality, survivorship, and burden of cancer that exist among specific population groups in the United States. Certain differences in cancer incidence and mortality have been noted in various ethnic groups. For breast cancer, white women have the highest incidence rate; however, the highest mortality rate is seen among African American women, making A incorrect. B is incorrect because for prostate cancer, African American men have the highest incidence and mortality rates of ethnic groups in the United States. For cervical cancer, Hispanic women have the highest incidence rate, making C incorrect; however, the highest mortality rate is seen among African American women. Asian and Pacific Islanders have the highest incidence and mortality rates of liver and stomach cancers.

9. *Answer:* C

Rationale: Tobacco use, whether alone or in combination with alcohol, is a risk factor for all oropharyngeal cancers. In addition, HPV-16 is detected in a substantial proportion of squamous cell carcinomas of the soft palate, tonsils, and base of the tongue and in 60% to 70% of all HPV-associated cancers of the oral cavity and oropharynx. A, B, and D are incorrect; none of the combinations is a risk factor for oral cancer. Consumption of red and processed meats is a risk factor for colorectal, prostate, and pancreatic cancers. A history of diabetes mellitus is a risk factor for pancreatic cancer. Although obesity is associated with overall cancer development, human immunodeficiency virus (HIV) infection results in immunosuppression that increases risk of Kaposi sarcoma and B-cell lymphomas. Asbestos is the single most important known occupational carcinogen leading to lung cancer and mesothelioma development. A history of exposure to ultraviolet radiation can lead to melanoma, and Epstein-Barr virus is associated with Burkitt lymphoma, some nasopharyngeal cancers, undifferentiated parotid carcinoma, Hodgkin disease, B-cell lymphoma, and gastric carcinomas.

10. *Answer:* B

Rationale: It is important to use sunscreen lotion with an SPF of 30 or higher to protect exposed skin whenever outdoors. Reapplication may be necessary after getting in the water or after extreme perspiration. Indoor tanning booths and sunlamps should not be used at all. Their use has been found to increase the incidence of all types of skin cancers including melanoma. Ultraviolet rays are most intense between 10 AM and 4 PM each day.

11. *Answer:* A

Rationale: B, C, and D are incorrect. Hepatitis B vaccination for newborns should be administered in three doses: the first at birth, the second between 1 and 2 months of age, and the third at 6 to 18 months of age. Hepatitis A vaccines are recommended beginning at 12 to 23 months, with a second dose 6 to 18 months later, but hepatitis A is not associated with an increased cancer risk.

12. *Answer:* A

Rationale: Guidelines on nutrition for cancer prevention include the consumption of a healthy diet with emphasis on plant sources. Some recommendations include eating smaller portions of high-calorie foods; limiting sugar-sweetened beverages; limiting consumption of processed and red meats; and choosing fish, poultry, or beans as alternatives to red meat. Guidelines also emphasize choosing at least 2½ cups of vegetables and fruit per day, choosing whole-grain instead of refined-grain products, and limiting alcohol intake to no more than 2 drinks per day for men and 1 drink a day for women.

13. *Answer:* C

Rationale: The choice of appropriate cancer prevention strategies is the main benefit to a person undergoing a cancer risk assessment. Documenting, recording, and verifying risk factors does not help the patient implement a healthier lifestyle. The purpose of cancer risk assessment is to use the information to make appropriate recommendations for cancer prevention and early detection.

14. *Answer:* D

Rationale: African American men have the higher rates (40%) of obesity than non-Hispanic white men (37%) and Hispanic men (37%). African American women have higher rates (59%) of obesity than non-Hispanic white women (32%) and Hispanic women (46%). Obesity is a major risk factor for cancer, second only to tobacco use. Overweight and obese patients contribute to 14% to 20% of all cancer-related deaths. Obesity is defined as a body mass index of 30.0 or above. Obesity is responsible for approximately one quarter to one third of all cancers in the United States. Obesity rates for men and women are similar; the obesity rate among men is 35.5%; among women, it is 35.8%.

15. *Answer:* C

Rationale: More advanced disease at diagnosis is found among poor populations and those who live in rural areas. There is increased, not decreased, tobacco use among poorer populations. Low SES is associated with increased risk of lung cancer, cervical cancer, stomach cancer, and cancer of the head and neck. High SES is associated with increased risk of breast, prostate, and colon cancers. Economic, social, and cultural factors can create barriers to accessing information and preventive services.

16. *Answer:* B

Rationale: The ACS guidelines encourage adults to have 150 minutes of moderate activity or 75 minutes of vigorous activity each week. The guidelines also emphasize that all physical activity above usual levels can have health benefits. The ACS recommends that children engage in at least 1 hour of physical activity each day, with vigorous activity on at least 3 days per week. Although special considerations should be followed for those undergoing treatment and cancer survivors, sedentary behavior should be limited for all populations. These populations should start with low-intensity activity for limited periods of time and work up to healthy activity levels. Cancer survivors should aim to engage in 150 minutes of exercise per week and at least two sessions of strength training per week.

17. *Answer:* A

Rationale: Cigar use is highest among African Americans. Adults without high school degrees are three times more likely to be current smokers than those with college degrees. Whereas approximately 21.6% of adult men smoke, 16.5% of adult women are current smokers.

18. *Answer:* B

Rationale: Occupational cancer risks account for about 4% of cancers. Introduction of effective regulation of workplace exposures, in the middle years of the 20th century, is believed to have reduced these risks substantially. The following workers have increased rates of certain cancers. Chemical workers have increased rates of bladder cancer, steel workers have increased rates of lung cancer, rubber workers have increased rates of prostate cancer, and miners with an increased exposure to uranium and radon have a subsequent increase in gastric cancer and birth defects.

19. *Answer:* D

Rationale: The first three options are incorrect because they do not ask questions related to lifestyle changes. D is an example of using motivational interviewing to determine if there is a way that patients will consider changing risky behaviors to decrease their cancer risk.

20. *Answer:* A

Rationale: Aging population, increased tobacco use, dietary factors, and reproductive and hormonal influences will increase the cancer risk worldwide by 75% in 2030. Fluoridated water and increased screening has not been linked to higher cancer incidence rates.

CHAPTER 2

1. *Answer:* C

Rationale: Cancer incidence is the number of new cases identified in the specified population and in a defined period of time (generally over a 1-year time frame). A and B are incorrect because they describe prevalence, the percentage of all individuals with disease at a given point in time in a specified population, including new and existing cases. Prevalence is often expressed as a proportion of disease cases per 100,000 persons. D describes mortality rates.

2. *Answer:* B

Rationale: Secondary prevention is early detection of cancer and consists of measures, such as a mammography and other screening tests, to identify the potential for developing cancer in asymptomatic individuals, with the goal of diagnosing cancer at a stage when cure is possible. A is incorrect; primary prevention aims to prevent the disease from occurring. Encouraging individuals to protect themselves from ultraviolet sun rays is an example of primary prevention of skin cancer. C, tertiary prevention, targets the patient who is already symptomatic by treating to slow disease progression and prevent complications from occurring. Tertiary prevention results in decreased morbidity and mortality. Quaternary prevention refers to avoiding the consequences of unnecessary or excessive interventions within the health care system.

3. *Answer:* A

Rationale: Sensitivity is improved as the experience and competency of the providers conducting and interpreting the study are increased. B and D are incorrect because they describe specificity, a measure of the probability that a test result will be positive if the disease is present. A test with high specificity will have few false-positive results.

4. *Answer:* C

Rationale: Currently, there is evidence to recommend screening for breast, prostate, cervical, lung, and colorectal cancer in certain populations, although there is controversy regarding the use of these screenings. Cervical cancer has the strongest evidence of the screening's

ability to decrease mortality. A, B, and D are incorrect because there is less rigorous evidence about the screening of those cancers.

5. *Answer:* B

Rationale: Screening biases can threaten the validity of screening tests and programs. B is the correct answer because it describes lead time bias, the appearance of improved survival resulting from a longer interval between diagnosis and death. A describes the definition of overdiagnosis. C defines length time bias, which occurs when a greater proportion of individuals undergoing screening have less aggressive disease. D is the definition of selection bias, which may occur when individuals participate in screening programs because they choose to do so and "select in." These patients may have easier access to care or better health habits than the general population. Better access or health habits may contribute to improved outcomes after a cancer diagnosis.

6. *Answer:* D

Rationale: According to the National Comprehensive Cancer Network (NCCN) guidelines, there is no high level evidence (RCTs) of the benefit of chest radiography with or without sputum cytology in screening for lung cancer risk. Low-dose computerized technology (LDCT) is the most sensitive test available, with the National Lung Screening Trial demonstrating a 20% reduction in lung cancer mortality using LDCT versus chest radiography in 53,454 high-risk participants.

7. *Answer:* C

Rationale: *BRCA1* and *BRCA2* mutations are responsible for approximately 20% to 25% of hereditary breast cancers (about 5% to 10% of all breast cancers in women and 4% to 40% in men). This genetic testing is not currently recommended for the general population because of the expense and low rate of return.

8. *Answer:* A

Rationale: *BRCA1* and *BRCA2* mutation testing may be offered to persons with features indicating an increased likelihood of a *BRCA* mutation. These include (1) multiple cases of early breast cancer in family; (2) strong family history of other cancers, such as ovarian and pancreatic cancers; (3) Ashkenazi Jewish heritage; (4) more than one primary cancer in the same person; (5) male breast cancer; (6) individual from a family with known positive *BRCA1* and *BRCA2* mutations; (7) triple-negative breast cancer; and (8) early age of breast cancer onset.

9. *Answer:* A

Rationale: According to the American Cancer Society guidelines, A is correct. B is incorrect because mammography should be started as soon as the patient is diagnosed with lobular cancer, because this abnormality is generally widely distributed throughout the breast and may occur in both breasts simultaneously. C is incorrect because all women aged 40 years and older should have an annual mammogram. D is incorrect; men with a genetic predisposition should consider baseline mammography at age 40 years. Different agencies have different guidelines for the prevention and early detection of cancer.

10. *Answer:* D

Rationale: Guaiac-based fecal occult blood test (gFOBT) is the only CRC screening method proven consistently effective in randomized clinical trials. The iFOBT is not affected by diet and medications, but gFOBT is. Three consecutive stool specimens is ideal. Specimens should not be procured by rectal examination.

11. *Answer:* D

Rationale: Based on observational studies, the average time required for a polyp to develop into an invasive colorectal cancer is 10 years. Therefore, the timing of screening is based on this biologic evidence. This is the interval recommended by the NCCN, ACS, and USPSTF.

12. *Answer:* C

Rationale: Computed tomography colonography is a noninvasive method to examine the colon and rectum for polyps and cancers requiring a bowel preparation before the examination. Because the exam is noninvasive, it is a good option for frail and elderly clients. It should not be used alone as a screening measure; typically, an annual stool test is recommended. If a lesion is noted, further testing will be required.

13. *Answer:* B

Rationale: PSA has limited sensitivity and specificity. PSA levels may be affected by age, presence of BPH, inflammation, urethral or prostatic trauma, and ejaculation within past 48 hours, as well as medications including androgen deprivation therapy, 5-α-reductase inhibitors (e.g., finasteride), and ketoconazole. NSAIDs and ethnicity are not factors that affect PSA level.

14. *Answer:* D

Rationale: D is the correct answer because men at high risk for prostate cancer have one or more of the following: (1) African American ethnicity and (2) a father or brother diagnosed with prostate cancer before age 65 years. These American Cancer Society screening guidelines are available to the general public. It is within the nurse's role to educate the public about screening guidelines, advocating for patients to understand prevention and detection techniques.

15. *Answer:* B

Rationale: According to the guidelines, B is the correct answer. A Pap test (otherwise known as the Pap smear) is the principle screening tool for cervical cancer. Women with persistent infection with an oncogenic HPV have a much higher risk of developing cervical cancer than do non–HPV-infected women. Thus, HPV testing is important to include when screening for cervical cancer. However, there is controversy regarding frequency, how to implement HPV testing into routine screening practices, and the lack of applicability in developing countries (because of expense and lack of equipment and clinicians). Yearly screening is no longer recommended because it generally takes 10 to 20 years for cervical cancer to develop. Thus, lengthening the screening interval is appropriate.

16. *Answer:* B

Rationale: B is the only correct answer. A, C, and D are incorrect because postmenopausal women, women who have had a surgery to remove cervical cancer or precancerous lesions, and women who are not sexually active can still develop cervical cancer. The choice to discontinue screening for cervical cancer is always made at the discretion of the healthcare provider and individual.

17. *Answer:* D

Rationale: D is correct because "overdiagnosis" happens when an individual receives a diagnosis he or she does not really need. If a patient has an indolent cancer that is not screened, it would not have been diagnosed nor have needed treatment. For very slow growing tumors, especially in older individuals, screening may not afford a survival benefit and instead may cause unnecessary treatment, anxiety, cost, and pain. PSA screening has not been correlated with decreases in prostate cancer mortality and has instead prompted the use of aggressive therapies, which may cause significant side effects in many men who would never have required treatment either because of age or tumor growth pattern.

18. *Answer:* C

Rationale: The best screening tool has the ability to discriminate between those with the cancer in question and those who are cancer free. Screening tools must be safe, reliable, valid, and inexpensive. Extreme sensitivity and specificity are key factors. A screening schedule strategy (timing and frequency) should reflect the cancer (i.e., designated ages to begin and end screening mirror the natural history of disease in the population at risk). A is incorrect because certain cancers have a slower doubling time and may not need to be screened as often (e.g., colorectal cancer). The benefit of screening should outweigh the risks, so B is incorrect. D is incorrect because the location of the screening will be dependent on the screening tool.

19. *Answer:* A

Rationale: Biomarkers are substances that may be produced by tumor or the body's reaction to the cancer and are detected in abnormal quantities in blood, body fluids, or tissues. The PSA is the only marker used in cancer screening programs; its efficacy (ability to decrease mortality) remains controversial. Although CA 19-9 and the CA-125 are both biomarkers, their sensitivity and specificity are limited. The result of CA 19-9, a test used to detect pancreatic or colorectal cancer, may be falsely negative in many cases or abnormally elevated in people who have no cancer at all (i.e., false positives). The CA-125 test is not accurate enough to use for ovarian cancer screening in all women because many noncancerous conditions (e.g., uterine fibroids, menstruation) can increase the CA-125 level. HPV is not a biomarker, but an HPV DNA assay is performed on a liquid based Pap specimen to identify if the oncogenic viral types are present (either as primary screening, or as a "reflex test" if an abnormal Pap result is reported).

20. *Answer:* A

Rationale: Although mammography is still the primary screening modality for breast cancer, there is considerable variability in screening practice, particularly in age of first screening and frequency of screenings.

145

Ultrasonography and MRI are used to evaluate any abnormality; they are not routinely used as screening methodologies. Digital mammography (uses digital receptors and computers to display images) is widely available, but randomized clinical trials have not shown digital mammography to be more effective than traditional mammography for screening to date. Breast self-examination is no longer widely endorsed and recognized as a reliable screening tool.

21. **Answer:** C

Rationale: Genetic testing for CRC is not used for screening the general population. The National Cancer Institute recommends genetic testing for those with one or more of the following factors: (1) strong family history of CRC and/or polyps, (2) personal history of adenoma or CRC, (3) multiple primary cancers in a patient with CRC, (4) family history of other cancers consistent with known syndromes causing an inherited risk of CRC (e.g., endometrial cancer), and/or (5) early age at CRC diagnosis. A personal history of ulcerative colitis or diverticulitis is not a risk factor. Early age for a CRC diagnosis is younger than 50 years old. CRC is typically a slow growing tumor, so screening starts at age 50 years.

22. **Answer:** B

Rationale: There is no direct evidence that colonoscopy improves mortality rates even though it is widely used. According to the guidelines, an annual Pap testing is not appropriate because of the slow growth rate of cervical cancer unless an abnormality is noted on previous screening. Screening does not commence until age 50 years. There is insufficient evidence to support breast cancer screening for women older than age 75 years.

23. **Answer:** C

Rationale: Those at high risk for developing lung cancer are current smokers with a 30-pack-year history of smoking, those with a history of more than 30 pack-years of smoking and who have quit within the past 5 years, those with a history of more than 20 pack-years of smoking and one additional risk factor (e.g., occupational exposure, family history of lung cancer in a first-degree relative, personal history of COPD or pulmonary fibrosis). A and B are incorrect because a family history of COPD or pulmonary fibrosis and a personal history of leukemia or hepatoma are not risk factors. Regional location is not a risk factor.

24. **Answer:** A

Rationale: Taking a personal history of patients incorporates many factors. The chief complaint is a brief description of the reason why the patient is seeking care, making A the correct answer. C is incorrect because it is not part of the personal history. A physical examination is an adjunct to taking a personal history of the patient and includes cancer-related physical assessment (examination of the skin, mouth, neck, lymph nodes, breasts, cervix, pelvis, testicles, rectum, and prostate). A physical examination should be conducted on all new and returning patients. A complete breast examination may not be applicable based on the need for the visit.

25. **Answer:** A

Rationale: A positive predictive value is the percentage of persons with a positive screening test result who actually have the disease. B, the percentage of persons with a negative result without the disease, describes negative predictive value. Specificity is a measure of the probability that a test result will be positive if the disease is present. Sensitivity is a measure of the probability that a test result will be negative if the disease is not present.

26. **Answer:** A

Rationale: Enlargement, darkening, or change in a mole may be indicative of a malignant melanoma; further evaluation is warranted promptly. Having a history of skin cancer and using tanning booths may increase the risk of melanoma, but these are not symptoms of melanoma. Dry, flaky skin is not a risk factor or symptom of melanoma.

27. **Answer:** C

Rationale: Assessing for barriers (cultural, religious, lack of knowledge, cost and transportation issues) to screening is a key opportunity to understand the reasons why someone may not want to adhere to recommendations and may assist you in teaching and problem solving with the individual.

28. **Answer:** A

Rationale: Determining the number of individuals offered screening and the number of individuals who participated, the number of preclinical cancers detected in persons with abnormal screens resulting in further testing and a definitive diagnosis, and cost per cancer detected are all short-term measures. The impact of early detection on cancer stage, symptom assessment and management and quality of life, and mortality rates are long-term measures of effectiveness.

29. **Answer:** A

Rationale: B, C, and D are incorrect because these symptoms may be suspicious for cancer in general or other bacterial or viral infections. Dyspnea, edema, and cough may be symptoms of a pulmonary problem; lung cancer should be ruled out. A lists findings that point specifically to brain tumors or metastases.

30. **Answer:** D

Rationale: Although A, B, and C are important to assess, a personal and family history of cancer is the most useful and necessary information to determine cancer risk—it is specific to cancer-focused risk assessment.

31. **Answer:** A

Rationale: A cancer-related physical examination will inspect for and palpate masses, lesions, discharge, and bleeding. The cranial nerves should be assessed to rule out nervous system cancers.

CHAPTER 3

1. **Answer:** A

Rationale: Hashimoto thyroiditis is associated with lymphoma development. Reflex sympathetic dystrophy is a chronic regional pain syndrome with clinical features of neurogenic inflammation. It has not been associated with brain tumor development. Lichen sclerosus is associated with vulvar squamous cell carcinoma.

2. *Answer:* C

Rationale: Carcinogenesis is synonymous with the term *oncogenesis*. It is a process by which normal cells are transformed into malignant cells through the action of biologic, chemical, or physical agents. Mutagens cause changes (mutations) in the genetic material of cells that may lead to cancer formation. Teratogens cause irreversible, damaging structural malformations in fetuses; cancer may not be caused. Cancer immunosurveillance is an important host protection process that decreases cancer rates by inhibiting carcinogenesis and preserving cellular homeostasis. Tumor necrosis factor is a cytokine that can have an antitumor effect in the process of immune surveillance.

3. *Answer:* C

Rationale: Tumor suppressor genes in normal cells control proliferation by preventing uncontrolled growth, but when mutated in cancer cells, tumor suppressor genes no longer suppress proliferation. Epigenetics describes a mechanism that can change the activity of a gene without changing the sequence of the DNA. An example of epigenetic mechanisms is DNA methylation. Adding or removing methyl groups from DNA affects the transcription of genes. Cancers are associated with both hypermethylation and hypomethylation of regulatory genes.

4. *Answer:* C

Rationale: Microscopic evaluation of cancer cells demonstrates various structural changes that are described in pathologic terms. Polymorphism describes enlargement of the nucleus and variation in shape. The term *pleomorphism* is used when the cells are variable in size and shape. Amplification is an increase in the number of copies of a DNA sequence. The term aneuploidy refers to an abnormal number of chromosomes.

5. *Answer:* B

Rationale: Clonal cells can be traced to a single origin and change over time, and different clones can arise from the same tumor.

6. *Answer:* D

Rationale: Certain tumor antigens are clinically useful and may be used as tumor markers (biochemical substances synthesized and released by tumor cells) to monitor response to therapy. Tumor antigens may be present in a variety of benign conditions and are not often used for screening because they lack specificity.

7. *Answer:* C

Rationale: Cancer arises from the combination of multiple mutations in a cell's genes, genomic instability, and inflammation. Normal cells experience apoptosis (programmed cell death). Contact inhibition is a process that limits cancer cell growth (cell growth and division stops on physical contact with other cells). Some cancer cells have mutations that disable gatekeeper proteins controlling mitoses, thereby inactivating contact inhibition.

8. *Answer:* B

Rationale: α-Fetoprotein and ß-human chorionic gonadotropin are tumor markers specifically used for germ cell tumors (e.g., testicular cancer). Carcinoembryonic antigen is used to track most gastrointestinal malignancies and pancreatic, lung, and breast cancers. CA19-9 can be elevated in many types of gastrointestinal cancer, such as colorectal, esophageal, and pancreatic cancers, and is not an ideal tumor marker for this disease. It may also be elevated in patients with pancreatitis or bile duct obstructions. ACTH is elevated in pituitary tumors or benign adenomas.

9. *Answer:* A

Rationale: EBV is associated with nasopharyngeal and upper airway cancers as well as gastric cancers. HBV and HCV are associated with hepatocellular carcinoma. HTLV-1 is associated with adult leukemias and lymphomas.

10. *Answer:* A

Rationale: Almost any cancer, if around for a long period of time, can metastasize to the brain; however, the more common ones include breast, colorectal, lung, kidney, and melanoma. Endometrial cancer, pancreatic cancer, and multiple myeloma do not commonly spread to the brain.

11. *Answer:* A

Rationale: Viruses, both RNA and DNA, have been linked to human cancer with DNA viruses more prevalent. Adenovirus is not associated with any human cancer. HTLV-1 is associated with adult leukemias and lymphomas, not primary liver cancer. BK virus is associated with prostate cancer. EBV is associated with nasopharyngeal and upper airway cancers as well as gastric cancers.

12. *Answer:* B

Rationale: Cancer arises from the combination of multiple mutations in a cell's genes. *Ras* is a commonly mutated oncoprotein, typically found in pancreatic and colorectal cancer. When proto-oncogenes are mutated, they can enable a cancer cell to be self-sufficient growth. *Ras* is not a mutated tumor suppressor gene or DNA repair gene. Thus, A and C are incorrect. Chromosome translocation results when pieces of one chromosome move to another chromosome as the cell divides. This type of genetic alteration can activate an oncogene; D is not a correct answer.

13. *Answer:* C

Rationale: Tobacco smoke is a very important risk factor, but the client has not smoked in the previous 43 years. Alcohol consumption is not implicated in lung cancer development. Because he was in the Vietnam War, the client may have been exposed to Agent Orange, but that has not been implicated in lung cancer development. Exposure to mustard gas (used in World Wars I and II) is a risk factor. Occupational exposure to coal for 45 years is the client's biggest risk factor for lung cancer.

14. *Answer:* D

Rationale: Adenocarcinoma and squamous cell cancers arise from epithelial tissue lining glands and ducts and stratified squamous tissue; therefore, A and B are incorrect. C, mesothelioma, is incorrect because it arises from endothelial tissue.

15. *Answer:* B

Rationale: Tumor markers are typically used to monitor disease progression or recurrence in particular cancer types. HVA/VMA is a marker for neuroblastoma, not hepatoma, and CA-125 is a marker for ovarian cancer, not endometrial cancer. Bence Jones protein is associated with multiple myeloma.

16. *Answer:* B

Rationale: Tumor growth rates vary widely. B is correct. When the tumor has gone through 30 doublings, it has reached roughly the size of a marble, about the size of the tip of your small finger. A tumor of this size contains approximately 1 billion cancer cells. This is the earliest point at which screening radiography can detect the cancer.

17. *Answer:* A

Rationale: In the TNM staging system, N denotes the absence or presence of regional lymph node metastasis. T denote the size or extent of the primary tumor, and M denotes the absence or presence of distant metastasis.

18. *Answer:* D

Rationale: A explains the theory of clonal evolution, B clarifies immune surveillance theory, and C describes epigenetics.

19. *Answer:* C

Rationale: Normal cells regulate proliferation with growth, signaling the start and stop of mitosis, whereas some cancer cells deregulate the signals, allowing for continued growth and spread of cancer.

20. *Answer:* A

Rationale: Differentiation refers to the extent to which tumor cells resemble comparable normal cells, both morphologically and functionally. B is not correct because the greater the degree of differentiation of a cell, the more likely it will have some part of the functional capabilities of its normal counterpart. The more anaplastic or malignant a tumor, the less likely any specialized function will be intact. C is incorrect because the tumor grade is an evaluation of the degree of differentiation of the malignant cells; staging is necessary to determine disease extent and treatment options. D is incorrect because grade 2 tumors are moderately differentiated. The higher the grade, the less differentiated the tumor.

21. *Answer:* B

Rationale: C and D are incorrect. Tumor cell growth actually slows because of faulty cell-to-cell communication and hypoxia. Tumor growth constantly doubles over time, not triples.

22. *Answer:* C

Rationale: Metaplasia involves replacement of one mature cell type by another mature cell type not usually found in the involved tissue.

23. *Answer:* D

Rationale: Normal cells regulate growth with tumor suppressor genes that cause cellular aging and apoptosis (programmed cell death). Cancer cells, not normal cells, secrete VEGF to stimulate angiogenesis (vascularization), and cancer cells use autophagy to survive in nutrient-deprived conditions.

24. *Answer:* B

Rationale: A and C are not correct because younger children are more susceptible to developing cancer after ionizing radiation exposure, and diagnostic radiography and computed tomography scans are medical sources of radiation exposure. D is incorrect because although they are tumors associated with radiation exposure, they are not the most common.

25. *Answer:* B

Rationale: Metastasis is regarded as a highly inefficient process in that fewer than 0.01% of circulating tumor cells eventually succeed in forming secondary tumor growths. C is incorrect; tumors can spread through the arterial and the venous system. Because arteries have thicker walls, they are less readily penetrated by tumor cells than are veins. Tumor cells often go to the first capillary bed encountered. D is incorrect. Liver and lung are the most frequent sites of metastasis even though common sites for metastasis include bone, lung, liver, and the central nervous system. The predilection for certain tumors to metastasize to specific sites is influenced by multiple factors.

26. *Answer:* C

Rationale: A is incorrect because it describes growth fraction (the fraction of proliferating cells in the tumor). B is not correct because TNM does not pertain to liquid tumors (e.g., lymphomas and leukemias). D describes the grading system of a tumor, not the staging system.

27. *Answer:* C

Rationale: As more is known about the biology of cancer, biomarkers are increasingly used to assist with establishing a diagnosis, staging, directing treatment options, and providing prognostic information about the cancer. They are not routinely used in all cancer types; certain biomarkers are present in certain cancers.

CHAPTER 4

1. *Answer:* B

Rationale: Physical barriers include epithelial cells of intact skin and mucus membranes.

2. *Answer:* D

Rationale: The inflammatory response has the described effect. It can be initiated when tissues are injured, burned, or infected. The damaged cells release chemicals such as bradykinin, histamine, and prostaglandins, causing blood vessels to leak fluid into the surrounding tissues, producing swelling.

3. *Answer:* C

Rationale: Tissue Associated Antigens (TAAs) can occur when a cell transitions from normal to malignant. Examples include HER2/neu, carcinoembryonic antigen, CA-125, and PSA. The other options would not point to the changes in this patient's cancer status and staging.

4. *Answer:* B

Rationale: Hematopoiesis is defined as the body's ability to regulate, produce, and develop blood cells to maintain the body's blood supply. Self-regulation is the body's ability to recognize and respond to physiologic changes. The ability of the human body to maintain a balanced blood cell supply is called homeostasis, but this does not include production and development of blood cells. Immune surveillance is the ability of the body to recognize and destroy malignant or altered cells.

5. *Answer:* C

Rationale: Interferons (IFNs) limit the spread of certain viral infections. They are produced early in response to infection and offer a first line of viral resistance. Mast cells are granulocytes with multiple mediators that produce an inflammatory response within tissues. Phagocytes internalize (engulf) and consume pathogenic microorganisms and debris. Platelets have some immunologic function; they can release inflammatory mediators via thrombogenesis or the formation of a thrombus.

6. *Answer:* C

Rationale: Blood cell development (hematopoiesis) begins with a single cell, the pluripotent stem cell. It does not begin with PMNs. Noncommitted stem cells are produced later in the process, as are B lymphocytes.

7. *Answer:* A

Rationale: Acquired immunity is not present at birth but is developed over time in response to the exposure of an outside threat to the body, such as antibodies produced to offset an infection.

8. *Answer:* A

Rationale: The monocytes and macrophages are distributed throughout the tissues of the body and are capable of phagocytosis. They do not produce antibodies specific to an antigen or release histamine or chemotactic factors. Macrophages cannot cause cellular lysis.

9. *Answer:* B

Rationale: Antibodies are blood proteins produced in response to a specific antigen. The other choices represent stimuli that require an immune response.

10. *Answer:* A

Rationale: Dendritic cells (DCs) travel from tissue to secondary lymphoid organs to present antigen to T cells. They function as APCs to initiate immune responses known as priming. Mature DCs are influenced by inflammatory stimuli, leading to migration through the lymphatic system to present antigen proteins to CD4+ and CD8+ T cells. Vaccines used in fighting cancer act through DCs to initiate an immune response.

11. *Answer:* B

Rationale: Lymphoid tissues are an organ of the immune system rather than a barrier to invasion. The remaining answers are barriers to bacterial invasion.

12. *Answer:* B

Rationale: Immunity that is not inherited is acquired immunity. It can be passive or active. Passive immunity results from the introduction of antibodies from another person or animal. Active immunity results from the development of antibodies in response to an antigen such as from vaccination. *Latent immunity* is a term not commonly used in healthcare today. Inherited immunity is a genetic or chemical immunity to a disease passed on from a parent to his or her offspring. Innate immunity is immunity possessed by a group (such as a species) that is present at birth.

13. *Answer:* A

Rationale: Inflammation is an innate immune process that is crucial in combating infection. Immune cells secrete protein cytokines and chemokines, causing inflammation. The infectious process describes how bacteria or viruses invade the body. A flare reaction is usually a skin reaction that occurs in response to exposure to an allergen. Photosensitivity is an oversensitivity of the skin to ultraviolet light.

14. *Answer:* C

Rationale: Primary lymphoid organs allow for the maturation of lymphocytes, including antigen receptors. A and D describe secondary lymphoid organs and tissues. B describes bone marrow.

15. *Answer:* D

Rationale: To be recognized by a B or T lymphocyte as a nonself, the antigen must have a high molecular weight (defined as > 8-10 K Daltons) and be composed of recurring molecules called epitopes.

16. *Answer:* C

Rationale: Dendritic cells function as antigen-producing cells for naïve T cells. The other types of cells play other roles in the immune response.

CHAPTER 5

1. *Answer:* B

Rationale: In humans, each cell normally contains 23 pairs of chromosomes, for a total of 46 chromosomes. Only a small number of cancers are considered hereditary, but genetics also plays an important role in the development of cancer and the response to treatment. There are three stop codons and RNAs that stop the growth of the amino acid chain.

2. *Answer:* B

Rationale: DNA base pairs are complementary on the double strand: purine A (adenine) attaches to pyrimidine T (thymine), and purine G (guanine) attaches to pyrimidine C (cytosine). The two types of bases are purines and pyrimidines. The nucleotide chains actually run in opposite directions and are held together by hydrogen bonds, which are coiled around one another to form a double helix. Messenger RNA, not DNA, contains the information about the order of amino acids in a protein.

3. *Answer:* D

Rationale: RNA is a single chain that represents a complementary copy of a strand of DNA. Transcription is the process of making RNA from DNA. Translation is the process of making protein from RNA.

4. *Answer:* B

Rationale: RNA, a template consisting of a single nucleotide that represents a complementary copy of a strand of DNA, is created in the process of transcription. Translation refers to the process of making proteins from RNA. The mRNA contains information about the order of the amino acids in a protein. The location of the nucleotide changes determines the likelihood it will cause an amino acid change.

5. *Answer:* C

Rationale: C identifies the three "stop" codons; these codons and associated RNAs are able to stop the growth of the amino acid chain. The codons are sets of three, not four, mRNA nucleotides. They consist of three common bases that correspond with matching bases on a tRNA anticodon. More than one codon will code for a specific amino acid.

6. *Answer:* B

Rationale: Genes are individual units of hereditary information located at a specific position on a chromosome and consist of a sequence of DNA that codes for a specific protein. Chromosomes are threadlike structures that contain genetic information. Exons are protein-coding segments of a gene; introns are the nonprotein coding segments or sequence interrupting piece of a gene. Genes code for a sequence of amino acids resulting in a protein that has a specific function. DNA is two nucleotide chains, running in opposite directions that are coiled around one another to form a double helix.

7. *Answer:* C

Rationale: Cancer usually has a multifactorial etiology with several genetic, environmental, and personal factors interacting to produce a malignancy. Genetic mutations and genetic instability are at the very core of cancer development.

8. *Answer:* D

Rationale: Frameshift mutations occur when one or more bases are added or deleted from the normal sequence, resulting in an altered form of the protein. Splicing mutations occur when DNA that should be removed from the coding sequence is retained or DNA that should not be added is spliced in. Nonsense mutations change an amino acid signal into a signal to stop adding amino acids to a growing protein. RNA-negative mutations result in an absence of RNA.

9. *Answer:* A

Rationale: Although most cancer is associated with a mutation that occurs in single cells during the lifetime of an individual, there are some hereditary cancers. An inherited mutation can be either autosomal dominant or recessive and results in an individual with a genetic predisposition to cancer.

10. *Answer:* C

Rationale: Microsatellite instability segments are chromosomal abnormalities. Translocations refer to segments of one chromosome that break off and attach themselves to other chromosomes, resulting in altered protein production. Loss of heterozygosity refers to the loss of a segment of both copies of a chromosome. Polymorphisms are changes in DNA sequence of a gene that often are not disease related.

11. *Answer:* C

Rationale: Proto-oncogenes are normal genes essential for normal cell growth and regulation. Mutations occurring in proto-oncogenes convert to oncogene activation, which can result in uncontrolled cell division. Tumor suppressor genes function as regulators of cell growth. Some tumor suppressor genes appear to play a role in cell cycle regulation; others have a role in DNA repair. Mutations of tumor suppressor gene may lead to uncontrolled cell growth.

12. *Answer:* D

Rationale: Mutations are variations in the sequence of DNA. Tumor suppressor genes, proto-oncogenes, and mismatch repair genes are different types of regulatory genes that control cell growth and proliferation.

13. *Answer:* B

Rationale: Autosomal dominant inheritance requires only one altered copy of a gene to result in cancer susceptibility. The risk of transmission to a first-degree relative is 50%.

14. *Answer:* B

Rationale: The decision whether to undergo predisposition genetic testing hinges on the adequacy of the information provided to the individual regarding the risks, benefits, and limitations of testing. Confirmation of the family history of cancer is a critical component of determining eligibility for predisposition genetic testing but is not part of the informed consent process. Insufficient data exist regarding the benefits and limitations of all cancer risk management strategies in individuals at high risk for cancer because of an alteration in a cancer susceptibility gene. The healthcare provider should outline the potential alternatives and limitations of cancer risk management as part of the informed consent process but should not recommend a particular strategy. Informed consent for predisposition genetic testing does not depend on the client's personal health status.

15. *Answer:* C

Rationale: The primary role of the nurse in predisposition genetic testing should be to provide the information necessary for an informed decision without steering patients toward a particular decision. The nurse should also be sure that the client understands that testing is completely voluntary and will not prejudice his or her future healthcare. The nurse can play a role in identifying family members who are eligible for testing, but testing is completely voluntary, and no healthcare provider should dictate who should be tested. Laboratories where predisposition genetic testing is performed should be Clinical Laboratory Improvement Act approved, but selecting a laboratory is not the primary role of the nurse.

16. *Answer:* D

Rationale: Apoptosis refers to the activation of a program that leads to normal programmed cell death and often occurs in response to DNA damage. A malfunction leads to uncontrolled proliferation of damaged or malignant cells.

17. *Answer:* A

Rationale: As cells age, telomerase is normally repressed, and the telomeres, the ends of the chromosomes, are progressively lost. In cancer, telomerase is reactivated, which keeps the telomeres intact, facilitating cell immortalization.

18. *Answer:* B

Rationale: Penetrance refers to the cancer risks associated with a specific genetic mutation, determined by whether the corresponding phenotype is expressed. The other answer choices are related to penetrance and are parts of assessing inherited risk, but they do not fit the definition of penetrance. The complex interaction between genes and the environment may affect the penetrance of a specific gene. The degree to which a single individual with a specific genotype will exhibit a specific trait is expression.

19. *Answer:* A

Rationale: Pharmacogenetics refers to drugs designed specifically for the genetic characteristics of the tumor. Introduction of a functioning gene into the somatic cells to replace missing or defective genes or to provide a new cellular function is somatic gene therapy. Introduction of a functioning gene into an egg or sperm to prevent transmission of a genetic mutation is germline gene therapy. The analysis of the structure, composition, and function of proteins is proteomics.

20. *Answer:* B

Rationale: Genome-wide association studies survey the entire genome for small nucleotide alterations. This technique detects small mutation to determine association with disease. Direct sequencing determines the sequence of the gene being tested and detects sequence changes in the regions being analyzed. Single-strand confirmation polymorphism analysis detects insertions or deletions of four or more bases of DNA; however, mutations exchanging one base for another without altering the length of the DNA fragment are difficult to detect. Microarray technique attaches large numbers (hundreds to thousands) of DNA, RNA, protein, or tissue segments to slides for analysis.

21. *Answer:* B

Rationale: The DNA Laboratory Proficiency Certification does not exist. CLIA is general certification but a useful one. The laboratory director should have certification. The NIH guidelines apply to research laboratories and studies.

22. *Answer:* B

Rationale: Cytogenetics is accurately described in answer B and is used in cancer diagnosis. Karyotype is a subtype of cytogenetics that offers a view of the number and structural appearance of chromosomal structures in the cell nucleus. Gene expression profiling uses multiple techniques to identify the expression of 10s to thousands of genes concurrently. It uses a personalized approach to cancer to diagnose, predict outcomes, or suggest the best treatment regimen for a person's cancer.

23. *Answer:* C

Rationale: Deleterious mutations in *BRCA1* are associated with an increased risk of breast, ovarian, and other cancers. Deleterious mutations in p53 are associated with an increased risk for cancers of the breast and

brain, as well as leukemias, sarcomas, and adrenal cortical tumors. Deleterious mutations in PTEN are associated with an increased risk for cancers of the breast, thyroid (most often follicular type), and endometrium, as well as benign skin lesions. Deleterious mutations in APC are associated with an increased risk for colon and rectal cancer, colon polyposis (adenomas), and other desmoid tumors.

24. *Answer:* C

Rationale: Multiple primary cancers in one individual is a hallmark sign of hereditary cancer, as is early age of cancer diagnosis. Telomerase plays a role in cellular aging and can be involved in carcinogenesis but is not a clinical feature of hereditary susceptibility. The presence of metastasis is not indicative of a hereditary susceptibility to cancer.

25. *Answer:* A

Rationale: Frameshift mutations occur when one or more bases are added or deleted from the normal sequence. Missense mutations are single-base pair changes that result in the substitution of one amino acid for another in the protein being constructed. Splicing mutations occur when DNA that should be removed from the coding sequence is retained or DNA that should not be added is spliced in. Translocations are segments of one chromosome that break off and attach themselves to other chromosomes, resulting in altered protein production.

26. *Answer:* B

Rationale: A negative test result for a known genetic mutation in a family indicates that the client is within the general population risk of cancer associated with that branch of the family. However, family history from the other parent and other personal risk factors still influence the risk of developing cancer.

27. *Answer:* B

Rationale: The cancer risks associated with deleterious mutations in MSH2 include increases in risk for the colon, ovary, and endometrium. Sarcoma is associated with germline mutations in p53. Lung cancer has not been seen with mutations in MSH2. Thyroid cancer in combination with breast cancer is associated with mutations in PTEN.

28. *Answer:* C

Rationale: The DPD protein of gene DYPD is involved in metabolism of 5-FU. DPD inactivates 80% of active 5-FU. Persons with a DYPD2A variant have a greater risk of a grade 3 or 4 toxicity, most commonly neutropenia. The explanation of pharmacodynamics and pharmacokinetics have been reversed in options A and B. Genetic testing can be used in many aspects of cancer treatment planning; the extent of disease present does not typically provide the key information for diagnosis of cancer type.

29. *Answer:* B

Rationale: B is correct as stated. Testing is recommended for irinotecan and nilotinib for colorectal cancer. It is regarded as informational only at this time for busulfan in CML and Arsenic trioxide for PML.

30. *Answer:* A

Rationale: A negative result when there is a known mutation in the family does not mean there is no risk but that the risk is similar to that of the general population.

31. *Answer:* B

Rationale: There are many recommended medical management considerations associated with the care of individuals harboring a mutation in a cancer susceptibility gene. Risk can be mitigated and surveillance is necessary. Those with a risk of transmitting a cancer susceptibility gene to children may benefit from counseling, but all decisions should be the patient's.

32. *Answer:* B

Rationale: HIPAA guidelines ensure that genetic information cannot be used to influence eligibility for insurance. The NCI site contains information for many common cancer genetic syndromes but is not as applicable for advocacy roles. The other options do not represent advocacy actions.

CHAPTER 6

1. *Answer:* C

Rationale: The term "clinical" implies that the research is done in the clinical setting. All research subjects must provide informed consent. Clinical research studies may be an interventional study with comparison groups, but they may also be observational or epidemiologic; they do not always involve the comparison of interventions. CTs can include prevention, screening, and early detection, which improve diagnostics, quality of life, supportive care, and treatment studies. Quality of life and supportive care studies are not always observational research; they may include a client-focused intervention. CTs do not always involve treatment; they may focus on screening and early detection.

2. *Answer:* C

Rationale: In an observational study, the researcher is assessing or describing biomedical and health outcomes in human subjects; the focus is not on changing the outcome for subjects. A phase IV clinical trial is a postmarketing study often used to further evaluate the safety of an intervention. An interventional study involves some type of an intervention or interventions that will be evaluated.

3. *Answer:* B

Rationale: The purpose of the institutional review board (IRB) review is to provide safeguards and protection, not to increase the paperwork of planning a research study. Failure to obtain appropriate IRB approval for research can result in institutional sanctions. All research involving human research must be reviewed and approved by the IRB. Data collection cannot be initiated until approval has been obtained. Use of electronic medical record data for research is not permissible without IRB approval.

4. *Answer:* D

Rationale: This body is independent of the primary investigator and is designed to ensure subject safety and the validity and integrity of the data. They report interim results and intervention-specific toxicity to the institutional review board. They are required by some National Institutes of Health–supported clinical trials but may not be required in minimal risk studies, especially behavioral interventions.

5. *Answer:* D

Rationale: The AEs include any unfavorable or unintended sign, symptom, or disease temporarily linked with the intervention being evaluated that is likely related to the study is *not* correct; they must include both those that may and may not be related to the study. The PI does have the primary responsibility regarding AEs; however, all clinical investigators share this responsibility. Clinical staff caring for subjects must also report findings and concerns. Assessment of adverse events is not determined by individual institutions.

6. *Answer:* B

Rationale: Informed consent involves the potential subjects being informed of their rights, having all questions answered, and feeling comfortable with the option to decline or even to withdraw in the future. Stating that Dr. M. would never recommend anything he thought was too risky puts additional pressure on J.B. to consent. Yes, research is needed to improve the outcomes of cancer care, but it should never be conducted at the expense of compromising clients' rights. Dr. M. may well be willing to return and re-explain the study, but that does not sound like the concern for J.B.

7. *Answer:* A

Rationale: Children are considered a vulnerable group because they may feel pressured to participate or not fully understand the study. Women are not considered vulnerable, but pregnant women have additional health concerns, and any trial must also adequately protect the fetus. English-language proficiency, if necessary, can be listed as eligibility among criteria.

8. *Answer:* B

Rationale: By definition, CER is the process of generating, synthesizing, and comparing the benefit and harm of interventions in typical patients to identify the most efficacious, safe, and cost-effective care for an individual. New medications and devices must undergo appropriate testing for use in humans before use in comparison studies.

9. *Answer:* A

Rationale: The oncology nurse serves as an advocate for both client safety and clinical trial integrity by promoting ethical care per state standards of professional practice. These standards are never to be violated for research. The nurse also promotes the informed consent process by validating that the client understands the clinical trial and has had all questions answered. The oncology nurse should also consult with the clinical trials nurse before administering any new medications; this is important because of the potential for interactions. Although clinical trial success is important, as is research for the advancement of cancer care, the nurse must always advocate for her or his patients. Hopefully, family members are supportive of the research, but it is important that they not tell their loved one what to do or discuss it in a coercive manner to influence them.

10. *Answer:* D

Rationale: Phase IV is postmarketing study of agents that had been evaluated in research. It allows comparison of the drug with another similar product that is already being marketed. The nurse's intent should be to clarify their misunderstanding and listen to their concerns but not to convince them to support the study.

11. *Answer:* B

Rationale: B is correct as stated. Expanded access allows investigational new drugs to be made available by manufacturers with Food and Drug Administration approval to clients who are too ill to participate in a clinical trial because of poor performance status, have a disease for which there is no approved treatment available, or have shown a therapeutic response at the end of the clinical trial. The intent is not to provide medicine to individuals without insurance coverage or give a principle investigator permission to alter eligibility criteria. It does provide for continued use by subjects who were responding when a trial ended.

12. *Answer:* B

Rationale: Even if the study involves minimal risk, D.F.'s rights should be protected. The legal representative for her care will be the one to work with her and make the decision regarding participation. A data safety and monitoring board will not focus on D.F.'s rights as a vulnerable subject; therefore, D is not correct.

CHAPTER 7

1. *Answer:* A

Rationale: Adipose tissue is a type of connective tissue in which fat is stored. Sebaceous tissues are microscopic glands in the skin that secrete an oily or waxy substance called sebum. Glandular tissue is the tissue that primarily comprises lactiferous lobes and milk ducts. This broad category of tissue contains the terminal duct lobular units, which produce fatty breast milk.

2. *Answer:* D

Rationale: Breast cancer is the most common cancer in women worldwide and is the second leading cause of cancer-related deaths in U.S. women. There has been a 7% decrease in breast cancer incidence between 2002 and 2003, primarily because of the decrease in the use of hormone replacement therapy. An estimated 64,640 women were newly diagnosed with in situ breast cancer in 2013.

3. *Answer:* D

Rationale: Patients who are diagnosed with breast cancer and who have the *BRCA1* gene mutation are also at increased risk for ovarian cancer. Elevations in CA-125 would reveal the presence of ovarian cancer. A pelvic examination might detect an ovarian mass or cancer. The Philadelphia chromosome and a complete blood cell count are used in the detection of leukemia and anemia.

A complete metabolic profile would reveal abnormalities in electrolytes, which are related to numerous medical conditions, including cardiac and renal conditions. Amylase and lipase levels are usually reviewed in regards to pancreatic issues such as pancreatitis, renal issues, and high cholesterol. Bence Jones urine is a diagnostic tool used in the diagnosis of multiple myeloma.

4. *Answer:* B

Rationale: Lobular carcinoma in situ (also called lobular neoplasia) is a nonmalignant tumor. It is often multicentric and multifocal, comprised of more than one tumor and occurring in more than one quadrant of the breast. A fine needle aspiration would not be appropriate. Trastuzumab is used in the treatment of Human Epidermal growth factor Receptor 2 (HER-2) positive breast cancer. The status of receptors for HER-2 and estrogen is not addressed in this patient.

5. *Answer:* A

Rationale: The *BRCA1* gene mutation is located on chromosome 17q21 and accounts for 20% of all familial breast cancers. Those who carry this gene mutation have a 50% to 85% lifetime risk of developing breast cancer, and men with this gene mutation have an increased risk for developing prostate cancer.

6. *Answer:* A

Rationale: A patient with it *BRCA2* breast cancer is at risk for all of these cancers. While in Florida, she will likely be exposed to high temperatures and increased ultraviolet rays, making malignant melanoma her most significant risk at this time.

7. *Answer:* C

Rationale: This patient's most significant risks for breast cancer include being female (breast cancer is 100 times more common in women than in men), breast cancer history in a first-degree relative (her mother), being an African American woman (diagnosed with breast cancer at an early age [before 45 years of age]) compared with Caucasian women, smoking at an early age, and continued tobacco use. Hyperthyroidism and hypothyroidism are not documented risk factors for breast cancer. The patient is taking Synthroid for hypothyroidism. Having a first pregnancy after the age of 30 years or being nulliparous increases one's risk of breast cancer, but the number of pregnancies one has decreases the risk of breast cancer. Breast cancer in her aunt is a risk factor for this patient, but less so than her mother's breast cancer history.

8. *Answer:* C

Patients are always advised to have proper healthcare, and regular visits with their primary care provider are essential. The primary care provider would likely be cognizant of the specialty training and practice of breast cancer professionals and follow their recommendations regarding the diagnosis and surveillance of breast cancer patients. Self-breast examination is a self-care modality that allows the patient to actively participate in her own wellness, but it is not meant to replace mammographic studies in patients who have a known breast abnormality. Obesity and a diet high in fat or polyunsaturated fats can increase the risk for breast cancer. Reducing those factors should decrease the risk but should not be a determining factor in mammography screening.

9. *Answer:* D

Rationale: Because the patient was diagnosed with breast cancer in her mid-70s, it is likely that she had other comorbidities before that diagnosis. She has also had a lapse in her therapy. The patient's symptoms of shortness of breath and back pain are suspicious for lung and spinal cord involvement. She has received trastuzumab, which can cause decreased left side ejection fraction or pulmonary problems such as interstitial pneumonitis or pulmonary fibrosis. Axillary involvement is caused by lymphatic spread, the symptoms described here are those of a patient in late stage disease with distant metastases. Spread to distant organs is likely owing to hematologic spread. Brain and liver metastases are seen in patients with breast cancer, but her symptoms do not describe disease in those areas.

10. *Answer:* B

Rationale: An echocardiogram would evaluate her cardiac ejection fraction, which is a concern because of her treatment with trastuzumab. A chemistry profile would include an alkaline phosphatase level that, if elevated, would indicate bone involvement. The bone pain exhibited makes chemistry a better choice than a complete blood count. A computed tomography (CT) scan of the chest would highlight mediastinal lymph nodes and any metastatic chest lesions and is a better tool than chest radiography. The bone scan is an important diagnostic tool for bone lesions or metastases. An electrocardiogram reveals heart irregularities, which are important but not the predominating factor for this patient. Magnetic resonance imaging is indicated, but the other choices in D are not. This patient's symptoms do not indicate the need for abdominal ultrasonography, a CT of the abdomen and pelvis, sentinel lymph node biopsy, mamma print gene assay, electrocardiogram, or pulmonary function tests.

11. *Answer:* A

Rationale: Overall, African Americans have the highest breast cancer incidence and mortality rates, usually because of decreased access to care. This is followed by whites, Hispanics, and Pacific Islanders.

12. *Answer:* D

Rationale: Patients who are estrogen receptor positive and progesterone receptor positive have a better overall prognosis and additional treatment options with aromatase inhibitors and selective receptor modulators. The greater the lymph node involvement, the poorer the patient's prognosis. More invasive tumors have an increased ability to metastasize, and high-grade tumors are more aggressive. Alcohol intake, history of other cancer treatment, and gouty arthritis are not prognostic factors in breast cancer prognosis or treatment.

13. *Answer:* D

Rationale: The Oncotype DX is a 21-gene assay used to predict chemotherapy benefit and estimate the 10-year risk of distant recurrence in women with early-stage, node-negative, estrogen receptor–positive invasive breast cancer. The recurrence score result is determined from gene expression. There is no measurement category indicating no risk of recurrence. A score of 0 to 17 indicates a low risk of recurrence, 18 to 31 is intermediate risk, and high risk is any score greater than 31.

14. *Answer:* C

Rationale: Stage IIIA breast cancer in this patient's case is T3 (a tumor >20 mm but <50 mm at its greatest dimension), N1 metastases to moveable ipsilateral axillary lymph nodes, and M0 (no evidence of distant metastasis).

15. *Answer:* A

Rationale: Basal cell breast cancers are not responsive to hormonal therapies such as Herceptin because they are estrogen receptor negative, (ER-); progesterone receptor negative (PR-); and HER-2 negative. These factors comprise the name) "triple-negative breast cancer." Men are not usually diagnosed with a triple-negative breast cancer. Because these cancers do not respond to targeted interventions against receptors for estrogen or HER2, they often are treated with a combination of surgery, chemotherapy, and radiation treatments.

16. *Answer:* B

Rationale: The Bloom Richardson grading system uses criteria to determine histologic grading of breast cancer. Grade 1 is low grade and well differentiated. Grade 2 is intermediate grade and moderately differentiated. Grade 3 is high grade and poorly differentiated.

17. *Answer:* A

Rationale: Lapatinib (Tykreb) is a kinase inhibitor used for locally advanced and metastatic HER-2–positive breast cancer, often in combination with chemotherapy. Potential side effects include a decreased left-sided ejection fraction, hepatic toxicity, nausea and vomiting, diarrhea, interstitial lung disease or pneumonitis, QT prolongation, palmar and plantar erythrodysesthesia, rash, and fatigue. Anemia and neutropenia are not side effects of lapatinib.

18. *Answer:* B

Rationale: The patient is distressed because of her upcoming surgery, which is complicated by the fact that a close family member underwent a similar procedure several years earlier with poor outcomes. It is also possible that these feelings are compounded by issues related to self-image, sexuality, and intimacy. Telling her that there is no guarantee she will not lose the function of her arm could terrify the patient, and she may not want to proceed. It is also inappropriate to suggest that her aunt's surgeon removed too much tissue when the nurse is not certain of that fact. A patient relation's department is a good resource, but it does nothing to allay K.L.'s concerns before her surgery. The best strategy in this situation is to explain how surgical techniques have improved. This can bring her some peace and build a relationship between the patient and the nurse for the future.

19. *Answer:* A

Rationale: It is much easier to prevent lymphedema postoperatively than to correct lymphedema after it has occurred. The most valuable tool is a baseline measurement of the affected arm preoperatively, which is compared with postoperative measurements. The patient should be instructed to keep accurate records of these measurements and to notify her healthcare provider if it increases. Guidelines should also be provided regarding preventing trauma and infection in the affected extremity, signs of which would include the color and warmth of the extremity and fever. Sodium restriction is not currently a component of monitoring or preventing lymphedema.

20. *Answer:* C

Rationale: Phantom breast sensation can occur because residual breast tissue can have nonpainful sensations and phantom pain caused by surgical trauma and damage to nerves during surgery. This syndrome can affect between 30% and 80% of patients having mastectomies. It can greatly impact the quality of life combined with the impact of physical disability and emotional distress. Symptoms can include pain, discomfort, itching, a pins and needles sensation, tingling, pressure, burning, and throbbing.

21. *Answer:* D

Rationale: The five subgroups categorized tumors as luminal A, luminal B, normal-like breast tumors, HER-2–amplified tumors, and basal tumors. Luminal A tumors tend to have the highest levels of ER expression, are PR positive, and tend to be HER-2 negative; they are low grade, tend to be less responsive to chemotherapy, and have a favorable prognosis.

22. *Answer:* B

Rationale: Aromatase inhibitors are used in breast cancer patients who are postmenopausal at diagnosis and who are hormone receptor positive. These medications are used to reduce the likelihood of disease recurrence and are usually given for a 5-year time span. This group of medications has the potential to cause a decrease in bone density.

23. *Answer:* A

Rationale: The patient is postmenopausal and may have had bone loss before starting Arimidex, which was then compounded. Initially, tests should include bone density and alkaline phosphatase followed by a bone scan if she voices increased complaints of pain or an increase in the number of areas where this discomfort occurs. Depending on these results, the drug may be contraindicated in this patient. A complete blood cell count is not indicated. Bence Jones urine is a diagnostic test for multiple myeloma.

CHAPTER 8

1. *Answer:* D

Rationale: Although he has had exposure to a chemically toxic work environment and a smoking history, the first response does not address his symptoms. A diagnosis of lung cancer should not be selected simply because of exclusion of other obvious comorbidities. In addition, the respiratory symptoms alone that the patient mentions could be caused by other respiratory ailments such as chronic obstructive pulmonary disease. Response D takes into account a more complete patient assessment, including chest radiography, both respiratory symptoms of cough and shortness of breath, the additional constitutional symptoms of weight loss and lethargy, as well as the risk factors of his chemical exposure at the paint factory and his previous smoking history.

2. *Answer:* B

Rationale: The multi-hit theory refers to continuous carcinogen exposure over an extended period resulting in DNA damage and mutation of cells.

3. *Answer:* D

Rationale: The symptoms of pallor and fatigue are closely related to anemia. Crackles in the lungs can be symptoms of a myriad of lung ailments. Although the history of heavy smoking in the patient's father is a risk factor for lung cancer, the most comprehensive response is D. This covers her long-term chemical exposure and addresses the current symptom of numbness in her arm, which could be related to spinal cord compression, as well as the classic cough. The cough could be caused by a tumor, nerve impingement of a tumor, or collection of fluid in the lung in space displaced by a tumor. The nerve involvement points to systemic spread.

4. *Answer:* B

Rationale: In the United States, lung cancer accounts for 14% of new cancer cases annually. Lung cancer accounted for 27% of all cancer deaths in both genders projected for 2013. The overall 5-year survival rate for localized disease is 52%. In the United States, African Americans have the poorest outcomes compared with other ethnic groups and are diagnosed with more advanced disease.

5. *Answer:* A

Rationale: Female gender, weight loss less than 5%, and good performance status are all positive indicators. Weight loss and performance status are associated with constitutional symptoms. Treatments are more effective when the disease is diagnosed in the early stages. Regional and metastatic lung cancer is more difficult to contain and treat compared with treating one primary lesion.

6. *Answer:* C

Rationale: Currently, there are no specific tumor markers available for disease status in lung cancer. Preliminary chest radiography would reveal a density or fluid in the lungs; however, a computed tomography (CT) scan of the chest provides a more detailed report. The positron emission tomography scan is useful in determining nodal disease and to identify metastatic sites. Magnetic resonance imaging (MRI) would be helpful in establishing advanced disease. Complete blood count (CBC), chemistry profile, a-fetoprotein, abdominal CT, and pulmonary function tests may be useful in determining treatment plans but are not used in diagnosis.

7. *Answer:* A

Rationale: All of these factors impact a poor prognosis for those with lung cancer, but the primary reason is because lung cancer is frequently diagnosed at a late stage.

8. *Answer:* B

Rationale: A positron emission tomography (PET) scan is a valuable tool in oncology, but its main purpose is to identify spread and metastatic disease, not to identify primary sites. It can be particularly helpful in identifying nodal involvement. Sputum for cytology can be used when cancer is suspected as well as in other lung ailments. A bone scan or a full-body bone scan is used to detect bone metastases. Thyroid transcription factors(TTF-1) and Cytokeratin (CK) stains are histology-sensitive markers that assist in differentiating the histology of a primary versus metastatic adenocarcinoma of the lung.

9. *Answer:* B

Rationale: Small cell lung cancer is staged as either limited or extensive disease. Limited stage disease is confined to one lung and lymph nodes on the same side of the mediastinum. Extensive stage disease is any of the following: spread widely throughout one lung; spread to a second lung; spread across the mediastinum to another lung; and/or spread to distant organs.

10. *Answer:* B

Rationale: The pack history is defined by the number of packs of cigarettes smoked in a day multiplied by the number of years the patient has smoked. Therefore, a man who smokes two packs per day for 30 years has a 60-pack-year history.

11. *Answer:* C

Rationale: Despite side effects and the potential for serious complications, in early-stage lung cancer, the only curative modality is surgery. Lung cancer is often detected at a stage with disseminated disease, and there are limited response rates for chemotherapeutic agents.

12. *Answer:* D

Rationale: It is commendable that J.J. quit smoking, particularly after he smoked for many years, and the nurse certainly wants to applaud his efforts and determination. Smoking cessation is associated with a gradual decrease in the risk of lung cancer. Symptomatic improvements may be noticeable immediately on smoking cessation. Five or more years must elapse before an appreciable decrease in risk occurs.

13. *Answer:* C

Rationale: The American Lung Association, based on the findings of the NLST Trial, recommends lung cancer screening with low-dose computed tomography (CT) for people who meet certain criteria. This includes current or former smokers age 55 to 74 years with a smoking history of at least 30 pack-years (an average of a pack a day for 30 years) and with no history of lung cancer. Chest radiography is not a screening tool for lung cancer. Sputum for cytology is also not diagnostic for lung cancer. The CT screening needs to be conducted in settings that have expertise in lung cancer screening, diagnosis, and treatment. Screening does result in increased detection of early stage lung cancer, which is more treatable, but screening can also result in the identification of many nodules that may be benign and may result in unnecessary procedures and psychological distress.

14. *Answer:* A

Rationale: Because of the patient's age and cardiac history, chest surgery could be risky and recovery could bring complications. Radiation therapy is used as a primary therapy for stage I and II disease if the patient is not a surgical candidate. Bruising from his tree limb injury would not have been a major consideration in selecting this treatment.

15. *Answer:* D

Limited stage disease is confined to one lung and lymph nodes on the same side of the mediastinum. Extensive stage disease is any of the following: spread widely throughout one lung; spread to a second lung; spread across the mediastinum to another lung; and/or spread to distant organs. Extensive stage disease is disease that has spread beyond the supraclavicular area and is too widespread to be included in the definition of limited disease. Patients with distant metastases are considered to have extensive stage disease.

16. *Answer:* C

Rationale: Prophylactic cranial irradiation (PCI) is an option for patients who have achieved complete response to chemotherapy or radiotherapy (RT) to reduce the risk of developing brain metastases. Patients whose cancer can be controlled outside of the brain have a 60% actuarial risk of developing central nervous system (CNS) metastases within 2 to 3 years after starting treatment. The majority of these patients relapse only to their brain, and nearly all of those who relapse in their CNS die of cranial metastases. The risk of developing CNS metastases can be reduced by more than 50% by the administration of PCI.

17. *Answer:* A

Rationale: The main toxicities that occur with cisplatin are nausea/vomiting and neurotoxicity, including numbness, tingling, hearing loss, tinnitus, difficulty with fine motor movements, and difficulty with ambulation.

18. *Answer:* A

Rationale: Targeted therapies affect molecular targets or pathways to reduce tumor growth and target specific genetic mutations in the tumor. This is not a systemic treatment such as chemotherapy. Specific cells are targeted, and normal cells are not impacted. Because of this selectivity, there are different side effects than are typically seen with chemotherapy. Targeted therapies have been approved for use in specific cancers and work in a variety of ways. Some interfere with the cell's growth and inhibit cell division, others decrease tumor blood vessel development in the cell, causing cell necrosis. Targeted therapies can also promote cell death of specific cancer cells, stimulate the immune system to destroy specific cancer cells, or deliver toxic drugs to cancer cells.

19. *Answer:* B

Rationale: Crizotinib is the most appropriate and efficacious in this case. It is a first-line therapy agent for persons with non–small cell lung cancer (NSCLC) who have advanced disease and are ALK (anaplastic lymphoma kinase) gene positive. Bevacizumab in addition to chemotherapy is recommended in select patients with advanced NSCLC but increases risk of bleeding. Erlotinib is first line therapy for individuals with advanced, recurrent or metastatic nonsquamous NSCLC. Gefitinib has been approved to treat advanced NSCLC that is epidermal growth factor receptor mutation positive.

20. *Answer:* B

Rationale: The best approach is to take the time to sit in private with the patient and her family support system to assess what they understand about the disease, noticing their nonverbal cues and facial expressions as they react to what is being said. This gives them the opportunity to ask questions or speak about topics they have been avoiding. The time that the nurse takes with the patient and family in private shows caring, respect, and builds trust with the patient and family. This over time will allow the nurse to nurture and guide the patient in appropriate decision making as the disease trajectory progresses.

21. *Answer:* B

Rationale: The nurse tells the patient that she honors and respects her decision but that it is important the patient is well informed regarding all of her symptoms. After explaining the treatment options to make sure she is aware, the nurse also mentions that palliative measures and symptoms management will be available to her if she changes her mind. She does not appear to be in any emotional or psychiatric crisis, and she should not be made to feel guilty if she does not consider a clinical trial. Notifying the crisis intervention team is not necessary and could undermine trust. The social worker can help the patient to make plans or changes to her living situation or support system as needed.

22. *Answer:* B

Rationale: According to the American Cancer Society (ACS, 2013), the average 5-year survival rate is only 16% for all persons diagnosed with lung cancer.

23. *Answer:* C

Rationale: The diagnosis of small cell lung cancer (SCLC) is associated with a more aggressive course than non–small cell lung cancer (NSCLC). SCLC accounts for approximately 15% of cases and is responsive to chemotherapy and radiotherapy. The prognosis is poor with an overall 5-year survival rate of 5% to 10%. Untreated, the median survival time is 2 to 4 months. Current evidence does not support maintenance chemotherapy outside of a clinical trial. Both SCLC and NSCLC are associated with an increased risk for metabolic emergencies.

24. *Answer:* D

Rationale: Despite standards of care for treatment, a clinical trial is a viable option for individuals with lung cancer because of the low cure rate and poor survival rate of the currently available regimens.

CHAPTER 9

1. *Answer:* D

Rationale: Helicobacter pylori is a bacterial infection that occurs in the stomach. It is present in about 66% of the world's population. It can cause peptic ulcers and gastric cancer. Currently, *H. pylori* is not associated with pancreatic, liver, or colorectal cancers.

2. *Answer:* C

Rationale: Oxaliplatin is a chemotherapeutic agent used in the treatment of gastric cancer and other gastrointestinal malignancies. It is given before his gastric resection to eradicate micrometastases at an early stage and improve resectability by reducing tumor burden. Oxaliplatin, a chemotherapeutic agent, does not treat nausea or pain, reduce gastric acid secretions, or treat *Helicobacter pylori* infection.

3. *Answer:* A

Rationale: The most common type of gastric cancer is adenocarcinoma, comprising approximately 90% of all gastric malignancies. Gastrointestinal tract tumors, neuroendocrine tumors, and lymphoma tumors together comprise only 5% of gastric malignancies.

4. *Answer:* B

Rationale: The normal signs and symptoms of gastric cancer include indigestion, nausea, vomiting, and anorexia (loss of appetite), things that we all experience on occasion and therefore may dismiss or ignore for a long time. This is not a reflection of denial. Alcohol and exposure to chemicals are both risk factors for gastric carcinoma but do not necessarily cause or negate symptoms.

5. *Answer:* C

Rationale: The main factor for the increasing incidence of hepatocellular cancer is the increase in incidence of hepatitis C infection. Although it is true that tobacco use is increasing in underdeveloped countries, it is not related to the increased incidence of hepatocellular carcinoma. The use of statin type drugs and exposure to chemical carcinogens are risk factors for hepatocellular cancers but at this time are not implicated as causing the increased incidence.

6. *Answer:* C

Rationale: Because G.J. has multiple tumors larger than 3 cm, he would be staged in T3a. Stage T0 is defined as having no evidence of primary tumor. Core needle biopsy is preferred for patients who have tumors larger than 2 cm. α-Fetoprotein is a tumor marker for hepatocellular carcinoma. It is usually drawn in conjunction with an abdominal ultrasonography every 3 to 6 months for those who are at risk for hepatocellular cancer.

7. *Answer:* B

The type of surgery the patient has depends on the location of the tumor. Because her tumor is located in the rectum, she will have a low anterior resection. This allows for sphincter preservation and continence. There is always the chance that some unforeseen emergency could occur during surgery, and a colostomy would be necessary. A right-sided hemi-colectomy is usually performed for a right-sided colon cancer. An extended right-sided hemi-colectomy is generally for patients with colon cancers in the transverse colon.

8. *Answer:* A

Rationale: The fact that the patient reports blood mixed with his stools, changes in bowel patterns, and symptoms related to an early bowel obstruction points to an advanced colon cancer located in the transverse colon. A cancer in the descending colon would cause the patient abdominal pain, obstructive symptoms such as nausea and vomiting, and constipation alternating with diarrhea. Ascending colon cancers exhibit a vague abdominal pain, weakness, weight loss, changes in the stool, and anemia. Symptoms related to rectal cancers include a rectal fullness, urgency, bleeding, and pelvic pain.

9. *Answer:* D

Rationale: The American Cancer Society (ACS) does recommend a colonoscopy every 10 years. However, ACS recommendations for other tests are a flexible sigmoidoscopy every 5 years, an annual fecal occult blood test (FOBT), or a double-contrast barium enema every 5 years. Recommendations from the National Comprehensive Cancer Network (NCCN) include a colonoscopy every 10 years, a flexible sigmoidoscopy every 5 years, or a guaiac-based or immunochemical-based testing annually (with a flexible sigmoidoscopy every ~5 years).

10. *Answer:* C

Rationale: Although the risk factors for several of the gastrointestinal malignancies include toxic chemicals, coal gases, tanning supplies, and pollutants from the transportation industry, exposure to dry-cleaning supplies and chemicals is specifically noted to increase one's risk for esophageal cancer.

11. *Answer:* C

Rationale: Achalasia is a rare disorder in which the muscle ring in the lower esophagus fails to relax during swallowing, resulting in decreased peristalsis of food into the stomach. This condition and tobacco use carry an increased risk for esophageal cancer.

12. *Answer:* A

Many of the answers contain risk factors for gastric cancer, including gastroesophageal reflux disease, physical inactivity (because of its link to obesity), and smoking. Choice A, which addresses the previous gastric surgery (likely because of a gastric ulcer) and her pernicious anemia, is the most complete answer.

13. *Answer:* E

Rationale: Gastric cancer carries the ability to spread directly into the perineum. Anal cancer extends directly into the pelvis. It can spread hematogenously to the liver and lung, and can spread with distant metastases via the lymphatics.

14. *Answer:* A

Rationale: Herceptin and docetaxel are appropriate choices in this case. Herceptin (trastuzumab) is used in HER-2–positive tumors in metastatic setting in combination with chemotherapy. The chemotherapy agent docetaxel is an option to use in patients with metastatic disease. Interleukin-2 is a cytokine that has been used in the treatment of melanoma and kidney cancer. It is not known as an active agent in gastric cancer. Epirubicin is used as a perioperative chemotherapy agent but not as a drug for metastatic disease. Rituxan/Rituximab, used in treatment of non-Hodgkin lymphoma and chronic

lymphocytic leukemia, is not indicated in the treatment of gastric cancer. Etoposide is not a chemotherapy agent normally used in gastric cancer. Leucovoran and 5-FU are older chemotherapy agents that have been used in patients with colon cancer.

15. *Answer:* C

Rationale: The liver is the most common site of metastatic spread. The patient has had a previous Whipple procedure, leaving very little pancreatic tissue for recurrence. Food poisoning may cause jaundice but more commonly causes diarrhea, nausea, and vomiting. Reactions to statin medications for control of cholesterol usually occur as elevations in liver enzymes shortly after the medication is initiated.

16. *Answer:* D

Rationale: The main risk factors for colorectal cancer are divided into those that can be modified, including smoking, alcohol use, and high-fat red meat diet, obesity, inadequate intake of fruits and vegetables, and physical inactivity. Risk factors for colorectal cancer that cannot be modified include age older than 50 years, personal or family history of colon cancer or inflammatory bowel disease, hereditary polyposis syndrome, familial adenomatous polyposis, hereditary nonpolyposis colorectal cancer, Lynch syndrome, or the presence of adenomatous polyps.

17. *Answer:* D

Rationale: Squamous cell carcinoma of the esophagus is common in developing countries and is usually found in the upper two thirds of the esophagus. Adenocarcinoma arises from glandular tissue in the distal (lower one third) esophagus. It is associated with the risk factors of GERD.

18. *Answer:* D

Rationale: Systemic chemotherapy for advanced liver cancer has long been known to produce low response rates and no survival benefit. Although patients with liver cancer can develop ascites, they may also have a decreased ability to metabolize chemotherapeutic agents in the liver, causing renal failure.

19. *Answer:* D

Rationale: Controversy regarding the correct number of lymph nodes to dissect is a concern when discussing anal cancer. For colon cancer, a minimum of 12 lymph nodes must be assessed to determine proper staging.

20. *Answer:* C

Rationale: The medications listed are all biotherapy agents approved for use in colorectal cancer. Avastin is usually used in combination with chemotherapy. Both Vectibix and Erbitux are used in patients with the KRAS mutation, and can be given in combination with chemotherapy or as a single agent. Stivarga is only used as a single agent.

21. *Answer:* C

Rationale: Although all of these educational topics could be of value to the patient, the most important one at this stage in his disease process is the care of the percutaneous endoscopic gastrostomy tube and the administration of the tube feeding. The patient has a loss of appetite and significant weight loss related to his diagnosis of pancreatic cancer. The patient has not complained of any dysphagia or odynophagia, nor is there any mention of constipation issues. His loss of appetite will not be improved with nutritional information.

22. **Answer:** C

Rationale: Carcinoembryonic antigen can be elevated in clients with colorectal cancer. It is generally used to monitor efficacy and as an indication of disease recurrence. CA 19-9 is often used as a tumor marker for pancreatic cancer. CA 27-29 is used in breast cancer, and a-fetoprotein is used for both primary liver cancer and testicular cancer.

23. **Answer:** D

Rationale: Signs and symptoms of late-stage colon cancer include weight loss, anorexia, and anemia. Blood in the stool, a change in bowel habits, and flatulence can be early signs of colon cancer.

CHAPTER 10

1. **Answer:** C

Rationale: Because the patient had cervical cancer (CIN2 disease), she is required to have Pap smears every 3 years for a 20-year time span from diagnosis even beyond the age of 65 years. It is unwise to presume that the patient is not sexually active because she is a widow. HPV testing in combination with Pap smears would extend the frequency to every 5 years. However, testing should still be continued for 20 years after diagnosis.

2. **Answer:** A

Rationale: Her symptoms describe the triad of unilateral leg edema, sciatic pain, and urethral obstruction, indicating recurrent disease. The most common pathway for metastatic disease related to cervical cancer is direct extension into the parametrium, vagina, lower uterine segment, the abdomen, and other pelvic structures. There is a possibility of metastatic disease to the liver; however, that is not usually the initial route of metastatic spread and does not account for her back pain, leg edema, and difficulty with ambulation. A diagnosis of arthritis could be responsible for back pain and difficulty walking but is not likely the cause of the patient's leg edema and abdominal bloating. Although she may have developed a deep vein thrombosis, that choice also would not account for her back pain or abdominal bloating.

3. **Answer:** A

Rationale: Smoking increases the risk of cervical cancer by two- to fivefold. Long-term use of oral contraceptives increases the risk for cervical cancer; a history of multiple sexual partners and a high parity rate also increases the risk.

4. **Answer:** D

Rationale: Certain subtypes of human papillomavirus (HPV) are known to be oncogenic including, but not limited to, HPV 16, 18, 31, 33, 35, 39, 45, 51, 52, 56, 58, and 59. Epstein-Barr virus is not implicated in cervical cancer but is implicated in other cancers such as Burkitt lymphoma, Hodgkin disease, and nasopharyngeal carcinoma. There is little evidence to suggest that oral contraceptives are protective against cervical cancer.

5. **Answer:** A

Rationale: Vaccination for human papillomavirus (HPV) does not alter the recommendations for screening against cervical cancer. Screening for cervical cancer is recommended to determine premalignant changes. Current recommendations include screening should begin at 21 years of age. Between 21 and 29 years of age, liquid-based cytology is recommended every 3 years. DNA testing is not required unless there is an abnormal Pap test. From age 30 to 65 years, recommendations include HPV testing and cytology (co-test) every 5 years (preferred) or cytology alone every 3 years. Those older than 65 years of age do not need screening after more than three consecutive negative Pap test results or more than two consecutive negative HPV and Pap test within the previous 10 years, with the most recent tests within the previous 5 years. The number of sexual partners does increase one's risk of cervical cancer. Homosexual women may perceive discrimination from healthcare providers regarding their sexual orientation and choose to defer healthcare screenings.

6. **Answer:** C

Rationale: The patient can expect the practitioner to swab the cervix with an acetic acid solution during the procedure. Patients should not douche, use any vaginal creams, or have intercourse within 2 days before the examination. Ideally, the patient should not be menstruating.

7. **Answer:** B

Rationale: Obesity is a risk factor for ovarian cancer because adipocytes convert androstenedione to estrone, which increases circulating estrogen levels. A history of abnormal Pap tests or cervical cancer does not increase risk. A personal or family history of ovarian cancer or colon cancer or a family history of endometrial cancer increases risk. Hormone replacement therapy increases risk.

8. **Answer:** D

Rationale: Exfoliated malignant cells from the endometrium are rarely detected on cervical sampling (the Pap test). A Pap test is a screening test for cervical intraepithelial neoplasia or cervical cancer. Endometrial cancer can be detected through bimanual pelvic examination to determine the size and shape of the uterus, or through endometrial aspiration or biopsy or fractional dilatation and curettage if previous endometrial biopsy results have been negative, stenosis makes endometrial biopsy impossible, or abnormal bleeding persists.

9. **Answer:** D

Rationale: The patient is encouraged to drink fluids unless contraindicated to promote free flow of urine, prevent urinary stasis, concentrated urine, and infections. The suprapubic catheter is a temporary postoperative measure, in which bladder training is a necessary step in gaining control of urinary function. Although the amount may vary slightly, it is usually the norm for suprapubic catheters to be discontinued after the patient has less than 50 mL of residual urine after voiding for several days in a row. When the suprapubic catheter is discontinued, the patient will void and rely on intermittent self-catheterization.

10. *Answer:* D

Rationale: Ovarian cancer is an aggressive disease. Local extension of the tumor can occur in adjacent organs such as the bladder and the colon. Exfoliated cancer cells can also be transported throughout the peritoneum by physiologic peritoneal fluid and disseminate throughout the intraabdominal cavity. Extensive seeding of the peritoneal cavity by tumor cells can be associated with ascites, especially in high-grade serous carcinomas. Metastatic spread can also take place in the pelvic and periaortic lymph nodes. Ovarian cancer, however, rarely disseminates via hematologic spread through the vasculature.

11. *Answer:* A

Rationale: Vulvar cancers comprise 5% of all female cancers, and the survival rates are 80% to 90% for stage I and II disease. Ovarian cancer is the leading cause of death from gynecologic cancer in the United States, and is the country's fifth most common cause of cancer death in women. Cervical cancer is the fourth most common cancer worldwide and the fourth most frequent cause of cancer-related deaths in women worldwide. Endometrial cancer is the most common gynecologic malignancy among women in the United States and the fourth most common cancer among women in the United States. Testicular cancer is a very rare cancer, but it is the most commonly occurring cancer among men ages 15 to 35 years of age.

12. *Answer:* C

Rationale: Patients who undergo radical hysterectomies have postoperative side effects of difficult urination and constipation. Narcotic analgesia, inadequate bowel cleansing, and lack of dietary intake can all impact bowel function to some extent. However, in patients undergoing radical hysterectomy, constipation is primarily caused by bowel manipulation.

13. *Answer:* A

Rationale: CA-125 is a tumor marker for ovarian cancer. It is usually elevated in approximately 80% of patients with advanced ovarian cancer. Carcinoembryonic antigen (CEA), CA 19-9, and CA 27-29 may be elevated in patients with ovarian cancer but are generally used to follow patients with other types of tumors. CEA is often used as a marker in patients with cancers of the colon, rectum, pancreas, stomach, lung, and gallbladder. CEA may also be elevated in patients with breast, head and neck, melanoma, lymphoma, liver, thyroid, cervix, bladder, kidney, and ovarian cancer. CA 19-9 may be elevated in colorectal, pancreatic, hepatobiliary, and gastric cancer. CA 27-29 is found in the blood of most patients with breast cancer but may be elevated by cancers of the colon, stomach, kidney, ovary, pancreas, uterus, and liver.

14. *Answer:* A

Rationale: A gynecologic oncologist at a large medical center would have more surgical experience with this patient population and could provide optimal tumor debulking or cytoreduction and complete surgical staging, as well as removal of all tumors or tumors greater than 1 cm in size so that minimal residual disease remains, to improve overall survival. Optimal versus suboptimal debulking with initial surgery is an important prognostic factor. Insurance options are very important in access to healthcare, but the most important consideration is the type and quality of care offered. Access to clinical trials is not limited to large medical centers. Although it is important for the patient to have surgery in a timely manner, it is most important that she obtains the proper surgical intervention.

15. *Answer:* B

Rationale: Vaginal cancer usually occurs in women older than 60 years of age. It is a very rare cancer, occurring in 1% to 2% of the population. The majority of vaginal cancers (85%) are squamous cell carcinoma. Vaginal cancer is associated with a personal history of maternal diethylstilbestrol use during pregnancy.

16. *Answer:* A

Rationale: Abdominal carcinomatosis is a common condition that occurs in late-stage abdominal malignancies. The ovarian cancer can spread to the peritoneum and grows rapidly throughout the abdominal cavity. This space-occupying lesion can cause uncomfortable abdominal swelling, weight gain, lower leg edema, shortness of breath, loss of appetite, nausea, fluid and electrolyte imbalance, malabsorption, constipation, and extreme fatigue. Bloating and constipation are not readily relieved with laxatives or other bowel regimens. Acute cholecystitis causes significant right upper quadrant pain and usually occurs after a meal, particularly a large meal. Crohn's disease is an inflammatory bowel disease that usually is diagnosed between the ages of 15 and 35 years of age. Metastatic disease from ovarian cancer usually occurs early in the disease and by direct extension into the bladder or the colon. This patient has had the disease for 4 years, so her symptoms do not likely represent metastatic disease to the colon.

17. *Answer:* B

Rationale: Intraperitoneal chemotherapy is administered through an intraperitoneal catheter directly into the peritoneal cavity and allows for the chemotherapy agents to come into direct contact with the tumor. It can cause more nausea because of the increased plasma level in the peritoneal cavity. Chemotherapeutic regimens are carefully calculated for disease status, drug efficacy, scheduled administration, and treatment tolerance. Dosing and frequency is not variable because of an intrapertioneal catheter. It is not administered at home.

18. *Answer:* B

Rationale: Risk factors for ovarian cancer include a personal history of breast, endometrial, or colon cancer;

a family history of Lynch syndrome, breast, endometrial, colon cancer, or *BRCA1* or *BRCA2* mutation; nulliparity; and infertility. Miscarriage is not a risk factor. The peak age for ovarian cancer incidence is age 60 to 64 years; ovarian cancer can also occur in premenopausal women commonly between the ages of 45 and 60 years. Serial CA-125 laboratory values along with transvaginal ultrasound are used as surveillance monitors in high-risk women. However a maternal history of CA-125 is not a documented risk factor.

19. *Answer:* A

Rationale: Gestational trophoblastic neoplasia (GTN) is a rare spectrum of oncology diseases that arise from the placental contents of the uterus. This disease group has the potential to metastasize to the lung, vagina, liver, and brain, not ovarian cancer. Treatment strategies include suctioning of the uterus to eliminate the mole and to preserve childbearing. If childbearing does not need to be preserved, a hysterectomy can be done. Chemotherapy is also extremely effective in managing GTN. Single-agent therapy with methotrexate or actinomycin-D is used in nonmetastatic or good-prognosis disease. If the patient receives chemotherapy as a treatment option, it is important to emphasize that the wife stay on treatment and follow the treatment course to completion. The couple will likely have concerns and questions regarding sexual intimacy and future birth control measures during and after treatment. Since the patient is more than 40 years old and has had one molar pregnancy, she is at high risk for a second. A regular pregnancy does not place someone at risk.

20. *Answer:* D

In general, when a patient wants to talk about a loss, the nurse's first objective is to listen. Suggesting a vacation that will help the patient "forget" belittles the pain that she is currently feeling. B and C are both disrespectful of the patient and chastise her unnecessarily. These choices also negate the loss and grief the patient feels. D acknowledges that the patient and her husband have experienced a devastating loss and that it is appropriate to weep and grieve but also shows confidence that they can overcome this and go forward.

21. *Answer:* B

Rationale: Pap smears are not a measurement of the length of time a patient has used oral contraceptives. Diethylstilbestrol use is a risk factor for cervical cancer and is not quantified by Pap smear results. Approximately 80% of cervical cancers are squamous cell carcinomas. However, closer examination and biopsy of the type of cancerous tissue would be determined by colposcopy, not a Pap smear.

22. *Answer:* A

Rationale: Testicular cancers commonly occur in men between the ages of 20 and 35 years. Risk factors include cryptorchidism (undescended testicle). Achondroplasia is short-limbed dwarfism and is not associated as a risk factor for testicular cancer. Seminomas occur in 50% of cases of testicular cancer; spread slowly, primarily through the lymphatics; and are responsive to radiation

therapy. Lynch syndrome is associated with an increased risk for colon, endometrial, and ovarian cancers.

23. *Answer:* A

Rationale: The cancer process affects the sperm, and clients may be sterile or subfertile at diagnosis. The likelihood of a successful pregnancy using sperm during or after chemotherapy treatment is markedly decreased or absent. Tumor markers should not be used as a determining factor in regard to timing of sperm banking.

CHAPTER 11

1. *Answer:* A

Rationale: Magnetic resonance imaging (MRI) is very useful in the evaluation of renal cell carcinoma in those patients for whom other radiologic tests were inconclusive, those who have significantly compromised renal function, and those who have a serious contrast allergy. If a patient had a large vascular mass, renal artery embolization may be considered. A KUB (kidneys, ureters, and bladder) radiograph is a basic radiograph showing the outline of kidneys, urethra, and bladder, not considered as diagnostically sound as MRI. Patients who have presented with low hemoglobin, low hematocrit, and hematuria often initially have intravenous pyelography ordered to determine the presence of a kidney stone.

2. *Answer:* C

Rationale: The role of radical nephrectomy has been challenged over the past decade because of equal oncologic efficacy compared with partial nephrectomy for tumors smaller than 4 cm. Thirty percent of patients have metastatic disease at diagnosis. Cytoreductive nephrectomy is used before systemic therapy in patients who have a surgically resectable primary with multiple metastatic sites. Active surveillance is considered in patients who have a limited life expectancy or those who have extensive comorbidities that put them at risk for more invasive treatments.

3. *Answer:* D

Rationale: Renal medullary carcinoma is a distinct type of renal cell cancer that occurs almost exclusively in children and young adults with sickle cell trait and sickle cell disease. The vast majority of patients are younger than 10 years old, and the male-to-female ratio is five to one. Papillary renal cell carcinoma comprises only 10% of cases. Clear cell carcinoma (also known as conventional or nonpapillary renal carcinoma) is the most common renal cell cancer overall, seen in 70% to 80% of cases. Chromophobe renal cell carcinoma only comprises 5% of cases.

4. *Answer:* B

Rationale: Cytoreductive nephrectomy is an option for patients who have T1 lesions and are not surgical candidates. Partial nephrectomy incurs less morbidity, is associated with less blood loss, and a shorter recovery time. Radiation therapy is not an effective treatment option in renal cell cancers. A partial nephrectomy is preferred in patients who may have limited renal function, have bilateral tumors, or have a solitary tumor.

5. *Answer:* C

Rationale: Although radical nephrectomy has been the primary method of treatment since 1960, partial nephrectomy is the preferred method of treatment, especially for patients with limited renal function.

6. *Answer:* D

Rationale: Kidney cancer comprises 3% of all cancers in the United States. There is an increased incidence because of improved detection with high-resolution imaging. Occupational risk factors include exposure to petroleum, heavy metals, and asbestos. Both incidence and mortality rates have increased since 1998.

7. *Answer:* A

Rationale: A radical nephrectomy is an invasive surgery. It has been the standard treatment since the 1960s. A partial nephrectomy is preferable to a radical nephrectomy, particularly in patients who have compromised renal function, bilateral tumors, or only one kidney. Cryosurgery and radiofrequency ablation is an option in patients with small lesions (T1) who are not surgical candidates. In this particular patient, active surveillance is the appropriate choice because he has limited support systems, challenged performance status, diabetes, cardiac comorbidities, and possible respiratory disease.

8. *Answer:* B

Rationale: Smoking is the most important risk factor in the development of bladder cancer, which occurs approximately four times as often in smokers than nonsmokers. Secondhand smoke is also associated with the development of bladder cancer. Coffee consumption of more than 5 cups a day is a moderate factor in men. Long-term use of acetaminophen is associated with renal cancer.

9. *Answer:* A

Rationale: The most common side effects after transurethral resection of bladder cancer (TURBT) are bleeding and infection. Urinary incontinence, urethral discharge, and passing of cloudy urine with sediment are possible but are not as commonly seen. Although patients also have issues concerning incontinence and urethral discharge, these are not common. Patients undergoing TURBT would not be expected to have cloudy urine containing sediment.

10. *Answer:* B

Rationale: The goals of treatment for non–muscle invasive bladder cancer are to prevent disease progression and invasion, avoid the loss of the bladder, and increase survival. Although comorbid conditions are of a concern and must be managed in any cancer patient, most patients who approach their late 60s and 70s have at least one comorbid condition and undergo treatment. Men should be followed for the risk of prostate cancer with prostate-specific antigen and digital rectal examination, but these do not reflect findings in bladder cancer.

11. *Answer:* C

Rationale: The ileal conduit would require a pouch or device for collecting urine through a stoma on the patient's abdomen. A double-barrel colostomy is used in patients with colon cancer, not bladder cancer. A radical cystectomy is removal of the bladder itself. The patient would likely prefer the continent ileal reservoir, as the "storage area" for the urine is located inside the abdominal wall. There is no appliance necessary, and urine is expressed only through self-catheterization.

12. *Answer:* C

Rationale: Blood cultures are not required as the patient does not have fever, has not received chemotherapy, and is not likely septic. Cystoscopy is not required at this time, however the groin swelling needs to be evaluated. A urine for cytology would examine cells from the lining of the bladder. Computed tomography (CT) of the abdomen and pelvis is required to determine lymph node metastasis.

13. *Answer:* C

Rationale: The 2013 guidelines from the U.S. Preventative Service Task Force do not recommend prostate-specific antigen (PSA) screening for men younger than 40 years of age. At-risk men 40 to 54 years of age may benefit from shared decision making with their physicians. Men 55 to 59 years old should definitely participate in shared decision making; screening is the most beneficial in this age group. PSA screening is not recommended for men older than 70 years of age or for those with life expectancy beyond <10-15 years. Digital rectal examination is not a good general assessment tool, but it can be used to assess for size, symmetry, lesions, and texture.

14. *Answer:* A

Rationale: Side effects of this surgery include incontinence, impotence, and postoperative hematuria. Incontinence occurs in 3% to 87% of men after radical prostatectomy. Myelosuppression is associated with chemotherapy, which is not an effective treatment for prostate cancer. Hot flashes, decreased libido, and elevated prostate-specific antigen are more often seen in advanced stages of prostate cancer. Cystitis and urethral strictures may occur after the surgery but are not as common as incontinence, impotence, and postoperative hematuria.

15. *Answer:* B

Rationale: The primary purpose of cystoscopy is to determine the presence of a tumor, location, size, and characteristics. Cystoscopy is not a tool to determine or measure urinary incontinence, nor would a cystoscopy be ordered for the sole purpose of collecting urine specimens.

16. *Answer:* D

Rationale: Digital rectal examination is an inexpensive and fairly easy diagnostic tool for prostate cancer, but DRE itself is not sufficient to make a diagnosis. DRE can help to assess symmetry of the gland, presence of nodules or texture of the gland, size, and any obvious lesions. The prostate gland can only be palpated on the lateral and posterior areas; large areas of the gland are inaccessible. Prostate-specific antigen is also a necessary screening procedure.

17. *Answer:* D

Rationale: It is unlikely that an exacerbation of the D.C.'s rheumatoid arthritis would cause immobility and urine retention. Chronic obstructive pulmonary disease can be a debilitating disease, but if this was the underlying problem, one would expect to see changes in his respiratory status. Neither D.C. nor his wife mentioned a fall. Patients who receive luteinizing hormone–releasing hormone can experience a flare-up of symptoms of prostate cancer, which can include bone pain, spinal cord compression, generalized fatigue, urinary symptoms, and even death in extreme cases.

18. *Answer:* A

Rationale: Eulexin (Flutamide) is an antiandrogen given orally, often in conjunction with luteinizing hormones such as Lupron, to prevent or reduce the risk of flare reactions. Dexamethasone is used in oncology care, usually to reduce pain, inflammation, and swelling. Leucovorin is used in the treatment of colorectal cancer; it is not indicated for use in patients with prostate cancer. Finasteride is an oral medication used in the treatment of benign prostatic hypertrophy and is not indicated for treatment of prostate cancer.

19. *Answer:* B

Rationale: Medical castration is used to control metastatic disease by decreasing the male hormone testosterone. Strontium is used in this patient population for bone pain caused by metastatic disease; it is not used to treat metastatic prostate cancer. Surgery and total-body radiation are not indicated in the treatment of advanced prostate cancer.

20. *Answer:* C

Rationale: Thirty percent of all male cancers are prostate cancers. The most common form is adenocarcinoma, comprising 95% of all prostate cancers. Sarcomas, mucinous or signet ring tumors, adenoid cystic carcinomas, and small cell undifferentiated cancers comprise the remaining 5%. Most prostate cancers develop in the peripheral zone. There is hematologic or lymphatic spread to the seminal vesicles, bladder, peritoneum, and pelvic lymph nodes. Bone metastasis usually takes place late in the disease process. Although metastatic spread to the lung is possible, local spread to the pelvic region is more likely. Survival rates for prostate cancer have increased since 1974.

21. *Answer:* D

Rationale: Transrectal ultrasonography is usually used as a guide in biopsy of the prostate gland. B.K. had a biopsy at diagnosis and is not complaining of any symptoms similar to urinary blockage, pelvic swelling, or edema. The most recent prostate-specific antigen (PSA) was drawn within the past few days; there is no need to repeat the test this at this time. Although the normal range for PSA varies by age, race, and prostate size, 0 to 4 ng/nl is considered the standard norm. B.K.'s result is well above the norm. Magnetic resonance imaging of the pelvis would be more useful in determining local penetration of the prostate cancer into the regional lymph nodes in the pelvis and seminal vesicles. The symptoms that the patient describes, along with his elevated PSA level, indicate that he may have developed metastatic disease to the bone, which would be best evaluated by bone scan.

22. *Answer:* C

Rationale: More than 75% of all prostate cancers are diagnosed in men 65 years or older. The mortality rate from prostate cancer is higher in developed than in developing countries. The highest incidence and mortality rates are among African Americans. There are genetic factors related to prostate cancer, such as hereditary prostate cancer-1(HPC-1) and some genetic mutations associated with breast cancer (*BRCA1* and *BRCA2*). There are tentative links with dietary factors. High-fat diets may promote prostate cancer. Diets high in vitamins E and D and selenium may inhibit or prevent prostate cancer. Diets high in lycopene are linked with a low incidence of prostate cancer. Prostate-specific antigen is a valuable tool in diagnosing and monitoring the progression of prostate cancer.

23. *Answer:* B

Rationale: At this point in time, it is not relevant to either provide literature on prostate cancer screening or to ask about his last prostate cancer screening. It is also premature to speak to the patient about hospice or wills. A visit by the orthopedic surgeon would have been requested as a consult and is important in EW's plan of care, but discharge planning is not an important initial intervention. The nurse should provide answers to the patient's questions and allow him to verbalize his feelings (perhaps with social work as an adjunct). The patient should be encouraged to report any symptoms and be assured that he will be made comfortable and that his pain will be managed.

24. *Answer:* D

Rationale: Gleason scores are a system of grading prostate cancer tissue and range from 2-10. The score indicates how likely the tumor is to spread. A low Gleason score means the cancer tissue is very similar to normal prostate tissue and is less likely to spread. A high Gleason score indicates that the cancer tissue is very different from normal prostate tissue and is likely to invade other areas. The Gleason score does not indicate how responsive the prostate cancer tissue will be to radiation or hormonal therapy.

CHAPTER 12

1. *Answer:* B

Rationale: Current practice is to obtain a sentinel lymph node biopsy in patients who have primary melanoma larger than 1 mm thick or those smaller than 1 mm thick that demonstrate adverse pathologic features such as ulceration or mitosis.

2. *Answer:* D

Rationale: Basal cell carcinoma starts in the basal cell layer of the epidermis. It is caused by a combination of cumulative ultraviolet (UV) exposure and intense, occasional UV exposure. Squamous cell cancer is caused by cumulative UV exposure over the lifetime, begins in the squamous cells in the epidermis, and has increased in incidence in women younger than the age of 40 years by 700% in the past 30 years. Melanoma arises from malignant proliferation of melanocytes, pigment-producing cells that originate in the neural crest and migrate to the skin. Overall, it is less common than basal cell or squamous cell carcinoma. Basal cell cancer is common in older adults, but the age at diagnosis is steadily decreasing. Melanoma is the most common form of cancer in young adults and the second most common form of cancer in those age 15 to 29 years.

3. *Answer:* A

Rationale: Superficial basal cell cancers are most commonly found on the trunk and typically present as a bright red to pink, often scaly, patch. Lesions are slow to progress. Micronodular basal cell cancers are an aggressive subtype; they may appear yellow to white when stretched. Nodular basal cell cancers most often appear on the neck and head and comprise 50% to 80% of all basal cell cancers; they typically appear as a round, pink, pearly, flesh colored papule with a depressed center. They often have telangiectasis (dilation of small blood vessels) within the lesion. Pigmented basal cell cancers are more common in darker pigmented individuals.

4. *Answer:* B

Rationale: The Breslow depth determines the depth of invasion of the melanoma, measured in millimeters. It is one of the most important prognostic features in localized melanoma. Lymph node involvement is determined by a sentinel lymph node biopsy, not by a biopsy of the lesion. The presence of telangiectasias occurs most often with basal cell cancers, not with melanoma. Examining the irregular borders is an important factor in screening, but the need to biopsy is not solely determined by the irregularity.

5. *Answer:* A

Rationale: The choice of biopsy technique depends on the size, location, and shape of the lesion.

6. *Answer:* A

Rationale: The involved lymph node requires dissection. The lymph node basin may or may not contain 12 lymph nodes. Radiation therapy is a treatment option but is not a tool for diagnosis and staging. Although the surgical excision of the melanoma lesion will likely be part of the treatment plan, doing so at this point and ignoring the results of the sentinel lymph node biopsy results does not address the potential metastatic characteristics of this lesion. There is not a standard criterion of leaving 5-mm margins.

7. *Answer:* A

Rationale: The most important factors in treatment decision making are the size and location of the lesion and whether it is a primary or recurrent lesion. A recurrent lesion points to the aggressiveness of the cancer. Perineural invasion is a rare complication that is more common in recurrent tumors. The physician should be involved with education and discussion of treatment plans, but the ultimate decision is the patient's. Many factors (e.g., patient's overall health, immune status) should be taken into consideration when planning treatment, but diabetic status is not the most important factor in treatment planning.

8. *Answer:* B

Rationale: A history of chronic exposure to ultraviolet radiation is important in the assessment of persons presenting with nonmelanoma skin cancers (NMSCs). Those at highest risk for the development of NMSCs are whites with a chronic exposure to ultraviolet radiation. A 60-year-old white grain farmer would have a longer cumulative exposure to ultraviolet light than a 35-year-old white ski instructor. Mexican Americans and African Americans have significant cumulative ultraviolet radiation exposure but have a slightly reduced risk of having skin cancer because of their skin types.

9. *Answer:* A

Rationale: Basal cell carcinoma is the most common form of skin cancer. In the United States, approximately 2.8 million cases are reported each year.

10. *Answer:* C

Rationale: Self-skin examination should start with the head and end with the feet but only needs to be done approximately every 3 months. Skin cancers can be dangerous and yet painless; a suspicious spot should not be ignored just because it does not hurt. The most common forms of skin cancer are basal cell, squamous cell, and malignant melanoma.

11. *Answer:* B

Rationale: The ABCDEs of melanoma recognition are asymmetry (one half is unlike the other), border (irregular, scalloped, or uneven border), color (more than one color present), diameter (larger than 6 mm), and enlarging (changing over time).

12. *Answer:* C

Rationale: Systematic assessment of the skin at regular intervals by a physician or a nurse is important because malignant melanoma is the most aggressive and virulent type of skin cancer. Monthly self-examination of the skin is taught and recommended for those who have had skin cancer. D is incorrect because protective clothing, sunscreen, and sun blocks are important year round, not just during the warm, sunny summer months.

13. *Answer:* B

Rationale: Superficial spreading melanomas (SSMs) comprise approximately 60% to 70% of malignant melanomas. It is the most common melanoma in fair-skinned individuals. In SSM, the lesions are asymmetrical, poorly circumscribed, often with notching and scalloping. Only 25% occur in association with a preexisting nevus, the remainder arise de novo (as a new lesion). SSMs usually start as a brown to black macule.

14. *Answer:* A

Rationale: Patients should be educated regarding all types of skin cancer, but some people are at higher risk for squamous cell cancer. These include persons with HIV disease and other immunodeficiency diseases, those who experience chronic infections, use chemotherapy or other antirejection drugs, and those who have had excessive sun exposure. Actinic keratosis are rough scaly patches that develop on the skin of the face, lips, ears, hands, scalp, and forearms after years of sun exposure.

15. *Answer:* D

Rationale: There is a possible link between severe sunburn in childhood and the risk of malignant melanoma in later life. Children should be protected from traumatic sunburn, and it is advisable to keep infants out of the sun.

16. *Answer:* C

Rationale: Metastasectomy is reserved for those with solitary metastases to multiple metastases to the lung, distant lymph nodes, or gastrointestinal tract with long disease-free intervals.

17. *Answer:* D

Rationale: Although all of the standard therapies may be used during the course of treatment for skin cancer, excision is used 90% of the time. In the treatment of malignant melanoma in particular, it may be necessary to remove nearby lymph glands, although this is controversial.

18. *Answer:* A

Rationale: Exposure to ultraviolet radiation should be limited between 10 am and 3 pm in high-intensity sun areas. Sunscreens (SPF of 15 or greater, reapplied regularly) and protective clothing and sunglasses are recommended during prolonged sun exposure. All of these are important in teaching about the prevention of skin cancers. B, C, and D are related to risk assessment and early detection activities, not prevention.

19. *Answer:* B

Rationale: Acral lentiginous melanoma is commonly found in persons of African, Asian, and Hispanic descent.

20. *Answer:* E

Rationale: Risk factors for melanoma include a personal history or family history of melanoma, the number of moles (typical and atypical), ultraviolet exposure, fair skin, red or blonde hair, freckling, immunosuppression, advanced age, genetics, and gender (women have higher incidence rates than men).

21. *Answer:* D

Rationale: The risk of death from cutaneous melanoma is determined mainly by the thickness of the tumor, as described by Breslow's depth, the presence or absence of tumor ulceration, and microdeposits of melanoma in sentinel lymph nodes. Micrometastases from primary tumors migrate through the lymphatics to the regional lymph nodes. Malignant melanoma can occur on almost any skin or surface in the body, including conjunctiva, mucosa of the oral, genital or rectal regions. Malignant melanoma accounts for 5% of skin cancers diagnosed in the United States but is also responsible for the majority of deaths due to skin cancer.

22. *Answer:* B

Rationale: Prevention of skin cancer starts with properly protecting the skin from exposure to the sun. Applying sunscreen properly, limiting exposure during periods of strongest sunlight (especially between 10 a.m. and 4 p.m.), and using a sunscreen with a high SPF value are all important steps in skin cancer prevention. A baseball cap only protects part of the face and not the neck. No tan is safe, so a base tan is not recommended.

23. *Answer:* D

Rationale: A sunscreen's SPF is a measurement of how long unprotected skin can be exposed to ultraviolet rays before burning compared with how long it takes to burn without protection. Sunscreens must be properly applied for full protection.

CHAPTER 13

1. *Answer:* C

Rationale: Although there are a variety of environmental allergens that we can be exposed to, patients who experience allergy symptoms are usually bothered for a period of 1 week to 10 days, while the allergen is blooming. Most people who have allergy symptoms experience swollen or itchy eyes or sneezing. Patients with allergies do not usually present with a sore throat from presumed postnasal drip. It would be unusual for the patient's symptoms to be caused by his radiation exposure 5 years earlier because he was not experiencing these symptoms until 3 months ago. Symptoms of strep throat infection usually consist of a sudden severe sore throat accompanied by coughing, sneezing, fever, and other cold symptoms. Those diagnosed with head and neck cancer are at an increased risk to develop other primary tumors in the region because of the prolonged exposure to carcinogens. The most likely cause of J.M.'s sore throat is a new primary malignancy in the head and neck area.

2. *Answer:* B

Rationale: Helicobacter pylori infection is a bacterial infection biopsied from stomach mucosa. It is not known to be a risk factor for head and neck cancer. A history of herpes zoster is the cause of shingles and usually occurs in those who have had chicken pox. Occupational exposures to petroleum, asphalt paving, and painting supplies are linked to risk of several cancers but not head and neck cancers. Lactose intolerance and gluten allergies are not currently known to cause any type of cancer. Human papillomavirus infections, heavy alcohol use, and all forms of tobacco use are linked to head and neck cancers.

3. *Answer:* D

Rationale: Tobacco use increases the risk of developing head and neck cancer 25-fold. Excessive alcohol intake increases the risk of developing oral or pharyngeal cancer 9-fold.

4. *Answer:* A

Rationale: In a hemilaryngectomy there is vertical excision of one true and one false cord as well as the underlying cartilage. The patient will be able to speak, but the voice may be hoarse. The patient should have no or minimal problems swallowing. There are exercises that could improve voice quality, pitch, and loudness. A complete laryngectomy leaves the patient aphonic, without a voice. The hemilaryngectomy does impact phonation. The patient will not have her previous, preoperative voice. Patients who undergo a hemilaryngectomy usually have a temporary tracheostomy, not a permanent tracheostomy. Discussing a tracheostomy as being unsightly and telling the patient to retire are not appropriate.

5. *Answer:* C

Rationale: Chemotherapy alone is not curative for head and neck cancers. The chemotherapy is believed to reduce tumor volume and can remove clinically detectable squamous cell carcinomas. Chemotherapy is given intravenously. It is a systemic therapy and does not stay localized in the lymph nodes. Numerous protocols combine radiation and chemotherapy, and they are used concurrently with radiation therapy, not afterward. Several chemotherapeutic agents have been used such as cisplatinum, Blenoxane, 5-fluorouracil, Taxol, and methotrexate. Chemotherapy acts to sensitize the cells to radiation. It is used as adjuvant or neoadjuvant therapy; single agents or a combination of agents have been used.

6. *Answer:* C

Rationale: The patient is having a total laryngectomy. After surgery, he will have a tracheostomy, which will be permanent. His recovery is very involved. The tracheostomy collar will be used for several weeks while swelling subsides and the stoma heals. He will not be going home within 24 hours after surgery. His care may require postoperative mechanical ventilation and intensive care placement. The patient will not be able to communicate verbally. It would not be safe for the patient to be placed in a room at the end of the hall; he needs to be close to the nurse's station. There is concern about his lack of ability to notify staff if he has a problem, and nursing staff will need to check on him frequently to see that his tracheostomy tube is securely in place. Because of his history of alcoholism, he could experience confusion delirium tremens and may require readily accessible observation and care.

7. *Answer:* D

Rationale: The patient should be closely observed, but it is not required that he be suctioned every hour postoperatively. Although coughing and attempting to raise secretions orally may aid in clearing his upper airway and oral cavity, it will not clear his airway because his airway is now via the tracheostomy. Suction catheters should always be inserted cautiously. Accumulation of crusty secretions should be prevented. Tracheostomy care and cleaning is used to clear away those secretions that are otherwise a source of infection and delayed wound healing. Suctioning is an essential part of the patient's care and should be provided as needed.

8. *Answer:* B

Rationale: Postoperative care includes all of these procedures and considerations. But those specific to wound care consist of assessing the surgical wound every 3 to 4 hours, noting the color, temperature, and capillary refill of the skin and muscle flaps; assessing for and avoiding excessive pressure; and assessing for integrity of internal (if applicable) and external suture lines as breakdown can be an indication of infection or formation of fistula.

9. *Answer:* A

Rationale: Assessing for nutritional status is very important because 60% of surgical patients with head and neck cancer initially present with malnutrition.

10. *Answer:* D

Rationale: To swallow food, the bolus moves through the pharynx and is propelled through the esophagus; the vocal cords close; and the larynx moves upward and forward, preventing aspiration.

11. *Answer:* C

Rationale: Indentation in the mouth and oral cavity is usually caused by a mechanical trauma or pressure to the oral mucosa. Fungal infections can occur after chemotherapy and are related to the immunosuppressive effects of the agents. Allergic reactions are typically systemic or regional. The oral mucosa has a high cell turnover rate and is home to diverse and complex microflora. Therefore, the mucosa, when treated, is very susceptible to treatment-related toxic side effects. Oral mucositis (also called stomatitis) is an inflammation of the mouth and throat lining. It is a frequent side effect of radiation treatments in clients with head and neck cancer, as well as a reaction to some chemotherapy treatments.

12. *Answer:* A

Rationale: The patient will likely receive a tracheostomy tube during the course of his radical neck dissection, but the purpose of the radical neck dissection is to remove cancerous masses, lesions, and lymph nodes. A percutaneous endoscopic gastrostomy tube, J tube, or G tube for nutritional support is often considered for patients with head and neck cancer, but these are not usually placed during a radical neck dissection. Head and neck cancer often spreads beyond the lymph nodes encountered in a head and neck resection. Tumors can be very large and invade adjacent tissue early in the disease process. At the time of initial diagnosis, 43% have nodal involvement and 10% have distant metastasis, most commonly to the lung, liver, or bone. The radical neck dissection cannot completely stop the spread of head and neck cancers.

13. *Answer:* D

Rationale: The 1-year survival rate for oral and pharyngeal cancers is 84%. All stages of laryngeal cancers have a 60% to 90% 5-year survival rate if localized at diagnosis. Thyroid cancer's overall 5-year survival rate is 98%. There is a 2% to 3% decrease in new cases of laryngeal cancer per year, most likely because of fewer people smoking.

14. *Answer:* A

Rationale: Panoramic radiography is a tool dentists use. It is possible that a panoramic radiography could reveal a tumor, but these radiographs are not considered a screening tool. Oral examinations are recommended and should be done every 3 years for persons between the ages of 20 and 40 years and every year for people older than 40 years but are not currently considered screening tools for head and neck cancer. Although a thorough patient history regarding one's digestive tract, dietary preferences, and practices is an important tool for assessing a patient's nutritional status and pinpointing areas of concern, it is not a screening tool for head and neck cancer. At this point in time, there are no definitive screening practices suggested for early detection of head and neck cancer.

15. *Answer:* A

Rationale: Xerostomia is a side effect of radiation treatments concerning a reduction in saliva production.

This leads to decreased lubrication of the food bolus, which will impact one's ability to swallow and taste changes. Hypoxemia refers to an abnormally low oxygen content in the blood; it can occur during suctioning or can occur due to an airway blockage, which requires suctioning. *Phonation* is a term referring to the rapid periodic opening and closing, separation, and apposition of the glottis through the vocal cords to create speech. Dysphonia is a voice impairment.

16. *Answer:* B

Rationale: The immunosuppressive side effects of radiation and chemotherapy treatments do place the patient at risk for opportunistic infection but not for malignancy. Human papilloma virus-16 is associated with oropharyngeal cancers but has not been linked specifically to an increase risk of developing additional primary tumors. Petroleum products are not a known risk factor for head and neck cancers and in particular not for additional primary tumors. Patients diagnosed with head and neck cancer are at an increased risk to develop other primary tumors because of prolonged exposure of the mucosal surface to carcinogens.

17. *Answer:* D

Rationale: For nasopharyngeal cancers, surgery is avoided because of the close proximity to vital structures of the brain. For any of the head and neck cancers, chemotherapy alone is not curative. It can be used to reduce tumor volume and as treatment for recurrent or metastatic disease. Seed implantation with brachytherapy is an option for lesions on the posterior and anterior of the tongue, floor of the mouth, and the nasal vestibule. Radiation therapy is the primary treatment of choice for nasopharyngeal cancer. Only carefully selected patients who have treatment failure with radiotherapy may be treated with base of the skull resection of the tumor.

18. *Answer:* C

Rationale: Patients with both human papillomavirus (HPV)-positive and HPV-negative oropharyngeal cancer can receive targeted therapies combined with radiation therapy. The patients who are HPV positive have a better prognosis than patients with HPV-negative oropharyngeal cancers. HPV-positive patients are able to receive less intense treatments. It is believed that these targeted therapies work by blocking the growth factor–based cellular signaling and interfering with angiogenesis-related pathways.

19. *Answer:* A

Rationale: Temporary tracheostomies are usually placed in the operating room and maintained for a minimum of 5 days. When patients receive a tracheostomy, it is usually one with a cuff tube inserted. The cuff gets inflated if the patient is on mechanical ventilation or if there is danger of aspiration. The physician usually changes the initial tracheostomy tube from a cuffed to a noncuffed version, not the nurse. If the patient is aspirating, a cuffed tube will remain in place. As the swelling and edema subside, the patient may be able to breathe without the tracheostomy tube. The

tracheostomy tube is downsized to a number 4 or 5 fenestrated tube and plugged for 24 hours. If the patient can breathe with the tube plugged for a prolonged period of time and can expectorate secretions through the mouth, the patient's cannula can be removed. Humidification will still be important for this patient and all patients with temporary tracheostomies to prevent mucus drying and crusting of secretions. Humidity also prevents secretions from becoming thick and tenacious, making it difficult to expectorate.

20. *Answer:* A

Rationale: Patients should be considered for nutritional support if they have greater than 10% body weight loss during any phase of treatment or if they are more than 20% below ideal body weight.

21. *Answer:* A

Rationale: Esophageal speech, a tracheoesophageal prosthesis, is a method of communicating after having a total laryngectomy. This patient had a partial laryngectomy. She has the ability to speak but needs to strengthen her muscles and vocal cords with exercises provided by the speech therapist.

22. *Answer:* A

Rationale: Signs and symptoms of cancer of the oral cavity are white or red patches on the gums, tongue. Swelling of the jaw that may cause dentures to fit poorly; and unusual bleeding or pain in the mouth. Sinuses are blocked sinuses, as well as chronic sinus infections that do not respond to antibiotics, are signs and symptoms of cancer of the nasal cavity and sinuses. A sign and symptom of cancer of salivary glands is swelling under the chin or around the jawbone.

23. *Answer:* A

Rationale: Aspiration is a major risk after a supraglottic laryngectomy. Most patients maintain a relatively normal voice.

CHAPTER 14

1. *Answer:* C

Rationale: The main structures of the brain are the cerebrum, cerebellum, and brainstem. The brainstem is located at the base of the brain and top of the spinal cord. It connects the cerebrum with the spinal cord. The cerebrum is the large outer part of the brain, two hemispheres comprising four lobes (frontal, occipital, parietal, and temporal). The cerebellum is located in the posterior fossa at the back of the head.

2. *Answer:* B

Rationale: Epstein-Barr virus is known to be a risk factor for central nervous system (CNS) lymphoma. The Anopheles B virus can cause malaria, septicemia, and gastroenteritis. The macropodid herpes virus affects kangaroos. Human papilloma virus is responsible for several sexually transmitted diseases in humans and is associated with some non-CNS cancers.

3. *Answer:* D

Rationale: Although there are suggested limits to the amount of radiation that technicians and radiologists should be exposed to during the course of their work, patients and the public rarely come into contact with significant amounts of radiation to put them at risk. In children younger than the age of 10 years, the use of Panorex dental radiographs is associated with an increased risk of meningioma.

4. *Answer:* B

Rationale: The Circle of Willis connects the anterior and posterior arteries if blood flow to single vessels is blocked off. The dural sinuses, also known as the cerebral sinuses or the cranial sinuses, are venous channels formed between the layers or dura mater in the brain. Ependymal cells are a type of neuronal support cell that forms the epithelial lining of the ventricles and the central canal of the spinal cord. The Broca area is one of the main areas of the cerebral cortex responsible for producing language.

5. *Answer:* A

Rationale: Meningiomas arise from the meninges of the brain and (more commonly) the spinal cord. The common symptoms are related to the pressure the tumor causes on the brain, such as headache and vision changes, or on the spinal cord, such as paresthesia.

6. *Answer:* A

Rationale: The hypothalamus regulates the sleep–wake cycle, body temperature, water balance, appetite, blood pressure, and coordination of all patterns of activity. The cerebellum is responsible for coordination, balance, and muscle tone. The temporal lobe maintains hearing, memory of what is heard and seen, and word recognition. The parietal lobe integrates sensory input, visual and tactile perception, and memory.

7. *Answer:* C

Rationale: Known intrinsic risk factors for central nervous system (CNS) tumors relate to gender, age, and ethnicity. Men are at higher risk for glioma; women have a higher risk of meningioma. Children and elderly adults are at higher risk. Whites and those of Northern European descent have increased risk, and African Americans have the highest risk for CNS tumors.

8. *Answer:* C

Rationale: Primary brain tumors are not classified according to the tumor, node, metastasis system because two of the three criteria measured essentially do not exist—nodes and extracranial metastases. Primary brain tumors can be diagnosed early. The Hooper Crane Staging Criteria does not exist. The Ann Arbor Staging system is used in lymphomas. The grading of brain tumors is based on the histologic appearance defined by the World Health Organization.

9. *Answer:* C

Rationale: The most important prognostic factors for primary brain tumors are the size of the lesion, whether it is a single or multifocal lesion, the location of the lesion, and the degree of malignancy. These same criteria would apply to persons with an astrocytoma or primitive neuroectodermal cell tumors. The degree of confusion or personality changes often alert family members to the presence of a new illness or condition; they are not prognostic indicators. Substances such as vinyl chlorides, petro chemicals, pesticides, inks, solvents, hair dyes, and dietary N-nitrose compounds are being investigated as risk factors for brain and central nervous system tumors but are not prognostic factors.

10. *Answer:* A

Rationale: Lung cancer is the most frequent source of brain metastases in men and women, and more than 90% of patients with lung cancer will develop brain metastases; therefore, they are very common. Metastases from lung cancer to the brain usually develop within 1 year of diagnosis. Metastatic disease in women with breast cancer often develops in the brain within 2 to 3 years of diagnosis but is not as common as brain metastases caused by lung cancer.

11. *Answer:* C

Rationale: All of the choices are positive outcomes of surgical resection for brain tumors. The surgery can allow for obtaining a tissue sample. The mass effect of the tumor—size, pressure, and swelling—causes symptoms (headaches, vision changes, pain) that can be reduced (not necessarily eliminated) by the surgery. In reducing the symptoms and the swelling, neurologic function is usually preserved. Future treatments are easier because the amount of tumor burden is reduced.

12. *Answer:* D

Rationale: Although computed tomography or magnetic resonance imaging could assess for the development of hydrocephalus, an intracranial bleed, tissue inflammation, and infection, the primary use is to assess for residual tumor burden and establish a baseline for treatment.

13. *Answer:* A

Rationale: A lumbar puncture, also called a spinal tap, is a diagnostic tool that could be used to determine the presence of any of the choices. In this case, however, the most likely reason for the patient's headache, confusion, and upper extremity numbness is metastatic disease to the central nervous system (CNS). Melanoma has the highest predilection to metastasize to the CNS, and this metastasis is usually associated with a poorer prognosis than other types of brain metastases.

14. *Answer:* B

Rationale: Computed tomography (CT) without contrast is helpful in the emergency department at initial presentation to decipher between a stroke and an intracranial or spinal cord tumor. The patient needs to be evaluated and stabilized quickly. CT without contrast is readily available in most communities, eliminates the risk of reaction to the contrast material, is less expensive than magnetic resonance imaging, and is most appropriate for diagnosing spinal metastases in some areas and to evaluate bony metastases. CT is also the modality of choice for patients who have metallic devices such as ports, implants, or pacemakers who would be unable to use magnetic resonance imaging. After the patient is stabilized, the examination could be repeated with contrast, which is optimal for visualizing malignant tumors. A radioisotope bone scan is used to evaluate the entire skeleton for the presence of multiple metastatic bone lesions. Plain radiographs are used to determine bone reabsorption and repair showing osteoblastic, osteolytic, and mixed lesions as well as defining the bone anatomy.

15. *Answer:* C

Rationale: The subacute effects of radiation therapy for brain tumors usually occur 4 to 6 months after radiation. These can appear as somnolence and exacerbation of previous tumor-related symptoms. The radiation therapy treatments can cause radiation-induced demyelination, inflammation, altered capillary permeability, and radionecrosis, all of which are subacute effects. Patients with spinal cord tumors are more likely to develop hydrocephalus. Focal seizures can occur at any time in patients who have brain tumors, but they are more often an acute effect during and immediately after radiation therapy.

16. *Answer:* D

Rationale: Radio-induced demyelination occurs in the white matter of the brain near the margins of radiation treatments and can cause cognitive deficits and headaches. Radiation necrosis is a serious complication of intracranial radiation that occurs 1-3 years after treatment is complete. Symptoms are produced by localized brain necrosis, depending on the location of the lesion. Global effects are the broad range of cognitive deficits that patients experience with radiation treatments. Pseudoprogression of the tumor refers to the symptoms caused by radiation therapy but may be mistaken for signs of tumor regrowth.

17. *Answer:* B

Rationale: High-grade astrocytomas infiltrate surrounding brain tissue and are usually not encapsulated. They rarely metastasize outside the central nervous system. Most chemotherapy agents do not cross the blood–brain barrier and are therefore not efficacious in treating astrocytomas.

18. *Answer:* B

Rationale: The patient was recently prescribed warfarin, an anticoagulant, and is complaining of a worsening headache. He is at risk for a cerebral hemorrhage, and a noncontrast enhanced computed tomography is used to evaluate for hemorrhage. It is the faster study of choice in patients being evaluated for trauma or acute neurologic disorders. Although the direction and velocity of blood flow in the brain can be detected by ultrasonography, the ultrasound waves do not pass through bone easily, so it is not a preferred test on adults. A myelogram is not a diagnostic test for intracranial bleeding.

19. *Answer:* D

Rationale: The functions of the occipital lobe include sight and visual identification of objects. The parietal lobe controls sensory input such as pain and temperature. The frontal lobe controls personality, mood, and intellect. The temporal lobe controls hearing, memory, and receptive speech.

20. *Answer:* A

Rationale: Some primary brain tumors become more aggressive or malignant over time. It is common for patients to undergo second and third craniotomies to restage the tumor, evaluate treatment decision making, or provide symptom control. Craniotomies are performed to remove or debulk tumors as part of an effort to improve treatment outcomes and provide symptom control. The amount of tumor removed varies depending on the individual patient's comorbidities, surgical risk factors, and what can be safely accessed at the time. It is rare for primary brain tumors to metastasize outside of the central nervous system; therefore, a craniotomy would not be performed to reduce metastatic spread to the lung. Vascular access devices are not placed via a craniotomy.

21. *Answer:* A

Rationale: Temodar (Temozolomide) is an oral second-generation alkylating agent that can permeate the blood–brain barrier. Temodar with radiation therapy is standard of care for high-grade gliomas and may be used as monotherapy in lower grade tumors. Trileptal (oxcarbazepine) is used to treat partial seizures in adults and children. Tarceva (Erlotinib) is first-line treatment, maintenance, and second- and third-line treatment of advanced non–small cell lung cancer. Topotecan (Hycamtin) is used in ovarian, cervical, and small cell lung cancer.

22. *Answer:* D

Rationale: This patient is in an emergent situation because of a sudden increase in intracranial pressure affecting her respiratory center. Mannitol has osmotic properties necessary to rapidly reduce the brain edema that developed because of leakage of plasma into the brain parenchyma through the malfunction of the cerebral capillaries. It is considered a last resort emergent measure. Glucocorticoids are also used to manage acute cerebral edema as well as managing the edema created by extradural spinal lesions causing compression of the spinal cord; however, these agents do not act as rapidly as intravenous mannitol infusion. Temodar is a first-line glioma treatment that can permeate the blood-brain barrier but is not used to reduce intracranial pressure. A high-dose methotrexate-based regimen is used to treat the central nervous system lymphoma, which in turn would optimistically improve the cerebral edema; however, methotrexate is not a first-line therapy for cerebral edema.

23. *Answer:* A

Rationale: Almost half of all malignant tumors arise from astrocytes, star-shaped cells that support the neurons of the central nervous system. Epithelial cells are present in many parts of the body and help protect organs. Mast cells (mastocytes) are found throughout the body and are part of the immune system. Glial cells are supportive cells in the central nervous system. They do not conduct electrical impulses.

24. *Answer:* B

Rationale: Given this patient's history, the most important nursing assessment is bowel and bladder function. Dysfunction in this area or deterioration of the lower extremity motor and sensory function could indicate spinal cord compression, requiring emergency intervention.

25. *Answer:* C

Rationale: Stereotactic radiosurgery uses the same type of head frame that is used for stereotactic biopsy. This allows the radiation to be focused on the tumor. The radiation is delivered in several arcs so that the tumor receives the full dose, but normal tissues are spared. Standard conventional radiation is generally given over 6 to 7 weeks. Brachytherapy involves implantation of radioactive seeds into the tumor bed, and these are left in place for 3 or 4 days. Fractionated stereotactic radiotherapy uses an adjustable stereotactic frame so that several focused fractions can be delivered over several days.

CHAPTER 15

1. *Answer:* A

Rationale: Almost 90% of leukemia is diagnosed in adults. The most common type of leukemia in children and teens is acute lymphocytic leukemia, accounting for 75% of the cases. In adults, the most common leukemia diagnoses are chronic lymphocytic leukemia and acute myelogenous leukemia.

2. *Answer:* C

Rationale: Risk factors for leukemia include previous treatment with radiation, exposure to radiation such as in Hiroshima, and exposure to radiation in the work setting. Additional risk factors include previous treatment with alkylating agents or medications such as chloramphenicol and work exposure to chemicals such as benzene, formaldehyde, Agent Orange, arsenic-containing pesticides, and Triazine herbicides. Alcohol, gasoline and petroleum products, coal tars, and paving blacktop materials are not known risk factors for leukemia.

3. *Answer:* D

Rationale: In patients with chronic lymphocytic leukemia, one of the heralding diagnostic criteria is the presence of more than 5×10^9 B lymphocytes (5000/µL) in the peripheral blood for at least 3 months. A diagnostic criterion for acute lymphoblastic leukemia is the presence of greater than 20% of myeloid blasts in the marrow. To confirm a diagnosis of chronic myelogenous leukemia, bone marrow biopsy is done and must show the presence of the Philadelphia Ph1 chromosome (BRC-ABL). Acute lymphoblastic leukemia in adults will display the presence of greater than 20% lymphoblasts in the marrow, and 25% of adults will have the + Ph (Philadelphia) chromosome.

4. *Answer:* B

Rationale: Symptoms related to bone marrow failure are recurrent infections from neutropenia and bleeding; easy bruising from thrombocytopenia; and fatigue, weakness, and shortness of breath from anemia. Lymphadenopathy; bone pain from increased pressure in bone marrow; early satiety, fullness, and abdominal discomfort secondary to splenomegaly and hepatomegaly; and seizures caused by central nervous system involvement are

symptoms related to organ and lymphatic infiltration by leukemic cells.

5. *Answer:* D

Rationale: The Modified Rai Staging System for chronic lymphocytic leukemia defines risk or extent of disease as low, intermediate, or high. There is no medium category. Those with lymphocytosis (lymphoid cells >30%); no lymphadenopathy, splenomegaly, or hepatomegaly, are considered low. The intermediate level is defined by lymphocytosis; lymphadenopathy in any site, splenomegaly, or hepatomegaly. In both the low and intermediate levels, red blood cell and platelet counts are near normal. A high level is associated with lymphocytosis; presence of anemia (hemoglobin <11 g/dL) or thrombocytopenia (platelet count <100 $\times$ 10⁹/L), with or without lymphadenopathy, splenomegaly, or hepatomegaly. M.F.'s lymphocytes are greater than 6000, which indicates a more than 30% of the total white blood cell count percentage. He has thrombocytopenia, with the platelet count below 100,000. He has two sites of lymphadenopathy, the groin and axilla area, and he is having early satiety, which is likely caused by splenomegaly.

6. *Answer:* B

Rationale: The recurrent infections that M.F. is experiencing are related to the neutropenia caused by his chronic lymphocytic leukemia. His blood white cells do not possess the ability to ward off infections. Previous tuberculosis can infect any organ, but the symptoms do not fit M.F.'s situation. Chronic sinusitis will display symptoms related to acute sinusitis but to a lesser degree, such as purulent or nonpurulent nasal drainage, rhinorrhea, postnasal drip, nasal blockage, or the sensation of swelling in the nasal passages. An individual's exposure to secondhand smoke can present itself as eye irritation, headache, increased nasal secretions, nasal congestion, headache, and cough.

7. *Answer:* D

Rationale: Side effects related to corticosteroids include weight gain caused by sodium and water retention (see pages 288-290).

8. *Answer:* B

Rationale: Patients with acute myelogenous leukemia (AML) produce an abundance of immature white blood cells, which can crowd the marrow and peripheral bloodstream and compromise the function of the red blood cells. These patients can experience early satiety, easy bruising, and gingival or nose bleeds. Enlarged lymph nodes are not a hallmark sign of AML but can be seen with the lymphocytic leukemias such as chronic lymphocytic leukemia (CLL) or acute lymphoblastic leukemia (ALL). Whereas patients with CLL can describe having repeating infections, those with AML may present with an initial overwhelming systemic infection. ALL, which is most common in young children, often produces bony pain, fever, night sweats, and fatigue.

9. *Answer:* A

Rationale: A bone marrow biopsy with a wide range of cytogenetic testing is considered an essential component in the diagnostic process for acute myelogenous leukemia (AML). Cytogenetics for the presence of the Philadelphia chromosome are of value in chronic myelogenous leukemia (CML) and acute lymphoblastic leukemia (ALL), the lymphocytic leukemias, not the myelocytic leukemias. Immunophenotyping for the T-cell antigen CD5 and any B-cell surface antigen is associated with the lymphocytic leukemias, chronic lymphocytic leukemia, and ALL. Florescence in situ hybridization is a test used to determine the presence of the BRC/ABL 1 chromosome, an abnormality on chromosome #22. It is a diagnostic test in patients who are suspected to have CML and can also be used in those suspected to have specific types of ALL.

10. *Answer:* C

Rationale: Children are the patients with acute myelogenous leukemia (AML) or acute lymphoblastic leukemia most likely to develop central nervous system (CNS) involvement, but it occurs in approximately 5% of adults. Symptoms can include headache, irritability, cranial nerve palsies, seizure activity, and papilledema.

11. *Answer:* C

Rationale: Chronic myelogenous leukemia is not described in stages, but three phases have been identified: chronic, accelerated, and blast phase. Acute lymphoblastic leukemia is categorized according to risk factors present at diagnosis, categorized into low, high, and very high risk. Chronic lymphocytic leukemia is staged using the Rai staging system (in the United States) and the Binet staging system (in Europe). Acute myelogenous leukemia has no staging system; the prognosis is determined by age at diagnosis and chromosome status. The international staging system is used in the diagnosis and surveillance of multiple myeloma.

12. *Answer:* D

Rationale: Acute lymphoblastic leukemia (ALL) patients are categorized as low or standard risk if patients have B-cell ALL, are children age 1 to 10 years, and have a white blood cell (WBC) count less than 50,000 μL at diagnosis. Those at high risk include patients with T-cell involvement (regardless of age or WBC count), children younger than 1 years or older than 10 years who have a WBC count of 50,000 μL or more at diagnosis. This patient is at high risk. There is no category defined at intermediate risk.

13. *Answer:* C

Rationale: Allogeneic stem cell transplant is conducted between individuals who are genetically similar if not identical. The process of matching the donor to the patient includes human leukocyte antigen testing, which identifies certain protein antigens and determines the likelihood of transplant rejection. Xenograft transplants are transplants from one species to another species. Scl-70 testing is a test detecting a specific antibody pertaining to scleroderma. Autologous stem cell transplant refers to a transplant in which the blood cells of the patient are harvested and readministered after chemotherapy or radiation treatments. A syngeneic transplant takes place between two identical twins. NAAT testing is used for viruses or bacteria.

14. *Answer:* D

Rationale: Tumor lysis syndrome (TLS) is an oncologic emergency seen in lymphoproliferative malignancies and can lead to severe electrolyte imbalances, including renal failure. It is most often seen just after the initiation of chemotherapy regimens in which large amounts of tumor cells slough off into the systemic circulation. TLS is most often seen in acute lymphoblastic leukemia. Although tumor lysis can take place in acute myelogenous leukemia, it is more likely to take place in the lymphocytic disorders.

15. *Answer:* C

Rationale: The FISH test is an additional test recommended for patients with CML and identifies when collection of bone marrow is feasible to determine the presence of the Philadelphia chromosome.

16. *Answer:* A

Rationale: Two factors that increase the risk of tumor lysis syndrome are elevated white blood cell (WBC) count and renal issues. A.B. has an elevated WBC count, creatinine, and blood urea nitrogen and a decreased glomerular filtration rate. Although deep vein thrombosis is prevalent in oncology patients because of the increased likelihood of clotting, these laboratory values do not relate to clot formation. The patient's renal compromise associated with his diabetes does not put him at increased risk for central nervous system involvement. A.B. is taking oral agents for his diabetes, so he probably has type 2 diabetes and is not insulin dependent. Diabetic ketoacidosis most often affects those with type 1 diabetes. The laboratory values described are not concerned with hyperglycemia, ketoacidosis, or ketonuria, hallmarks of diabetic ketoacidosis.

17. *Answer:* C

Rationale: Induction is the initial treatment with chemotherapy agents given at high doses to eradicate leukemia and achieve complete remission (CR), resulting in repopulating the bone marrow with normal cells (represented by less than <5% blasts and normal blood counts). Current induction therapies include cytarabine (cytosine, arabinoside, Ara C, Cytosar-U) plus an anthracycline (Idarubicin, or daunorubicin). Interleukin therapy is used for patients with malignant melanoma and advanced metastatic renal cell carcinoma. *Salvage therapy* is a loosely defined term used in oncology to describe treatment prescribed for patients after standard treatments have failed. Consolidation therapy is treatment (usually chemotherapy) given to the patient after the induction therapy has attained a complete remission to reduce leukemic cell population and achieve long-term disease-free survival.

CHAPTER 16

1. *Answer:* C

Rationale: A history of previous infections within the past 3 months that causes enlarged lymph nodes can be attributable to several infectious processes, not just Hodgkin lymphoma. Fever and night sweats can be presenting symptoms for other illnesses such as eosinophilic pneumonia, chronic pneumonia, endocarditis, or tuberculosis. Chest radiography or computed tomography of the chest will certainly be used in the workup of a patient suspected to have Hodgkin lymphoma; however, the definitive factor is presence of Reed-Sternberg cells.

2. *Answer:* B

Rationale: The client has raised an important issue for which the nurse should provide more information. He will likely need some private time to think and make a decision. He will possibly want to call significant others for help with the decision. Sperm banking should be done before the first chemotherapy session if at all possible. Telling the patient to not worry about it or ignoring the obvious silent response is avoiding the issue and not addressing the patient's concerns.

3. *Answer:* B

Rationale: The patient should be assessed for lymphadenopathy to evaluate diseases status clinically. His symptoms should not be delayed for a week. Enlarged lymph nodes may cause venous obstruction that may result in swelling, but other etiologies for leg swelling, such as deep vein thrombosis, should be considered in the absence of lymphadenopathy. Dietary intake of sodium is an unlikely cause of unilateral leg swelling.

4. *Answer:* D

Rationale: Computed tomography (CT) scans and a lymph node biopsy should be done initially to restage the disease and determine correct pathology. When recurrence of non-Hodgkin lymphoma occurs, a lymph node biopsy is crucial to determine the type of lymphoma. Sometimes the cell type is different at the time of recurrence compared with the initial diagnosis. The type of chemotherapy used will depend on the CT scan and lymph node biopsy results. Because Mr. H is afebrile, infection is unlikely, and a consult to a peripheral vascular physician is not indicated.

5. *Answer:* C

Rationale: Lytic bone lesions are the most common cause of pain in multiple myeloma. Although the marrow may be involved, this is not a common cause of pain. Neural infiltration and intestinal obstruction are not common in multiple myeloma.

6. *Answer:* C

Rationale: The physician was referring to the myeloma (M) protein levels in the patient's blood. The patient needs a nutritious, well-balanced diet and should not be encouraged to lose weight during chemotherapy treatments. The nurse should clarify the misconception and then provide referral or information on a nutritious diet. Giving the patient a pamphlet without clarifying issues would not be helpful.

7. *Answer:* D

Rationale: The fact that D.B. has received chemotherapy in the past increases his risk for lymphoma. Assessment of lymphadenopathy should include a review of systems. When assessing symptoms of enlarged lymph nodes, it is important to determine the timing of the development of lymphadenopathy and both the alleviating and aggravating factors. All areas of the supraclavicular, cervical, inguinal, and the axilla region should be checked for lymphadenopathy. Evaluation of other associated symptoms such as nausea and vomiting may lead to further physical assessment of abdominal lymphadenopathy. Fever, night sweats, and weight loss are considered B symptoms in staging of lymphoma that may indicate more systemic disease and a poorer prognosis. Although individual patients can exhibit a myriad of symptoms, joint pain in the lower extremities is not typically included in the presenting symptoms of lymphoma patients.

8. *Answer:* A

Rationale: To complete staging for non-Hodgkin lymphoma, computed tomography scan of the chest, abdomen, and pelvis must be completed. In addition, a bilateral bone marrow biopsy and aspirate are done to determine whether bone marrow disease is present. To diagnose lymphoma, a lymph node biopsy is required to determine pathology. If the pathology reveal CD 20+ tumor, the client may receive rituximab (Rituxan), a monoclonal antibody specific for CD 20+ cells, as part of the chemotherapy regimen. A, 24-hour urine is not necessary in staging of Hodgkin lymphoma.

9. *Answer:* A

Rationale: Although it is possible that the weight loss the patient describes could be related to a loss of appetite as a result of apprehension and anxiety regarding his upcoming appointment, increased activity related to his occupation, or an improvement of his diet, those situations do not explain the additional complaint of night sweats. The combination of these two symptoms is most likely a recurrence of his Hodgkin disease. Fever, weight loss, fatigue, and night sweats are B symptoms that are present in approximately 40% of patients. A thorough review of systems is necessary to determine the most likely cause.

10. *Answer:* B

Rationale: The most likely reason for the patient's arm pain is fracture. Patients with multiple myeloma are at risk for pathologic fracture caused by bone disease. Although the other answers listed are possible, they are not the most likely cause of this patient's pain, and evaluation for fracture must be considered.

11. *Answer:* A

Rationale: Because of the bone disease and lytic lesions associated with multiple myeloma, these patients are at high risk for pathologic fractures. Bisphosphonates such as pamidronate disodium (Aredia) and zoledronic acid (Zometa) have been used monthly for bone strengthening. In general, multivitamins and herbal supplements have not been shown to promote bone strengthening. Aspirin and aspirin-containing products should be avoided because of the risk of bleeding and interference with platelet counts. The nurse should also broach with her the possibility that she may need some help at the farm.

12. *Answer:* D

Rationale: The patient with multiple myeloma will likely have bone lytic lesions caused by the osteoclast-activating properties that the myeloma cells produce. Anemia is caused by the abundance of plasma cells, which crowd out the normal red blood cells. Serum calcium levels can be elevated because of the tendency for increased bone reabsorption. The abundance of light chain proteins over time reduces the ability of the kidney to filtrate, and creatinine levels will decrease, often as low as 0.2 mg/dL.

13. **Answer:** A

Rationale: Mononucleosis is a contagious disease caused by the Epstein-Barr virus. Symptoms include fever, malaise, fatigue, and sore throat. Patients with polymyalgia rheumatica describe muscle aches, stiffness in the neck, extremities, and across the buttocks. Rheumatoid arthritis is a serious autoimmune disorder that affects the joints, usually in a bilateral fashion. None of these three diseases typically presents with enlarged lymph nodes. This student athlete has on ongoing enlarged lymph node, nontender in the supraclavicular region. There is a tendency for spread to adjacent nodes, and this student has discovered an additional enlarged node in his axilla. Many of the symptoms he describes are classic B symptoms, including fever, weight loss, fatigue, and night sweats, which are present in approximately 40% of patients.

14. **Answer:** B

Rationale: Staging is determined by size and placement of involved lymph nodes. J.H. is not considered having stage I disease because his disease involves two or more lymph node regions. J.H. is at stage II, which can also be described as IIB, because of his night sweats.

15. **Answer:** C

Rationale: Risk factors for Hodgkin lymphoma (HL) include a family history of lymphoma (not leukemia) and a previous history of Epstein-Barr virus. A combination of chemotherapy and radiation therapy cures more than 80% of all newly diagnosed HL patients. The disease is usually diagnosed early and boasts longer survival rates with fewer treatment failures than classic HL. The U.S. death rate has decreased more rapidly for HL than for any other malignancy in the past 5 decades.

16. **Answer:** D

Rationale: Aspirin could be helpful in relieving any pain the patient has from his wrist fracture. It is well known that aspirin is a preventive measure to reduce cardiac events. There has been some discussion regarding aspirin's preventive effect against colon, esophageal, stomach, and rectal cancer. However, in this particular scenario, the best response is D because the MPT treatment consists of melphalan, prednisone, and thalidomide, the latter of which carries significant risk for deep vein thrombosis, and patients are required to use a thromboprophylaxis agent.

17. **Answer:** B

Rationale: Steroids, such as dexamethasone, can block the action of insulin, and patients often develop insulin resistance. Therefore, they need to check their blood sugar levels frequently and adjust their dosage accordingly, with the guidance of their endocrinologist. It is not common to stop using insulin. Steroids such as dexamethasone tend to cause insomnia, not hypersomnia.

Steroids are also likely to be responsible for water retention and weight gain, not weight loss.

18. **Answer:** A

Rationale: The cause of most cases of non-Hodgkin lymphoma (NHL) is unknown. Documented risk factors include a history of immunodeficiency, whether inherited, acquired, or from a solid organ transplant. Although high-fat diets and use of tobacco products are known to be a risk factor for several cancers and should be discouraged, these are not risk factors for non-Hodgkin lymphoma. There is a risk factor for MALT (mucosa-associated lymphoid tissue) lymphoma associated with a stomach bacteria called *Helicobacter pylori*. Barrett esophagus is associated with esophageal cancers.

19. **Answer:** C

Rationale: IPI risk factors include:

- Age: >60 years is unfavorable
- Number of extranodal sites: <1 is favorab , >1 is unfavorable
- Performance status (ECOG): <1 is favora e, >1 is unfavorable
- Ann Arbor Staging: I or II is favorable, III or is unfavorable

20. **Answer:** D

Rationale: Follicular lymphoma can be in lent for a long time, showing few symptoms until th bulk of the tumor displaces an organ or presses on erve. Because the patient is elderly and many no s are likely involved in the chest cavity, surgery is iot an option. MOPP therapy (Mustargen, Oncovin, pr rbazine, and prednisone) is an older regimen used i al- vage treatment after recurrence when other opt s have failed. Monoclonal antibodies such as Rituxi (rituximab) are mainstays of treatment in lymphoma, but they are most often used in combination with chemotherapy and radiation.

21. **Answer:** A

Rationale: Lymphoid cells are initially produced from a pluripotent stem cell in the bone marrow. This pluripotent cell has the capacity for continuous self-renewal. There is not a limited number of lymphoid cells. A portion of the cells migrate to the thymus and mature into T cells. The B-cell line involves plasma cells and produces immunoglobulins (antibodies). B cells continue to mature in the marrow. T cells have the capability of maturing peripherally.

22. **Answer:** A

Multiple myeloma is the second most common hematologic malignancy in the United States, but it comprises just 1% of all cancers. There is a higher incidence of multiple myeloma among African Americans, not the Hispanic population. Multiple myeloma produces lytic bone lesions, which contribute to fractures, but not osteoporosis.

23. **Answer:** C

Rationale: Although persons with multiple myeloma can experience anemia because of the disease process and treatment, multiple myeloma does not impact the coagulation cascade and clotting factors. Multiple myeloma does not affect the white blood cell line or produce neutropenia or leukemia. Multiple myeloma is a disease of the B-cell line, affecting production of mature, functioning immunoglobulins. Patients who have multiple myeloma are often treated with steroids. If a patient with multiple myeloma treated with steroids also has diabetes, the steroids will affect insulin dosing and will require special attention. However, the disease of multiple myeloma itself is not known to damage the β cells of the pancreas.

CHAPTER 17

1. **Answer:** C

   Rationale: Osteosarcoma is described accurately. Chondrosarcoma begins in the cartilage, occurs in the pelvis and upper leg, and is seen in patients 50 to 60 years old. Ewing sarcoma emerges from immature nerve tissue, usually found in the bone marrow. The pelvis, upper legs, ribs, and arms are likely sites. Ewing sarcoma usually occurs in young people from the age of 10 to 20 years old. A myoma is a benign tumor that grows in the muscle layer of the uterus, usually of women age 40-60 years.

2. **Answer:** D

   Rationale: Primary bone cancer, which originates in the bone tissue, is rare, but it can grow in any of the 206 bones in the adult body. The most common sites for primary bone cancer are the lower extremities (41%), pelvis (26%), the chest wall (16%), upper extremities (9%), spine (6%), and skull (2%).

3. **Answer:** A

   Rationale: Metastatic disease of the lung could account for his weight loss, fatigue, cough, and shallow respirations, and the lung is a common metastatic site for Ewing sarcoma. Pneumonia usually also causes fever and patients have a productive cough. A diagnosis of mononucleosis would account for his fatigue but not other symptoms.

4. **Answer:** B

   Rationale: Chest radiography would show a shadow, possible nodule or fluid in the lung. A bone scan would definitely be appropriate to determine further metastatic bone disease, but given the patient's symptoms, it would not be the initial test ordered. Sputum for cytology examines cells under a microscope to see if abnormal cells are present. Although chest radiography, bone scan, and sputum for cytology could be requested in J.T.'s workup, the best of the four choices is the computed tomography scan, which would reveal an in-depth examination of the lungs and provide additional characteristics about the tumor.

5. **Answer:** D

   Rationale: Ewing sarcoma is primarily a disease of the lower extremities (41%) and pelvis (26%). It occurs most often in children, is highly malignant, and 20% to 30% of patients have metastatic disease at diagnosis. Because of multimodality therapy and precision surgery,

40% to 70% of the patients become disease-free survivors. Radiation therapy is often used as an adjuvant therapy, but surgery, including amputation, is usually considered the primary treatment. Ewing sarcoma spreads to adjacent tissue via the cancer's many round cells with indistinct borders.

6. **Answer:** C

   Rationale: Rhabdomyosarcoma usually occurs in children, from infants to those 19 years of age. Rhabdomyosarcoma arises from striated muscle tissue. These tumors usually present in the head, neck, genitourinary tract, arms, legs, and neck. They are not usually found in the trunk.

7. **Answer:** C

   Rationale: Skipped metastases are smaller areas of the same tumor occurring in the same bone but anatomically separated from the primary lesion. They are usually smaller, but there may be multiple tumors found. The other definitions do not fit skip metastases. Metastatic disease can appear initially, resolve with treatment, and reoccur late. Punched-out areas of severe bone loss are often called osteolytic lesions and are common in metastatic lung cancer, breast cancer, and multiple myeloma.

8. **Answer:** C

   Rationale: Although the chondrosarcomas can occur anywhere in the body, they most often occur in the legs. A leiomyosarcoma is a soft tissue sarcoma that involves involuntary smooth muscle. Chondrosarcomas typically occur in children 10 to 14 years of age. Chondrosarcomas usually present with dull, aching pain.

9. **Answer:** A

   Rationale: Patients with osteosarcoma usually exhibit elevated alkaline phosphatase levels because of the increased osteoblastic activity. Radiographic changes are often not identified until the disease is advanced. The pain is described as an achiness that increases at bedtime, and the pain increases in intensity as the tumor burden increases. Pathologic fractures can occur and are experienced as acute, sudden pain. It would be very rare for an osteosarcoma to occur bilaterally.

10. **Answer:** A

    Rationale: Chondrosarcoma is more common in men and in patients 30 to 60 years old than in other populations. Bence Jones urine is a diagnostic test for multiple myeloma; it is not currently included in the chondrosarcoma workup. Chondrosarcoma most commonly metastasizes to the lungs, lymph nodes, and other bones. Surgery is one component of a multimodality approach, but wide resections are preferred.

11. **Answer:** B

    Rationale: A leiomyosarcoma is a tumor that arises from smooth muscle. It is most often found in the digestive tract and the uterus. The gastrocnemius is located in the calf, and the biceps muscle is in the upper arm. The bladder is not a common site of sarcomas.

12. *Answer:* A

Rationale: Fibrosarcomas are usually seen within the bone on radiographs. Low-grade fibrosarcomas have well-defined margins, but high-grade lesions have poorly defined margins with a moth-eaten pattern. Synovial sarcomas occur within the joint. Chondrosarcomas are usually extraskeletal, occurring in the soft tissue. Lymphangiosarcomas begin in the lymph vessels and are usually found in the arms.

13. *Answer:* B

Rationale: The term *extraskeletal* means occurring outside of the bone, but it is not an official term used to describe a form of Ewing sarcoma. Primitive neuroectodermal cell tumor is a type of Ewing sarcoma. Dermatofibrosarcoma is a type of tumor that arises from fibrous tissue, not a form of Ewing sarcoma. When a tumor begins in the muscles and soft tissue, it is called extraosseous, and there is a particular rare form of Ewing sarcoma which is called extraosseous Ewing sarcoma.

14. *Answer:* C

Rationale: Ewing sarcoma is a serious diagnosis that is usually considered after other malignant cell possibilities have been eliminated. The symptoms of Ewing sarcoma can be extremely vague. Complete blood count results would likely reveal anemia, not thrombocytopenia. Patients with Ewing sarcoma usually have increased swelling and pain in the affected area, and the patient may also feel heat.

15. *Answer:* C

Rationale: In patients who are diagnosed with soft tissue tumors, 50% are found in the early stages. Smaller lesions are usually benign. There is an extensive workup for soft tissue tumors, but a spinal tap is not generally part of this workup. A soft tissue tumor usually begins as a painless, swollen mass (>5 cm). Pain can occur if the tumor affects blood vessels or nerves, which does not happen with most tumors. The primary goals of treatment are to remove the tumor, avoid amputation, and preserve function.

16. *Answer:* A

Rationale: Radiographic results are not a dependable means of determining classification of soft tissue tumor subtypes; often radiographic changes are not observable until the disease is advanced. Knowing the tissue of origin can point to the type of tumor, but it does not determine tumor classification. There are different levels of intra- and extracompartmental involvement of soft tissue tumors (e.g., the amount of a particular muscle involved). This characteristic could impact mobility or range of motion but does not relate to tumor classification. Obtaining cell histology is now widely used to classify subtypes of sarcoma tumors.

17. *Answer:* A

Rationale: Soft tissue sarcomas arise from the mesodermal layer of cell origin in the following anatomical areas: extremities, 45%; trunk and retroperitoneum, 23%; and viscera, 18%.

18. *Answer:* D

Rationale: The patient and family are having a great deal of distress over this diagnosis. Their current thoughts are on the immediate issue of surgery. Although rehabilitation is an option, telling K.C. he will definitely play basketball again is unwise. K.C. needs to believe that he can speak about his shock and grief in a safe environment. It is normal for him to be depressed, anxious, and distraught. Darkness and refusing visitors could make him feel more isolated, hopeless, and alone. Although at some point a psychiatric consult may be helpful, suggesting it early on may create distrust and prevent K.C. admitting his true feelings. The most important action is to create a rapport and encourage K.C. to talk about his feelings.

19. *Answer:* C

Rationale: Patients may experience phantom limb pain between 1 and 4 weeks after surgery. It usually subsides in a few months. Symptoms of phantom limb pain may include itching, pressure, tingling, severe cramping, throbbing, and burning. Symptoms of phantom leg pain do not include fever, diaphoresis, nausea, and loss of appetite. The intensity of phantom limb pain is greater when the amputation is more proximal. Stress, emotional upset, excitement, and fatigue have been known to trigger episodes of phantom limb pain.

20. *Answer:* A

Rationale: Although it is natural for patients to be visibly upset at losing a portion of a limb, the patient had said that she was fine with it, and obviously her tears reveal otherwise. She should not be left to deal with it on her own because this may lead to depression, isolation, and a possible downward spiral. Pursuing interventions such as calling pastoral services or suggesting support groups can be helpful but should emerge from a discussion with the patient. Pushing her toward these options would be detrimental to the relationship and prevent future effective communication. The best action is to encourage her to discuss her feelings and to ensure that she knows the nurse will listen and advocate on her behalf.

21. *Answer:* A

Rationale: Postoperative patients who have lost a limb should be dangled over the edge of the bed and helped to transfer to a chair on the first postoperative day. To prevent hip contractures, the patient should be placed in a prone position for 15 minutes three to four times a day. The stump should be elevated for at least 24 hours postoperatively to prevent edema and promote venous return. Stump wrapping is important to promote long-term healing.

22. *Answer:* B

Rationale: The decision between amputation and limb-preserving surgery is an especially delicate one in children younger than the age of 10 years. Limb salvage surgery is usually followed by radiation therapy. The aim of the surgical technique selected is to obtain acceptable disease-free margins. Tumors involving blood vessels or nerves are challenging because of a possible compromised blood supply for postoperative healing or lack of innervations for return of function. Comorbid conditions, such as diabetes or peripheral vascular disease, impact healing and must also be considered.

23. *Answer:* C

Rationale: Osteosarcomas appear differently as the disease progresses. Slow-growing tumor meets nontumor tissue. In moderately aggressive tumors, there is extension of the tumor into soft tissue areas. Aggressive osteosarcomas can appear as perpendicular striated tissue in a sunburst pattern. Fibrosarcomas of high grade have poorly defined margins with a more moth-eaten pattern. On physical examination, chondrosarcomas present as firm and swollen, with high-grade tumors appearing soft and viscous. Ewing sarcomas appear onion-like on radiographs from multiple layers of subperiosteal new bone reacting to tumor invading the bone cortex.

24. *Answer:* B

Rationale: Usually, external-beam radiographic therapy is used before or after surgery for soft tissue tumors to debulk or remove a localized tumor.

CHAPTER 18

1. *Answer:* D

Rationale: HIV-1 is more virulent than HIV-2. HIV typically has a long incubation period with a gradual disease progression. The average time from the development of HIV infection to a diagnosis of AIDS is relatively short, only 2 to 3 years. The average life expectancy is 11 to 14 years.

2. *Answer:* D

Rationale: Multiple cofactors are implicated in disease progression, including the presence of many viruses, inadequate nutrition, general poor health, and smoking. There is an increased risk of HIV infection in uncircumcised males related to dendritic cells on the foreskin.

3. *Answer:* C

Rationale: Heterosexual women comprise only 15% of HIV diagnoses per year. African Americans and Latinos are excessively affected, not Asians. The fastest growing HIV positive patients at increased risk are older than 40 years.

4. *Answer:* B

Rationale: B-cell lymphoma is the most frequently diagnosed malignancy associated with AIDS. Since the advent of combination antiretroviral therapy, the incidence of Kaposi sarcoma has decreased significantly. Women with HIV are at increased risk for cervical cancer, but its incidence is not as high as for B-cell lymphoma. Head and neck cancer is not classified as an AIDS-defining malignancy.

5. *Answer:* C

Rationale: Malignancies associated with viral infection are more common in men and whites and are less likely to be related to viral load or CD4 count than AIDS-defining malignancies.

6. *Answer:* C

Rationale: There is a large list of antiretroviral agents that have diverse interactions with non-oncologic medications. Antiemetic use and diuretics are not on that list.

7. *Answer:* D

Rationale: Factors associated with shorter survival include CD4 cell count below 100 cells/mm^3, stage III or IV disease, age older than 35 years, history of injection drug use, and elevated lactate dehydrogenase.

8. *Answer:* C

Rationale: Body fluids for which universal precautions do not apply include urine, feces, vomitus, perspiration, nasal secretions, tears, and sputum or saliva. Body fluids for which universal precautions apply include blood (including any secretion or excretion contaminated with blood), cerebrospinal fluid, semen, vaginal secretions, synovial and amniotic fluid, pericardial fluid, pleural fluid, and peritoneal fluid.

9. *Answer:* A

Rationale: Small cell lymphomas are more likely to involve the bone marrow and meninges. The other statements are accurate.

10. *Answer:* D

Rationale: Primary central nervous system lymphoma is usually resistant to systemic chemotherapy because few agents cross the blood–brain barrier. Exceptions are high-dose methotrexate (>3 g/m^2) and high-dose cytarabine (Ara-C) (>2 g/m^2). Rituximab is also recommended and is usually well tolerated.

11. *Answer:* C

Rationale: The prognosis in patients with Kaposi sarcoma (KS) depends on multiple factors, including the location of the presenting KS lesions. The survival time is shorter in patients with gastrointestinal tract lesions, B symptoms, and prior opportunistic infections. Survival has increased dramatically in the era of combination antiretroviral therapy and may last several years.

12. *Answer:* B

Rationale: For cleanup of emesis or other body fluid spills, wear gloves and use a solution of one part household bleach to 10 parts water. A latex condom with a water-based lubricant should be worn during intercourse to reduce risks of the condom breaking (as seen with petroleum-based lubricants or cosmetic creams). Abstinence of intercourse during chemotherapy is not necessary.

13. *Answer:* B

Rationale: Organizational recommendations for cancer screening are not well described for HIV-infected patients despite their increased risks for developing specific cancers. Pap testing is recommended every 6 to 12 months (not every 2 years) for early detection of cervical cancer in HIV-infected women. Computed tomography of the chest, rather than chest radiography, is indicated to assess high-risk individuals for lung cancer. Professional organizations have not adopted routine anal screening with cytology or high-resolution anoscopy for early detection of squamous cell cancer. Digital anal examination is a proven cost-effective method to screen for this cancer in high-risk individuals.

14. *Answer:* B

Rationale: Although warfarin and aspirin may interfere with platelet function and cause undesired bleeding, patients may need to take these medications to prevent clotting.

15. *Answer:* D

Rationale: Hepatocellular cancer is more common in patients with hepatitis C and HIV dual infection than hepatitis B and HIV infection. Lung cancer, not anal cancer, has the highest incidence of mortality among HIV-related cancers and asserts an increase in survival if receiving concomitant combination antiretroviral therapy.

16. *Answer:* C

Rationale: Low health literacy has been linked to a delay in diagnosis, low adherence to medical instructions, lack of understanding one's condition, and increased mortality risk. It is a major healthcare issue. Although having a family caregiver present to hear and be part of the discussion about the patient's diagnosis and treatment may be helpful, the family caregiver's health literacy must also be assessed. The family caregiver may have difficulty understanding the discussion as well and should not be used to translate. Low health literacy is associated with only 17% to 40% of patients maintaining regular medical care.

17. *Answer:* B

Rationale: Enzyme-linked immunosorbent assay (ELISA) is used for screening and has high sensitivity and specificity. Certain conditions may lead to a false-positive result, such as syphilis, lupus, or Lyme disease. Therefore, ELISA is often repeated. A second positive ELISA test result is typically followed by a Western blot test. If the Western blot result is positive, it confirms an HIV infection. A negative Western blot test result means the ELISA test was a false-positive result. Epstein-Barr virus infection does not mean that the patient has HIV.

18. *Answer:* C

Rationale: There is no stage IV in the Centers for Disease Control and Prevention guidelines. Both stages I and II have a laboratory confirmation of HIV infection; however, the CD41 T-lymphocyte count in stage I is 500 cells/mcL or greater and in stage II is between 200 and 249 cells/mcL.

19. *Answer:* B

Rationale: Patients with simultaneously diagnosed HIV and malignancy, particularly lymphoma, should delay combination antiretroviral therapy because of the possible risk of developing severe immune reconstitution syndrome, an inflammatory response evidenced by a rapid increase in white blood cell count. Intrathecal administration of chemotherapy is considered when treating lymphomatous meningitis and is not useful in patients with bulky disease. Ongoing studies continue to evaluate the usefulness of stem cell transplant but do recommend it as first-line therapy.

20. *Answer:* D

Rationale: Assessment should include determination of JT's past experiences with HIV disease, concerns about his diagnosis and treatment, and previous coping behaviors to develop interventions specific to J.T.'s psychosocial needs. J.T. does not currently have a consistent significant other and has specified that he does not want anyone to know about his diagnosis. Focusing on his psychosocial needs is more appropriate at this time.

21. *Answer:* A

Rationale: There is a causative association between Kaposi's sarcoma associated-herpes virus (KSHV) and Kaposi sarcoma (KS).

22. *Answer:* A

Rationale: If oral thrush is present, the patient has at least stage 5 or 6 HIV. When chronic lymphadenopathy is present, the patient is stage 2 or greater. A skin test within normal limits is a stage 0, 1, 2, or 3.

23. *Answer:* A

Rationale: Risk stratification into good- and poor-risk categories can be helpful to determine patient response to therapy and overall prognosis. Good risk factors include Kaposi sarcoma is confined to skin or lymph nodes, the patient has minimal oral disease, the CD4 count is greater than 200/mcL, no oral thrush or B symptoms are exhibited, and Karnofsky performance status is greater than 70. Poor risk factors include edema or ulceration of tumor; extensive oral, gastrointestinal, or non-node visceral tumors; CD4 count less than 200/mcL; history of oral thrush or B symptoms; poor performance status; and presence of other HIV illness.

24. *Answer:* B

Rationale: Atazanavir and bevacizumab administered in combination can cause hypertension and idiosyncratic bleeding. The other statements are accurate.

25. *Answer:* C

Rationale: Antiretroviral medications are known inhibitors and inducers of enzymes that can affect levels of non-HIV medications, in particular chemotherapy agents. The only drug that is an inducer and speeds up the metabolism of other drugs is nevirapine. The other drugs are antiretroviral inhibitors.

26. *Answer:* B

Rationale: Cognitive changes and headache are neurologic signs. Malabsorption and diarrhea are associated with gastrointestinal tract lesions. Human herpes virus type 8, not Epstein-Barr virus, is associated with primary effusion lymphoma. Cough and dyspnea are common, and the patient may present with a pleural effusion.

28. *Answer:* A

Rationale: Chemotherapeutic agents can decrease the CD4 count. CD4/T4 counts also decrease in the absence of highly active antiretroviral therapy. B2 microglobulin (a serum marker for immune activation) and core antigen p24 (a major structural core protein of the HIV virus that is a highly specific predictor of disease progression) indicate progressive infection, so serum levels will increase.

CHAPTER 19

1. *Answer:* C

Rationale: A core needle biopsy is described as using a large needle, guided into a suspicious area and a core, or small piece of tissue is removed. In an excisional biopsy, the entire suspicious mass is removed through an incision. Aspiration biopsies are conducted using very fine needles guided into suspicious tissue. Tissue fragments are aspirated to obtain a sample. An incisional biopsy consists of making an incision and removing a piece of tissue from a larger mass.

2. *Answer:* B

Rationale: J.B. probably has a gallstone blocking his common bile duct. Endoscopic retrograde cholangiopancreatography will allow the gastroenterologist to remove the stone and place a stent in the duct to allow for drainage of bile. *Multimodality therapy* is a term used to describe a group of treatments (e.g., in oncology, chemotherapy, surgery, and radiation) used in combination to treat a disease. An upper endoscopy is an endoscopic outpatient procedure used to examine the upper gastrointestinal tract, primarily the esophagus, stomach, and duodenum. A Swans-Ganz catheter is a device used in cardiology, usually in critically ill patients to monitor and stabilize blood pressure.

3. *Answer:* C

Rationale: Radiologists who specialize in interventional radiology offer many options for patients at all phases of their disease or illness trajectory. Interventional radiology could be used to place a stent in the common bile duct. An Ommaya reservoir is a small soft domed device placed under the scalp connected to a catheter, threaded into a ventricle. It can be used to obtain samples of cerebrospinal fluid or to administer chemotherapy, monoclonal antibodies or antibiotics. A Groshong catheter can be either a tunneled or nontunneled catheter placed for central venous access. Brachytherapy is a form of radiation therapy that places radioactive sources in or adjacent to the target tissue.

4. *Answer:* D

Rationale: Ablation therapy is the use of thermal-based energy (cryoablation, radiofrequency ablation, or microwave) to destroy small lesions with direct application for cellular destruction. Because the patient has several small tumors scattered over both the left and right lobes, ablation therapy would be appropriate. Preoperative radiation is generally used to downsize a tumor. Carrier testing is a genetics-related test, not a treatment. Robotic surgery is helpful in that it produces little scarring and blood loss. Because this patient has numerous small tumors scattered across two lobes of the liver, the ablation therapy is the best option for her.

5. *Answer:* A

Rationale: Three of the choices are components in the surgical safety checklist recommended by the World Health Organization and mandated by The Joint Commission for American Hospitals. Sign in occurs before the patient receives anesthesia. The patient's identity, the planned procedure, and monitoring equipment are reviewed and checked. Review of systems is a component of the assessment in a history and physical examination. Time out takes place before the skin incision and includes an introduction of each member of the surgical team and his or her individual role, a review of the surgery taking place, ensuring the identity of the patient, the surgical site

and laterality, and an opportunity for any questions. Sign out occurs after the first closing count to ensure proper documentation is completed, counts are complete, specimens labeled, and any operational issues are discussed.

6. *Answer:* A

Rationale: The American Society of Anesthesiologists (ASA) classification system is used by anesthesiologists to describe preoperative health status and operative mortality risk. There are six categories defined as follows: ASA physical status 1, a normal healthy patient; ASA physical status 2, a patient with mild systemic disease; status 3, a patient with severe systemic disease; ASA physical status 4, a patient with severe systemic disease that is a constant threat to life; ASA physical status 5, a moribund patient who is not expected to survive without the operation; and ASA physical status 6, a declared brain-dead patient whose organs are being removed for donor purposes. B.C.'s type 2 diabetes and COPD would be categorized as mild systemic disease, which puts her at a ASA physical status 2 level.

7. *Answer:* A

Rationale: Peripheral nerve blocks can provide significant pain relief and can be used solely or combined with general anesthesia. Long-acting local anesthetics, such as bupivacaine, can provide a nerve block duration of 12 to 18 hours. Certain additives such as methylprednisolone can provide an additional 6 to 10 hours of analgesia. Peripheral nerve blocks do not cause a decrease in blood pressure or narcotic-related adverse effects such as urinary retention, nausea, or itching.

8. *Answer:* D

Rationale: The patient had major abdominal surgery 3 days ago, so she is quite immobile. There is a strong possibility that she has developed atelectasis or pneumonia. Most of her symptoms relate to her respiratory status. Therefore, the most appropriate choice is chest radiography, which would reveal any lung abnormalities. Also, being an inpatient puts her at risk for nosocomial infections such as pneumonia. Blood cultures would be important to determine any sepsis, but the results would not be as immediate of a finding as chest radiography, and often people who become septic are confused or delirious, and this patient was not confused. Tylenol 500 mg orally every 6 hours could be used for pain management and fever, but determining the cause of her change in breathing and temperature is more of a priority. Simply increasing her intravenous fluid rate to 150 cc/hr could cause fluid overload and cardiac issues, such as congestive heart failure.

9. *Answer:* A

Rationale: The purpose of most postoperative drains is to prevent the accumulation of fluids. Drains also allow for inspection of the wound fluid and early identification of blood, pus, or other signs of infection, such as serosanguineous fluids. Drains do not allow for wound granulation, but a wound that is accumulating fluids would be less likely to form granulation tissue and progress in the healing process. Drains are used to facilitate drainage exiting a wound; they are not used as an orifice to inject silicone or administer antibiotics.

10. **Answer:** A

Rationale: Lumpectomy is the removal of the primary tumor in total and is thus considered the primary treatment for this patient. External-beam radiation is additional therapy at the tumor site that is done to eliminate any local undetectable microscopic disease left behind. This is considered adjuvant therapy and can increase the disease-free time for patients. Palliative care is used for patients with more extensive disease. Many cancer treatment plans include a combination of treatments to produce the most positive outcomes, but one treatment has the greatest projected impact and is considered the primary therapy.

11. **Answer:** B

Rationale: Poor circulation would decrease the availability of nutrients and oxygen to the wound, which is a factor in healing. Age-related changes, such as mobility and physiologic function, impact wound healing, as well as the delayed healing response common in elderly adults. Healthy elderly adults are able to heal as well as younger adults, but the process takes longer. A person's immune response determines his or her ability to fight off opportunistic infections that would place the patient at risk for wound infection and other deteriorating conditions.

12. **Answer:** D

Rationale: Infection is a potential postoperative complication. The incision site must be assessed to rule out a local infection, abscess or fistula formation, impending wound dehiscence, or the occurrence of lymphedema (a complication of lymph node removal). The client may need antibiotic or other additional therapy to resolve the complication. The other options do not appropriately address the patient's problem.

13. **Answer:** B

Rationale: The surgical removal of a particular body tissue is recommended if that tissue has a very high risk for the development of cancer. A history of 10 or more years of chronic ulcerative colitis, along with the patient's age, significantly increases her risk for colorectal cancer. Such surgery is done prophylactically to preemptively eliminate the source of the likely cancer. Reconstructive therapy, described in A, cosmetically and functionally improves the defect left from the initial cancer surgical procedure. C and D describe common rationales for specific surgical procedures, but these are not preventing a cancer occurrence as in prophylactic surgery.

14. **Answer:** B

Rationale: Pain management and providing a means of communication are very important. However, maintaining an effective airway would be of foremost importance to prevent a life-threatening emergency. Providing adequate nutrition is essential over time and becomes more of an issue during the rehabilitation phase after surgery.

15. **Answer:** D

Rationale: Although speech therapy, the ability to swallow, emotional support, and nutritional assessment are all very important components of the patient's postoperative care, the most immediate and crucial educational component to pass on includes safety issues regarding the care of the stoma. Protecting the stoma from water, dust, dirt, and small objects and relaying other safety recommendations will keep the patient from harm and provide emergency airway access.

16. **Answer:** C

Rationale: Cytoreductive therapy is the reduction of tumor volume to improve the effect of other cancer treatments, as well reducing the toxicities of all the therapies used. Although cytoreductive surgery may add to client comfort and improve the patient's quality of life without curing the disease, this definition is more applicable to palliative care. Establishing a tissue diagnosis is done by biopsy. Prophylactic surgery is the removal of tissues or nonvital organs to reduce the risk of cancer regrowth.

17. **Answer:** C

Rationale: En bloc resection involves the removal of bulky cancer with contiguous tissues, nodes, and vascular structures required to attain safe margins. Debulking resection involves removal of a significant part of the tumor, ablation uses thermal-based energy to destroy small lesions, and local excision is the removal of cancer and a small margin of surrounding tissue.

18. **Answer:** A

Rationale: This patient's wound has opened up weeks after surgery and cannot be approximated. It will have to be managed using packing or dressing or possibly a negative pressure device. Cleaning wounds with closure at skin level using glue, staples, and stitches is primary intention. Tertiary intention is planned delayed primary closure because of wound contamination or unstable patient condition. This was not a planned outcome for this patient.

19. **Answer:** D

Rationale: Cancer patients are at greater risk after surgery for venous thromboembolism (VTE) if they have had previous VTE; have been treated with thalidomide or lenalidomide; arc immobile; or have received previous cardiotoxic chemotherapy such as doxorubicin, 5-FU, or cyclophosphamide. Rifampin and St. John's wort are associated with treatment issues in the care of patients with hepatitis C. A positive Tine test result indicates latent tuberculosis in a person with no other symptom of active tuberculosis.

20. **Answer:** A

Rationale: Ideally, radiation therapy can shrink the tumor to a more resectable size with more easily discernible margins. This will reduce the impact on surrounding tissues. The goal is optimum cancer treatment outcomes with minimal associated disability.

21. **Answer:** C

Rationale: Patients who have general anesthesia and analgesia may experience hypoxia, which can put them at risk for myocardial infarction. The patient has received methotrexate and previous radiation treatments to the torso area, placing him at risk for interstitial pneumonitis and pulmonary fibrosis. Because of his previous surgery and exposure to radiation, he is more likely to experience skin breakdown and impaired wound healing. Diarrhea and dehydration are not likely postoperative sequelae of his colon resection because his remaining bowel would be inactive, and it would take some time for peristalsis to return.

22. *Answer:* D

Rationale: Primary intention means a clean postoperative wound with closure at the skin level using glue, staples, or stitches. A laparoscopic approach is also called minimally invasive surgery or band-aid surgery. Incisions that are very small, usually 0.5 to 1.5 cm in size, are made in the abdomen compared with larger incisions as with laparotomy. Secondary intention is when the wound borders are not able to be approximated or there is significant tissue loss that then requires packing, dressing, or negative-pressure device. Tertiary intention means closure of the wound is intentionally delayed for 2 or more days after surgery because of wound contamination or an unstable patient condition.

3. *Answer:* A

Rationale: All options include strategies to promote positive rehabilitation for specific client populations with specific needs, but a multidisciplinary discharge plan is critical. A comprehensive assessment of the patient's short- and long-term needs using a multidisciplinary team approach is most helpful in determining the best plan of rehabilitation for the specific patient involved.

CHAPTER 20

1. *Answer:* D

Rationale: Infections remain a leading cause of mortality and morbidity associated with hematopoietic stem cell transplantation (HSCT). But, advances in antibiotic, antifungal, and antiviral therapies, along with better understanding of preventing cytomegalovirus pneumonia have reduced the risk significantly. The doses of antitumor treatment cause the marrow ablative effect of the treatment in HSCT. This effect is actually desirable in allografting. The cells that are used to recover the hematopoietic system are stem cells; they may come from peripheral circulation or directly harvested from the marrow. Tumors that are resistant to chemotherapy are not usually considered for HSCT; the underlying condition must be responsive to chemotherapy or to radiation therapy. The increased doses delivered can increase the effectiveness of the treatment.

2. *Answer:* C

Rationale: Syngeneic transplant involves receiving marrow from an identical twin and is beneficial because there is no concern about rejection. The mixed chimerism state that can occur with the coexisting of donor and recipient cells sets up a graft-versus-tumor type of response that can help to suppress tumor cell recurrence. That effect of graft-versus-host disease with allografting can include significant risk, especially for older individuals and those with comorbidities; autografting, although not free of risk, is regarded less risky. Allografting does involve transplanting stem cells from a donor who is

genetically different; the match however, is determined by human leukocyte antigen (HLA) typing or human leukocyte antigen. HLA is a protein, or marker found on most cells in the body, including white blood cells. Although it does require the testing of blood samples, it is not the same as blood type. Autografting can carry the risk of reinfusing malignant cells, but routine purging, even in diseases that involve the marrow, is not proven to be beneficial.

3. *Answer:* B

Rationale: The goals of pretransplant conditioning regimens are to eradicate any malignant cells that may remain in the recipient. Although marrow ablation increased the likelihood, the new cells will engraft and grow, the conditioning regimens cannot prevent graft-versus-host disease. Colony-stimulating factors, granulocytic colony-stimulating factor, granulocytic-macrophage colony-stimulating factor, and sometimes chemotherapy are used to mobilize marrow stem cells to the peripheral blood. Conditioning regimens cannot minimize comorbid conditions but rather may actually exacerbate them.

4. *Answer:* C

Rationale: Umbilical cord blood and placenta, bone marrow, and peripheral stem cells all are rich stem cell sources. Animal studies have not supported the use of animal sources for human hematopoietic stem cell transplantation. Although the stem cells present in donated blood can place an immunocompromised client at risk for graft-versus-host disease if the product is not irradiated, this is not a rich source of stem cells for a planned transplant. In addition the spleen is not a source of stem cells for transplantation

5. *Answer:* C

Rationale: Nonmyeloablative hematopoietic stem cell transplantations (HSCTs) are currently reserved for older clients (older than 60 years) and those with comorbidities because the risk of acute toxicities from the conditioning is less. Nonmyeloablative HSCTs are performed primarily in the allogeneic recipient. One of the goals of a nonmyeloablative HSCT is to create a graft-versus-tumor effect. Young individuals who are newly diagnosed clients can usually withstand the toxicities of HSCT and are restricted to an umbilical stem cell donor, but their size makes them better candidates for that as a source of the stem cells.

6. *Answer:* B

Rationale: Aplastic anemia causes pancytopenia, thereby destroying the client's marrow supply. Recipients of hematopoietic stem cell transplantation (HSCT) for aplastic anemia require a matched donor to replace the failing marrow of the client. Although patients with aplastic anemia can be treated with HSCT, they must have a matched donor source. The national marrow donor registry does support unrelated allogeneic transplants for treatment of aplastic anemia. We are not given the client's age, the concern is the presence of the underlying disease process in the marrow.

7. *Answer:* B

Rationale: The likelihood of a cure with transplant is increased when any remaining malignancy in the recipient has been eliminated; reduction will not produce a cure. If the immune system is not suppressed, it will interfere with marrow engraftment when allografting is required. Additionally, marrow ablative therapy serves to "clear out" space for the engraftment of the stem cells. The target of the conditioning is remaining malignancy and may actually increase the risk of infection from the current state. Although some transplants do combine high-dose chemotherapy with total lymph node or total body irradiation, this is not always the situation and not the goal of the conditioning regimen.

8. *Answer:* A

Rationale: Allogeneic hematopoietic stem cell transplantations (HSCTs) are performed with a matched donor, an autologous HSCT is performed using the client's own marrow, and donor cells for a syngeneic transplant are donated from a twin. Cadavers are a source of donor cells, although the first attempts in the early 1980s were unsuccessful and are no longer done.

9. *Answer:* A

Rationale: Underlying major organ (kidney, liver, lung, cardiac) system problems, psychosocial dysfunction, and previous infections can interfere with the success of transplant. Previous infections can cause complications; the critical information in that case would be the type of infection and the outcome of the intervention. Combination chemotherapy and radiation therapy is not necessarily a major risk factor; prior toxicities and response to management are the important components. The administration of chemotherapy may actually be a component of the decision process based on evaluating the responsiveness of the underlying disease to treatment.

10. *Answer:* B

Rationale: Among the early complications resulting from hematopoietic stem cell transplantation (HSCT) are nausea, vomiting, and infection. Chronic graft-versus-host-disease and herpes varicella zoster occur around 80 days after HSCT. Impaired growth and development in children will not be seen during the acute phase but should be followed closely.

11. *Answer:* A

Rationale: The target organs of acute graft-versus-host disease (GVHD) are the skin, liver, and gastrointestinal tract. Chronic GVHD affects the vagina but not the heart or spleen. The skin is a target organ of acute GVHD but not the pancreas or brain. Acute GVHD targets the gut, and chronic GVHD targets the eyes and mouth.

12. *Answer:* D

Rationale: Veno-occlusive disease/hepatic sinusoidal obstruction syndrome is an early complication of hematopoietic stem cell transplantation (HSCT), occurring between 3 and 21 days after the transplant. It is seen in both allogeneic and autologous recipients. This complication affects the liver, which can then impact the function of other organs, and is seen in both allogeneic and autologous HSCT.

13. *Answer:* B

Rationale: The classic symptoms of veno-occlusive disease (VOD) are sudden weight gain, mental confusion, and right upper quadrant pain. Clients with acute gastrointestinal graft-versus-host-disease may have some abdominal cramping, but right upper quadrant pain is typical of VOD. Treating Mr. O with nonsteroidal antiinflammatory agents for his pain is contraindicated because of hematopoietic immunosuppression from the conditioning regimens of HSCT. VOD occurs in both allogeneic and autologous recipients.

14. *Answer:* B

Rationale: Hand-washing has been shown to be the most effective way to reduce the spread of infections. It is important to maintain a clean environment and to avoid exposure to individuals with known infections; however, handwashing has been shown to be the most effective way to reduce the spread of infections. The client and family needs to be aware of the presence of a fever but would not need to monitor it as frequently as every 2 hours unless it has been elevated; then it should be watched closely because it is an indicator of infection that may be life threatening.

15. *Answer:* A

Rationale: Although anxiety is a complication of hematopoietic stem cell transplantation that should be addressed prophylactically, and rest is important, encouraging the client to comply with protective isolation requirement focuses more on infection than anxiety. Reducing the risk for complications from cyclophosphamide-induced hyponatremia is not addressed through the administration of mesna as ordered; mesna is to decrease the risk of hemorrhagic cystitis as a potential complication. The client should be monitored closely for the hyponatremia caused by the syndrome of inappropriate antidiuretic hormone secretion from the cyclophosphamide. Also, administering graft-versus-host-disease prophylaxis and monitoring symptoms is important, but it is not regarded as prophylaxis to reduce the risk of veno-occlusive disease.

16. *Answer:* B

Rationale: The use of cryotherapy (ice chips) is an important evidence-based mucositis prevention nursing intervention for high-dose melphalan, which has a very short half-life and is usually administered over a short enough time frame to maintain the cooling effect of the intervention. Clients receiving etoposide need to be monitored closely for cardiac-related problems. Thiotepa recipients benefit from frequent bathing 4 times a day while receiving this agent that is excreted via the integumentary system and can lead to skin problems. The half-life of thiotepa and etoposide are too long for cryotherapy to be effective. Voriconazole is actually an antimicrobial, not a chemotherapy drug.

17. *Answer:* D

Rationale: A history of chest irradiation or bleomycin therapy appears to increase the likelihood of further interstitial lung disease during hematopoietic stem cell transplantation. Idiopathic pulmonary interstitial pneumonitis occurs most frequently in clients older than 30 years of age. Encouraging activity, turning, coughing, and deep breathing are important interventions to improve respiratory status and decrease the risk of this pulmonary complication. Hemorrhage can occur with this pulmonary complication; intravenous or aerosolized antimicrobial therapy is important to treat any infectious component.

CHAPTER 21

1. *Answer:* C

   Rationale: Photons (not protons) are examples of electromagnetic radiation. Protons are examples of particulate radiation. DNA, not RNA, is the most important target for radiation damage. *Ionizing radiation* is a term that describes both electromagnetic and particulate radiation, and includes all examples in C.

2. *Answer:* C

   Rationale: The level of DNA damage determines the biologic effect of the radiation therapy on tissues. Other factors include oxygen effect and sensitivity of the cell to the radiation; well-oxygenated tumors tend to show greater response, and certain types of tumors are more sensitive, but others are more resistant. A buildup of toxins in the body can cause other problems but does not directly influence the biologic response to radiation.

3. *Answer:* B

   Rationale: All normal and cancer cells are vulnerable to the effects of radiation therapy, although some cell types are more sensitive to radiation. Radiosensitivity is not one of the 4 Rs; these are repair, redistribution, repopulation, and reoxygenation. Redistribution is forcing more cells into the mitosis phase of the cell cycle. Reoxygenation occurs as decreased tumor burden allows better blood flow in the tumor (rendering it more radiosensitive). The time in which biologic changes appear and the sensitivity of effects depend on the amount of radiation absorbed, fractionation, and the rate at which it is administered. The time and severity of biologic changes is determined by the amount of radiation absorbed, fractionation, and the rate at which it is administered, not the four Rs.

4. *Answer:* A

   Rationale: A is correct as stated. Neoadjuvant radiotherapy (RT) is given before, not after, definitive treatment. Adjuvant RT is given after definitive therapy to ensure local control. Control RT is given at any point of the treatment continuum to limit the growth and spread of cancer with the intent of a period of symptom-free time.

5. *Answer:* D

   Rationale: Total-body irradiation (TBI) is not used for bacterial control. Its purpose is to eliminate remaining cancer cells and to suppress the immune system in an effort to prevent graft rejection. TBI is not given to the stem cell donor. Donor stem cells are instead mobilized using once- or twice-daily colony-stimulating factors. T-cell depletion to prevent graft-versus-host disease is achieved by other methods.

6. *Answer:* D

   Rationale: The standard of care established by the American College of Radiology requires a weekly physical assessment and evaluation of possible side effects of therapy. The degree of myelosuppression is directly related to the percent of bone marrow in the radiation field. A lumbar spine field would not be large enough alone to cause a rapid significant anemia. Nausea is an unlikely side effect in this scenario because the field does not include the stomach or significant small bowel. Hematuria, although possible, would also be unlikely because of present-day treatment planning sparing the bladder.

7. *Answer:* C

   Rationale: Grays were initially used in Europe but are becoming more universal. Centigray (cGy) is the unit of absorbed radiation dose equal to one hundredth of a Gray. LDR is the abbreviation used for low-dose-rate as it applies to brachytherapy using a sealed source. Rads were used historically especially in the United States, but are now being replaced by Grays or Centigrays. HVL is the abbreviation for half-value layer or the amount of shielding needed to block half of the radiation.

8. *Answer:* D

   Rationale: Treatment with radiopharmaceutical therapy is carefully planned and regulated to treat the tumor but also to limit undesirable exposure. The principle of time, distance, and shielding applies to all forms of radioactive therapy. Even though it is regarded a pharmaceutical, it must be handled with caution according to regulations. The method of delivery and uptake determine if the distribution is fairly uniform over the body or concentrated in specific organs; this is a critical component of safety with these agents. ⚠

9. *Answer:* A

   Rationale: A is incorrect because distance is not a factor, but length of treatment, fractionation, and volume of tissue irradiated are factors that influence side effects. Radiosensitivity does affect reactions to radiotherapy; the different sensitivity of tissues determines both acute and delayed effects. Clients need to be able to maintain adequate nutritional intake for healing and may require enteral supplementation. Radiation type, energy, and depth of treatment influence tissue exposure and normal tissue sparing and thus the side effects.

10. *Answer:* D

    Rationale: D is the only option that complies with radiation therapy safety regulations. Rather than using biohazardous containers to transport linens, the linens and wastes should be kept in containers in the room and monitored for radiation before being removed. When the toilet is used for disposal of body fluids, it should be flushed three times after each use to dilute radioactive urine, stool, or vomitus. If the dressing securing the source becomes displaced, the physician should be notified immediately.

11. *Answer:* B

    Rationale: The oral mucosa, vagina, bone marrow, ovary, testis, larynx, lymph node, salivary gland, small bowel, stomach, colon, esophagus, arteries, skin, bladder, and capillaries have been identified as acute-responding tissues. Subacute-responding tissues are the lung, liver, kidney, heart, spinal cord, and brain. Late-responding tissues are lymph vessels, thyroid, pituitary, breast, bone cartilage, pancreas, uterus, and bile ducts.

12. **Answer:** A

Rationale: Diarrhea is a common side effect of radiation therapy to the pelvis because of inflammation of the mucosal epithelium and loss of villi, thus making it a primary side effect. With decreased gastrointestinal transit time, watery diarrhea occurs, and electrolytes can be lost. Any resulting electrolyte imbalances are secondary side effects. Hypokalemia is correct because stools have a high concentration of potassium. If dehydration occurs, decreased renal blood flow may result in calcium resorption, causing increased serum levels. Calcium and phosphorus have an inverse relationship, making phosphorus levels low whenever calcium levels are high. Hypermagnesemia is incorrect because magnesium is also excreted in diarrhea stools.

13. **Answer:** B

Rationale: Delivery of the same total dose is possible by other methods, not just brachytherapy. But fractionation with smaller doses allows for repair and repopulation of surrounding healthy tissues, decreasing toxicity. Time between fractions also allows for recruitment of the malignant cells into the cell cycle, making these cells more radiosensitive. The presence of oxygen (not the process of deoxygenation) enhances the effects of ionizing radiation.

14. **Answer:** D

Rationale: Options A, B, and C are all important considerations when planning an educational program. Educational programs need to be tailored to the needs of the patient and family and need to consider the planned therapy, the health literacy of the patient and family and safety considerations.

CHAPTER 22

1. **Answer:** D

Rationale: The cell life cycle is a highly regulated five-stage process of reproduction that occurs in both normal and malignant cells: gap 0, gap 1, synthesis, gap 2, and mitosis. Cell cycle, or cell cycle time, is the amount of time required for a cell to move from one mitosis to another mitosis. A shorter cell cycle time results in high cell kill with exposure to cell cycle–specific agents. Growth fraction is the percentage of cells actively dividing at a given point in time. Tumor burden is the volume of cancer present. As the tumor burden increases, the growth rate slows, the number of cells actively dividing decreases, and the heterogeneity of the tumor cells increases; these decrease the responsiveness to therapy.

2. **Answer:** C

Rationale: Having different biologic effects increases the likelihood of an effect on the tumor. The location of the tumor is a characteristic that influences response caused by the likelihood of being able to get an adequate dose of therapy to the tumor. Tumor burden and growth fraction also influence the response to therapy. The physical and psychosocial status of the client are important to assess and know as part of planning treatment in general more so than choice of specific agents.

3. **Answer:** B

Rationale: Cardiac toxicity is the dose-limiting toxicity of doxorubicin. Fluorouracil can cause diarrhea, mouth sores, and some nausea/vomiting. Myelosuppression is dose limiting for nitrogen mustard, and nephrotoxicity is dose limiting for cisplatin administration.

4. **Answer:** A

Rationale: Control-focused therapy acknowledges that a cure is not realistic but that additional quality of life is possible. The theoretical goal of adjuvant chemotherapy is to eradicate remaining micrometastases after primary treatment. The goal of palliation is to relieve or alleviate symptoms. Combination therapy uses more than one agent or type of therapy.

5. **Answer:** B

Rationale: Cell cycle–specific agents are schedule dependent and most effective if administered in divided doses or by continuous infusion. *Cell cycle specific* indicates they are more effective during a specific phase or phases of the cell cycle. Divided doses allow time for additional cells to progress to the sensitive phase.

6. **Answer:** D

Rationale: If extravasation is suspected, discontinue the infusion, leave the needle in place, aspirate for residual medication, and apply cold. Dexrazoxane is regarded an antidote for doxorubicin, it should be infused via a fresh intravenous line within 6 hours. Do NOT continue the infusion; doxorubicin extravasation can cause extensive damage.

7. **Answer:** C

Rationale: The most common toxicity associated with bleomycin is pulmonary toxicity. Risk increases with cumulative doses and high fractional inspirational oxygen (FiO2) concentrations.

8. **Answer:** C

Rationale: Dexrazoxane is a cardioprotectant for use with doxorubicin. Amifostine is a cytoprotectant that is bound in tissue and has seen limited use. Mesna is used to protect against hemorrhagic cystitis with ifosfamide and cyclophosphamide. Anthracyclines are a classification of chemotherapy agents.

9. **Answer:** D

Rationale: Any agent can cause an allergic reaction during any cycle of therapy even if not listed as a potential side effect. Nurses must always be alert for signs and symptoms of a potential reaction. Reactions to paclitaxel and docetaxel occur most frequently in the first or second infusion, and reactions to platinum agents occur most often during the fifth (oxaliplatin), sixth, or later infusion (carboplatin). Skin testing of lymphoma patients with bleomycin before the first dose may not be predictive of a reaction.

10. **Answer:** B

Rationale: Although another provider may order the chemotherapy, the nurse is responsible to maximize client safety by performing each of the steps identified, except for answer B. Wearing the required personal protective equipment is important, but it applies to the safety of the nurse administering the agents.

11. *Answer:* D

Rationale: There is sufficient evidence available to justify these items as the correct answers. Although a lack of compliance with administration times can lead to serious complications, these effects are important to patient safety rather than the safety of the nurse.

12. *Answer:* A

Rationale: Idarubicin is a vesicant chemotherapy agent. It has the potential to cause cellular damage or tissue disfunction if leakage into cellular tissue occurs. Carboplatin and ifosfamide are both irritants, not vesicants. These can cause local inflammation but not tissue necrosis. Cisplatin is a vesicant if greater than 20 mL of 0.5 mg/mL concentration extravasates. However, sodium thiosulfate is used for an antidote, not dexrazoxane.

13. *Answer:* D

Rationale: Chemotherapy agents have been known to permeate gloves during drug preparation, administration, and the handling of contaminated wastes, thus placing staff at risk for exposure. Surgical masks are not respirators and thus do not protect against vapors or aerosols. Regular eyeglasses do not protect against splashes that can occur from the side. Gowns should never be re-used even if only one provider is using them.

14. *Answer:* B

Rationale: Monitoring central or peripheral intravenous administration requires that nurses verify presence of blood return before, during, and after administration of therapy.

15. *Answer:* A

Rationale: Infection is a potential complication of intraperitoneal chemotherapy. Peritonitis (infection) may present with temperature elevation and abdominal pain. The chemotherapy may cause abdominal cavity irritation, but the fever is most likely related to an infection.

16. *Answer:* A

Rationale: Clients receiving paclitaxel are at risk for a hypersensitivity reaction. An early sign of hypersensitivity is generalized uneasiness.

17. *Answer:* A

Rationale: A neuropathic side effect of vincristine is constipation. Stool softeners and laxatives are used to prevent constipation. Vincristine can lead to foot drop, but muscle relaxants are not indicated for prevention.

18. *Answer:* D

Rationale: Carboplatin reactions generally occur after 6 cycles of therapy and midway through the infusion. Prodromal symptoms include perioral and palmar itching.

19. *Answer:* B

Rationale: Evaluation of the client's right ventricular function (cardiac ejection fraction) should be performed before the first cycle of doxorubicin. This is done with a multiple gated acquisition scan or radionuclide ventriculography. Ejection fraction results should be communicated to the physician before initiating doxorubicin. Normal values for ejection fractions are above 50%. Normal values for lactate dehydrogenase are 105 to 333 international units/L; thus, 135 is within normal limits. The CA 125 would not warrant a change in this regimen, and the hematocrit of 34% is slightly less than a normal value of 36.1% to 44.3% in women and would not, by itself, necessitate a change in the regimen.

20. *Answer:* D

Rationale: A dose-limiting toxicity of irinotecan is early- and late-onset diarrhea. Prophylactic intervention; it should be a priority.

21. *Answer:* A

Rationale: Liposomal doxorubicin is an irritant. The rest are vesicants.

22. *Answer:* C

Rationale: Capecitabine, an oral antimetabolite, is converted to 5-fluorouracil (5-FU) when metabolized. Thus, it exhibits toxicities similar to those of 5-FU. Vinblastine is a vinca alkaloid, tamoxifen is a hormone antagonist, and prednisone is synthetic glucocorticoid.

23. *Answer:* B

Rationale: Powder-free, disposable gloves that have been tested for use with hazardous drugs should be worn when administering chemotherapy. Appropriate PPE requires nurses to double glove for drug preparation, administration, and handling of contaminated waste. Gowns should be disposable, lint free, and low permeability, with a solid front, long sleeves, tight cuffs, and back closure. Surgical masks are not respirators and do not protect against vapors and aerosols.

24. *Answer:* C

Rationale: Occupational Safety and Health Administration guidelines identify that the long-term effects of partial alopecia, chromosomal abnormalities, increased risk of cancer, and reproductive risks can occur within months to years after exposure to antineoplastic agents.

25. *Answer:* C

Rationale: Potential routes for the nurse to be exposed to antineoplastic agents include absorption through the skin or mucous membranes after direct contact, inhalation of drug aerosols, or ingestion with contaminated food or tobacco products. Extravasation of drugs, flare reactions, and hypersensitivity reactions are a result of client exposure to antineoplastic agents.

26. *Answer:* C

Rationale: Oncology Nursing Society Chemotherapy and Biotherapy Guidelines and Recommendations for Practice state that spill kits should be available wherever antineoplastic agents are stored, transported, prepared, or administered. In the event of a spill involving an antineoplastic agent, a spill kit containing personal protective equipment should be obtained and the area cordoned off to prevent others from being exposed. This requires the filing of a report and notification of a safety officer. But the initial priority is to locate a spill kit and cordon off the area to limit the risk of exposure of others to the spill.

27. *Answer:* D

Rationale: When preparing antineoplastic agents, a biologic safety cabinet or a compounding aseptic isolator should be housed in an area with negative pressure, not positive. Vents should be directed outside with exhaust emitted through a high-efficiency particulate air (HEPA) filter. Vertical unidirectional airflow is optimum, as is a fan operating continuously.

28. *Answer:* C

Rationale: Every effort needs to be made to reduce potential exposure. Needles should never be recapped to prevent accidental needle sticks and clipping could lead to aerosolization. Chemotherapy is a hazardous agent that should not be put in a drain and gowns could have chemotherapy contamination that could lead to exposure in others if they are disposed of in a regular trashcan. Chemotherapy should be disposed of in biohazardous containers and contaminated equipment in a sealable polypropylene bag so it is clear it is hazardous and to protect others from accidental exposure.

29. *Answer:* B

Rationale: Occupational Safety and Health Administration guidelines suggest that extremes of positive or negative pressure in medication vials should be avoided. Venting devices or dispensing pins allow outside air to replace the withdrawn liquid, thus preventing extreme pressure changes. Diluent should be added to vials slowly, and any excess solution should be expelled into a closed container within the biologic safety cabinet. When reconstituting agents packaged in ampoules, the American Society of Health System Pharmacists Technical Assistance Bulletin suggests that the contents of the ampule should be gently tapped down from the neck of the ampule before it is opened. The outside of the ampule should be wiped with alcohol, and a sterile gauze pad should be wrapped around the neck of the ampule when it is opened. The ampule should be broken away from the preparer. Gowns worn as personal protective equipment when handling chemotherapy are not to be used by multiple individuals; they should be discarded.

30. *Answer:* B

Rationale: Occupational Safety and Health Administration guidelines suggest that contaminated personal protective equipment should first be removed after direct contact with an antineoplastic agent. The affected area should then be thoroughly cleansed with soap and water. After these initial interventions, the nurse should then seek medical attention and document the exposure in an incident report or per the institution's policies and procedures.

31. *Answer:* D

Rationale: Occupational Safety and Health Administration guidelines state that splattering, spraying, and aerosolization can occur during the withdrawal of needles from drug vials and during the transfer of drugs using syringes and needles. It can also occur when ampules are opened and when air is expelled from a drug-filled syringe. Spiking a bag, discontinuing an infusion, and discarding contaminated materials are examples of when exposure can occur during the administration of antineoplastic agents.

CHAPTER 23

1. *Answer:* D

Rationale: Monoclonal antibodies are larger molecules than kinase inhibitors, and they do have less potential for drug-to-drug interactions; however, they have a greater potential for immune system activation. They are injected and have both extracellular and intracellular sites of action. The kinase inhibitors are small molecules that are taken orally. They have much shorter half-lives (i.e., a few hours) and do have a greater likelihood for drug-to-drug interactions.

2. *Answer:* D

Rationale: Monoclonal antibodies are used in the differential diagnosis of cancer such as classification of leukemias or lymphomas with flow cytometry. In neoadjuvant treatment, these therapies are given to achieve a pathologic response or to downstage the tumor. Cetuximab can increase radiotherapy benefit of the treatment of squamous cell cancer of the head and neck. Additionally, hematopoietic growth factors after antineoplastic therapy decrease the incidence and severity of neutropenia, anemia, and thrombocytopenia. Capillary leak syndrome is an adverse effect of interleukin-2.

3. *Answer:* D

Rationale: Chimeric monoclonal antibodies are made primarily of mouse protein with a human protein component. Humanized monoclonal antibodies include only a small percentage of the variable component of the antibody from the species used for immunization (e.g., mice), and the rest is human in composition. Whereas murine monoclonal antibodies consist of mouse variable and constant regions, primatized antibodies are created from monkey isotypes.

4. *Answer:* C

Rationale: Rituximab is a chimeric agent, and trastuzumab is a humanized agent; however, the indication for rituximab has been the treatment of DC20-positive B-cell non-Hodgkin lymphoma and chronic lymphocytic leukemia, not breast cancer. The mammalian target of rapamycin (mTOR) pathway regulates cell survival, proliferation, and growth; thus, the mTOR agents can affect these processes. The targeted therapies are classified into two groups, unconjugated or naked, which work by themselves with no drug or material attached, and those that are attached to a drug or other agents; they are not primarily conjugated, and both have an important role in improving cancer outcomes.

5. *Answer:* C

Rationale: Allergic reactions against murine antibodies may occur in humans, making C the correct option. Monoclonal antibodies are designed to work in conjunction with the host immune system. Previous reaction to chemotherapy would have no bearing on this because chemotherapy agents are not designed to modify immune responses. Tumor burden can increase the risk for sequelae such as tumor lysis syndrome but not an allergic reaction. Steroids are frequently excluded from the monoclonal antibody regimen with increased risk of anaphylaxis.

6. *Answer:* A

Rationale: Noninfectious pneumonitis is documented as a class effect of these inhibitors. The mammalian target of rapamycin agents have immunosuppressive properties even as nonconjugated agents. Gastrointestinal perforation with these agents is potentially fatal but fortunately rare with these agents. Current medications must be reviewed carefully to avoid problems with CYP450 substrates.

7. **Answer:** A

Rationale: Standard high doses of intravenous interferon used in the adjuvant treatment of stage 3 melanomas are known to be associated with increases in alanine aminotransferase (ALT) and aspartate aminotransferase (AST) (elevated AST reported as high as 63% in melanoma induction therapy), making A the correct option. Although a client with previous hepatitis exposure could have an increase in transaminases, this is not the general reason this is seen with high-dose interferon. Hepatic metastasis may also cause increases in ALT and AST; however, this would not be the most likely reason to see this in stage 3 clients who do not have evidence of distant metastasis before initiating interferon therapy.

8. **Answer:** A

Rationale: Dosing is used to determine the optimal biologic dose, the lowest dose in which the biologic activity of an agent is maximally stimulated. Increasing the dose of a biotherapy agent will not necessarily improve its efficacy. A minimally toxic dose may be insufficient to stimulate the desired immune response.

9. **Answer:** D

Rationale: One of the side effects seen during administration of the radioimmunoconjugate Zevalin is a significant delay in myelosuppression. The client's complaints are very consistent with myelosuppression, and therefore blood count evaluation would be the first step in client management with this therapy for non-Hodgkin lymphoma.

10. **Answer:** A

Rationale: Although the possibility of allergic reactions can exist with interferons and colony-stimulating factors, it is a rare occurrence with interleukins but may be seen with much greater frequency in monoclonal antibodies. This is especially true in monoclonal antibodies that are derived primarily from the mouse or murine isotype.

11. **Answer:** C

Rationale: Fatigue is by far the most common and most difficult to manage side effect seen with administration of interferon. Central nervous system alterations such as altered memory, decreased attention span, and difficulty concentrating are, along with fatigue, extremely difficult to manage. Diarrhea may occur but is less frequent and generally well managed by administration of antidiarrheals. Flulike syndrome and headache symptoms are commonly seen as part of the interferon tachyphylaxis response. They are generally controlled with acetaminophen or nonsteroidal antiinflammatory drugs in the early phase of treatment.

12. **Answer:** B

Rationale: Measures to decrease the severity of rashes include sun protection, tetracycline, topical steroids, and skin moisturizers. Controlling hypertension to reduce the risk of bleeding is supported in the ONS evidence-based guidelines for decreasing the risk of bleeding. Although tetracycline may be used to decrease the severity of rashes, culturing the rash is indicated if bacterial infection is suspected. It may be necessary to reduce the dose administered; however, this may impact likelihood of optimal response

13. **Answer:** A

Rationale: In this question, the client is indicating both a fear related to the side effects of a particular pharmacologic treatment for his malignancy and a lack of understanding related to risks involved. It is the responsibility of the health care team to make certain that patients have the information needed to provide informed consent for a particular treatment protocol. As the nurse, it is important to act as an advocate on the client's behalf. The remaining options all fail to address the need for the client to have his fears addressed and to completely understand his personal risks associated with the pharmacologic agent.

CHAPTER 24

1. **Answer:** C

Rationale: Advancement of surgical oncology techniques has led to an increased number of procedures and refinement of existing procedures. Client demand would not be an appropriate reason to increase the use of blood component therapy (BCT). There are specific established guidelines for appropriate use of BCT. Unfortunately, there is rarely an abundance of donations of blood products, and if there were excessive blood supplies, it would not be an appropriate reason for increasing BCT. Providing BCT is a supportive, not a curative, cancer treatment.

2. **Answer:** C

Rationale: Autologous donors are those who have their own blood preserved for later use. The risk for incompatibilities is very low or nonexistent with autologous transfusion. Tissue, not blood, has to be human leukocyte antigen matched. Blood is matched according to blood type. Bone marrow can be collected during organ harvesting, but blood cannot. The location of the blood donation and transfusion is not relevant to compatibility of the blood.

3. **Answer:** D

Rationale: Random donor plates are indicated to control or prevent bleeding in an individual with a platelet count less than 10,000 to 20,000/mm^3 or the client is bleeding and will be having major surgery. Although single-donor platelets may delay alloimmunization and lower the risk of infection, the current situation does not warrant their use. There is no indication that the client has a history of severe reactions to blood products, and the hemoglobin of 9 g/dL does not justify red blood cells at this time.

4. **Answer:** B

Rationale: A, C, and D are client-related factors (not treatment-related factors) that are known to increase the likelihood that blood component therapy (BCT) will be needed. Chemotherapy drugs that are known to suppress the bone marrow can increase the likelihood of needing BCT.

5. *Answer:* A

Rationale: Blood component therapy (BCT) exposes the client to components that are foreign to the individual's system and can lead to allergic reactions as well as the destruction of blood cells (hemolysis). Although fluid volume overload may occur, and the nurse should monitor the client closely, deep vein thrombosis is not a common reaction. Other coagulation problems are not seen as acute reactions to blood component therapy. Blood components can contain hematopoietic stem cells, and there have been cases of graft-versus-host disease in individuals with impaired immune system function; however, this is not seen as an acute reaction. Protocols will indicate when a client may require irradiated blood products to decrease this risk.

6. *Answer:* C

Rationale: To evaluate the effectiveness of teaching or any intervention, the outcome must be measurable and observable. The ability of the client to describe signs and symptoms of reactions to therapy reflects these qualities by incorporating the verb "describes." Although the other options are desirable outcomes, they are subjective and difficult to evaluate. Evaluating cognitive behaviors depends on a measurable and observable response that verifies that the client understands the intended message.

7. *Answer:* B

Rationale: Stopping the infusion immediately is critically important to decrease the severity of the reaction. A functioning intravenous line will be needed if the symptoms continue or worsen. You should also replace the tubing that contains blood product to decrease the infusion of additional blood component therapy; however, do not discard this tubing. Notifying the provider is also required, but the safety of the client depends on the action of stopping the infusion immediately. The reaction should be reported to the appropriate blood transfusion monitoring body, but again the client's safety is important now. The use of the diphenhydramine and meperidine will serve to treat the symptoms, but if this is an acute allergic reaction, stopping the infusion is the first priority. ⚠

8. *Answer:* D

Rationale: Two licensed healthcare professionals must verify that the blood component therapy product is correctly labeled and dated and that it matches the information on the client's blood identification band, usually worn as a bracelet. The client's name must be spelled correctly and the blood group and type identified on both the product and client identifiers. Using a gravity flow infusion line is not the priority intervention to maximize safety. Gravity infusions, although not the preferred method, may be used if controlled infusion pumps are not available. Slowly adding medications through the Y-port is incorrect; never add medications to blood component therapy BCT infusions. Intravenous therapy guidelines recommend larger catheters for viscous infusions such as BCT products. BCT products must be infused within 4 hours' maximum time to prevent degradation of the components.

9. *Answer:* B

Rationale: There is no indication at this time the client will be receiving intravenous therapy requiring long-term access. Midline catheters are intended for intermediate-term use and may be kept 2 to 6 weeks, and this option is the best one for this client. Peripheral catheters are intended for short-term use. Implanted ports and tunneled catheters are catheters for long-term use. Inserted surgically, these catheters may remain in place and be used for months or years if no complications such as infection develop.

10. *Answer:* A

Rationale: The client errs in believing that peripherally inserted central catheter (PICC) lines are inserted in arteries. Although the misunderstanding is not critical, the client needs more teaching. The other answers are true. Because the PICC line insertion is above the antecubital fossa and the catheter is threaded through the brachial vein, it is correct that there is a decreased risk for pneumothorax. The introducing needle remains in the antecubital fossa as the catheter is threaded into the superior vena cava. One of the advantages of PICC lines is their long-term viability, which decreases intravenous sticks, so this information is also correct.

11. *Answer:* D

Rationale: Maintaining aseptic technique does not guarantee that extravasation of a vesicant will not occur, but it does decrease the risk of infection at the insertion site of the intravenous catheter, promoting safety for the client. Using a computer-controlled infusion pump for accuracy promotes the correct rate of infusion but does not prevent extravasation of the medication. Until tissue pressure becomes significant, the pump will continue to introduce vesicants into interstitial space unless the client alerts the nurse to stop the infusion. Warming vesicant medications does not prevent extravasation from a vein. Extending the time over which the vesicant is infused will not safeguard against extravasation and may increase the risk of harm to the vein and possible infiltration.

12. *Answer:* D

Rationale: Radiographic validation must confirm that the tip of the catheter is in the superior vena cava (not in the right atrium of the heart, where it might trigger ectopic beats) before the infusion can be increased. Computed tomography scans are expensive and not necessary to confirm catheter placement. Endoscopy is a fiberoptic examination of the gastrointestinal tract, not the thoracic vasculature. Blood return does not guarantee correct placement of the catheter tip. Blood may backflow into the catheter at any point during insertion.

13. *Answer:* D

Rationale: Although most individuals can be taught to care for the commonly used access devices, those who are not good candidates should be considered for an implanted device as they require less self-care. Demonstration of the ability to care for the device is critical for all of the external access devices. The need for chemotherapy infusions and blood samples is a clinical indication for all of the access devices. The client expressing concerns about the implantation is an indication to provide additional education.

14. *Answer:* A

Rationale: Entering the skin by inserting the noncoring needle carries the risk of infecting the vascular central line; aseptic technique is important. The dressing should not obscure; a clear view of the insertion site is needed to assess for redness, discharge, or migration of the catheter. Performing the activity as a clean procedure is incorrect because the risk for infection needs to be addressed with strict aseptic technique. It is not necessary for the client to hold his or her breath while the needle is being inserted. It is a good idea for the client to turn his or her head away from the insertion site while the dressing is changed to prevent the introduction of respiratory microbes onto the site.

15. *Answer:* B

Rationale: The client should be able to assess the system to determine that the power is on and the infusion is occurring. The line should be flushed not with water but with normal saline. Flushing is unnecessary while infusion is ongoing. Flushing the line with sterile water every 12 hours is incorrect. Normal saline solution would be used, and when the infusion is ongoing, there is no need to flush the line. These systems should be used only for their intended purpose; only a nurse should assess the system and determine whether a second line is appropriate. Doses are programmed on the ambulatory infusion pumps with a sequence intended to prevent accidental or uninformed alteration by lay individuals. Changes in dose need to be made by the nurse when an order is changed or the infusion is complete.

16. *Answer:* C

Rationale: The push-stop method during routine flushing is recommended because it causes swirling, decreasing the risk of clots in the line. Applying too much pressure during an infusion would potentially rupture the line, which would necessitate removal of the catheter. Inadequate flushing after blood draws can contribute to a clot in the line, interfering with future use of the catheter, but these are not infectious clots. A line that has been partially pulled out is at risk of becoming displaced even further. External access devices should be secured adequately to decrease the likelihood of this problem.

17. *Answer:* C

Rationale: Fortunately, implanted access devices are sturdy. To prevent excessive pressure, infusions are made with large-volume syringes and with slow, steady rates. Nonsteroidal antiinflammatory drugs do not damage the catheter if they are administered in liquid form or tablets are powdered and dissolved in solution. Clients with implanted devices can and should bathe regularly. Because the lines are centrally implanted, care must be taken to prevent infection or displacement, but clients are able to participate in ordinary activities of daily living. These catheters may go unused for extended periods of time without deteriorating or being damaged. Care must be taken to prevent obstruction with blood clots, but they can be dormant for long periods.

CHAPTER 25

1. *Answer:* B

Rationale: Although renal function can require dose adjustments for antimicrobials, this finding itself does not increase the risk of infection. Mouth care is important because mucous membrane breakdown increases the risk for systemic infections. The surgical incision, which is not yet healed, is an example of a disruption of a primary barrier to organisms and demonstrates that the family likely realizes that this is a risk factor. Rituximab, fludarabine, alemtuzumab, and antithymocyte globulin cause alterations in B- and T-cell function and can increase the risk of infection.

2. *Answer:* A

Rationale: Penicillins, cefepime, and meropenem are all used as front-line therapy for neutropenic fever. An antifungal, voriconazole is first-line treatment for aspergillosis and is used as empiric therapy in febrile neutropenia. Echinocandins, also a type of antifungal, are used as first-line therapy for candidiasis and empiric therapy in febrile neutropenia.

3. *Answer:* B

Rationale: Although infections are the leading cause of problems in immune-suppressed individuals, hand-washing and temperature monitoring are critical interventions that make a difference. Because many of the infections are caused by organisms that are in the body already, not all can be prevented; early recognition is important for prompt initiation of treatment. Focusing on the newer antibiotic and the time since her father's death does not place the appropriate emphasis on proactive interventions that can make a difference. Experience can make it easier to recognize problems earlier, but it does not replace the need for and benefit of handwashing.

4. *Answer:* D

Rationale: Because many alternative therapies and practices are not closely regulated, they can actually be a source of infection and other problems. Keeping an open line of communication regarding all agents she is giving him is important. Although some adults may have the "desire to be mothered," this is not universally true and does not address any concerns regarding alternative therapies commonly used in Mr. T.'s culture. Encouraging Mr. and Mrs. T. to have his mother come to the clinic so the staff can provide personalized teaching may be beneficial, but it is important to be careful not to appear defensive regarding her approach to caring for her son. Motivation and increased activity are important, but nurses still need to be alert to potential concerns with culture-specific remedies that may interact with the treatment being administered.

5. *Answer:* A

Rationale: Amphotericin B and fluconazole are antifungals that are indicated for a fungal infection such as *Candida*. Caspofungin (Cancidas) is an antifungal, but ciprofloxacin is an antimicrobial for gram-negative bacteria. Voriconazole (Vfend) is used for *Candida* infection, but imipenem is for gram-positive infections. Cidofovir is an antiviral agent.

6. *Answer:* C

Rationale: The major toxicity of aminoglycosides is nephrotoxicity. Careful monitoring of antibiotic levels (peak and trough), serum creatinine levels, and urine output is indicated to maximize treatment while minimizing toxicity to the kidneys.

7. *Answer:* A

Rationale: Cephalosporins such as cefepime can cause allergic reactions, which are manifested by shortness of breath, hives, and itching. The other options are not associated with allergic reactions.

8. *Answer:* C

Rationale: Intravenous doses and schedules are designed to provide bactericidal serum levels for as long as possible between each dose interval for optimal coverage. Broad-spectrum (not gram-negative) coverage is vital to cover common infectious organisms. Antiviral (not antifungal) therapy should be considered for patients with a past history of outbreak (e.g., herpes simplex) during chemotherapy.

9. *Answer:* D

Rationale: Doses are based on ideal, not actual, body weight. Ganciclovir, not acyclovir, is the antiviral regarded effective preemptive therapy for cytomegalovirus in high-risk clients with cancer. Probenecid is given to prevent renal reabsorption of cidofovir.

10. *Answer:* A

Rationale: The mechanism of action of nonsteroidal antiinflammatory drugs involves the inhibition of cyclooxygenase and thus the production of prostaglandins. This break in the cascade in turn suppresses the inflammatory response of white blood cell and macrophage migration to the site of injury and results in or contributes to symptom relief. Antiinflammatory agents do not work centrally by blocking opiate neurotransmitters. Prostaglandins mediate nociceptive pain from inflammation.

11. *Answer:* A

Rationale: The combined interaction and potential side effects of aspirin, naproxen, and dexamethasone put Mr. P. at higher risk of gastrointestinal ulceration, bleeding, and fluid retention and urinary insufficiency. Constipation and immune suppression are not common side effects.

12. *Answer:* D

Rationale: Nonsteroidal antiinflammatory drugs (NSAIDs) have the potential to increase the effects of phenytoin, sulfonamide, and warfarin; clients' current medications should be reviewed carefully. NSAIDs should be avoided if a client is taking intravenous methotrexate because they can decrease renal clearance of this medication.

13. *Answer:* D

Rationale: Acne, weight gain, and a moon face would potentially be of greater concern for teenagers because they affect body image. Although the others are potential side effects of this combination of agents and are essential components of the education discussion, they may not be of as much concern to a teenage client.

14. *Answer:* B

Rationale: Nonsteroidal antiinflammatory drugs (NSAIDs) are associated with fluid retention caused by an inhibition of the renin–aldosterone system; thus, weight gain can occur while a patient is taking an NSAID. Most opioid analgesics inhibit peristalsis and therefore may lead to constipation.

15. *Answer:* B

Rationale: Naproxen is an over-the-counter (OTC) long-acting nonsteroidal antiinflammatory drug (NSAID). Other NSAIDs are also available OTC. The food indication and drug interaction with warfarin are not specific to this NSAID.

16. *Answer:* A

Rationale: In addition to tumor lysis fever, antiinflammatory agents are effective in pain related to bone metastasis. NSAIDs serve as excellent adjuvants with opiates. Few clients with cancer have adequate pain control with only antiinflammatory agents throughout the course of their disease. Potential adverse effects include gastrointestinal bleeding, renal toxicity, bleeding, cardiac toxicity, and confusion. These are seen especially in older adults, not younger.

17. *Answer:* D

Rationale: Their lack of an antiplatelet effect can provide advantages in clients with a lower platelet count. Few antiinflammatory agents have truly demonstrated gastrointestinal safety, and hepatic adverse effects must be monitored closely in this classification of agents. The long half-life of piroxicam allows for once-daily dosing.

18. *Answer:* A

Rationale: The major advantage of intermediate-acting corticosteroids is that they have minimal sodium-retaining activity; long-acting corticosteroids have no sodium-retaining activity.

19. *Answer:* A

Rationale: The neuromuscular and skeletal effects of corticosteroids include arthralgia, myalgia, fatigue, muscle weakness, myopathy, osteoporosis, muscle wasting, and fractures. Nursing implications include monitor muscle strength, pain medication as needed, regular exercise to promote bone development, and safety measures to prevent falls and injuries.

20. *Answer:* D

Rationale: On the Hesketh scale of emetogenic potential, dacarbazine is a level 5 (>90%) emetogen and is as severe as cisplatin and doxorubicin–cyclophosphamide in causing nausea and vomiting. Etoposide, melphalan, and busulfan are moderate (30%-90%). Ifosfamide greater than 2 g/m2 is high (>90%). Vinorelbine, bleomycin, and vincristine are very low (<10%). Docetaxel and paclitaxel are both low (10%-30%).

21. *Answer:* C

Rationale: Dexamethasone improves antiemetic efficacy by approximately 20% for both moderately and highly emetogenic chemotherapy. It is also used before taxanes (docetaxel and paclitaxel) for preventing and treating hypersensitivity reactions. It has no effect on allergic reactions to cisplatin.

189

22. *Answer:* C

Rationale: The use of a 5-HT3 antagonist (e.g., ondansetron, granisetron, or dolasetron plus dexamethasone) produces approximately 60% complete control (no emesis, no rescue) in clients treated with highly emetogenic chemotherapy. Substance P–neurokinin-1 receptor agents are also often added for improved outcomes. Prochlorperazine and metoclopramide are indicated for breakthrough nausea and vomiting or low-emetogenic agents. Lorazepam serves as an antianxiety agent and enhances the other antiemetics.

23. *Answer:* B

Rationale: Factors that increase the risk of nausea and vomiting are history of chemotherapy-induced nausea and vomiting, female gender, younger age (<50 years), anxiety, and history of motion sickness. Less alcohol intake history also increases the risk. The history of delayed nausea and vomiting increases the risk of acute nausea and vomiting in the next cycle of treatment.

24. *Answer:* B

Rationale: Prochlorperazine is an effective treatment for breakthrough emesis. 5-HT3 antagonists and lorazepam or diphenhydramine do not have proven efficacy. Lorazepam is useful for anticipatory nausea or vomiting, and diphenhydramine is useful to prevent dystonic reactions from metoclopramide.

25. *Answer:* A

Rationale: The client is experiencing both acute and delayed vomiting. The addition of a dexamethasone to the 5-HT3 antagonist might improve both acute and delayed episodes. In addition National Comprehensive Cancer Network guidelines encourage the addition of a substance P – neurokinin-1 receptor antagonist such as aprepitant. Prochlorperazine is used for treatment of nausea, not prevention. Lorazepam is not a proven effective antiemetic. It is useful for preventing anticipatory emesis and anxiety. Aprepitant (Emend) is effective for acute and delayed emesis but should be added to a 5-HT3 antagonist plus dexamethasone, not given as a separate regimen

26. *Answer:* C

Rationale: 5-HT3 antagonists can cause headache, which can be effectively treated with acetaminophen. Extrapyramidal side effects do not occur with selective serotonin antagonists (5-HT3). Principles of nursing management include the administration of prophylactic antiemetics to cover the onset, peak, and duration of action of each antineoplastic agent. Waiting to administer antiemetics only when a client vomits is not recommended.

27. *Answer:* B

Rationale: Selective serotonin antagonists, although more expensive than substituted benzamides and phenothiazines, do not have extrapyramidal side effects as a notable adverse side effect. Thus they have a major advantage over metoclopramide and phenothiazines, which also are sedating and have anticholinergic side effects.

28. *Answer:* D

Rationale: Diphenhydramine, dexamethasone, and lorazepam are all often used to augment antiemetics. Cimetidine is an H2 blocker that is not indicated for augmentation of antiemetics.

29. *Answer:* C

Rationale: Anticipatory nausea and vomiting is not uncommon in individuals who have had prior episodes of poorly controlled nausea and vomiting. It is important to prevent nausea and vomiting so that clients are less likely to develop problems with anticipatory nausea and vomiting. Anticipatory nausea arises from the cortex and limbic regions of the brain.

30. *Answer:* D

The serotonin antagonists include ondansetron (Zofran). Prochlorperazine is a D2 antagonist. Aprepitant is an NK-1 antagonist.

31. *Answer:* A

Rationale: Acute nausea and vomiting involves a chemotherapy-mediated release of serotonin from enterochromaffin cells; substance P and other mediators are also released. Late nausea and vomiting are not well understood and requires additional study. It occurs 24 to 120 hours after chemotherapy administration. Anticipatory nausea and vomiting arise from the cortex and limbic regions of the brain. Anticipatory nausea and vomiting can become a conditioned response. Prevention of nausea and vomiting is a priority for antiemetic therapy.

32. *Answer:* D

Rationale: The prevention of nausea and vomiting is the goal of medical management because it will decrease the likelihood of poor side effect management with future rounds of chemotherapy. Prophylactic treatment for delayed nausea and vomiting (when it is a known risk) is important for optimal outcomes. Selection of antiemetics should be based on the emetogenic potential of the chemotherapy and client-related risk factors. The complete follow-up assessment is also important, but option D is more important.

33. *Answer:* C

Rationale: The added sedation may be a side effect of the antiemetics and should be evaluated, but the safety concern would be that D.F. not be left home alone because of fall risk. The comment about expenses and the one in B about side effects as an indication need to be addressed but are not the safety concern at this time.

34. *Answer:* B

Rationale: Major neurotransmitter targets are as follows: serotonin (5HT3 antagonists, e.g., ondansetron), neurokinin (NK-1 antagonist e.g., aprepitant), dopamine (D-2 antagonist, e.g., prochlorperazine), histamine (H-1 antagonist, e.g., promethazine), acetylcholine (muscarinic, e.g., scopolamine), and cannabinoid (cannabinoid agonist, e.g., dronabinol).

35. *Answer:* C

Rationale: A neurokinin-1 inhibitor is added to the others in the protocol for moderately emetogenic agents; metoclopramide and prochlorperazine are used with the low-emetogenic agents.

36. *Answer:* B

Rationale: Prochlorperazine is known to cause extrapyramidal symptoms, including akathisia, which may appear as an inability to remain seated; diphenhydramine will decrease this effect. The remaining responses are not as relevant for this side effect.

37. *Answer:* C

Rationale: Pain is caused by the tumor itself about 70% of the time and diagnostic or therapeutic approaches about 20% of the time. Paraneoplastic syndromes and pain unrelated to the malignancy comprise the final 10% of reported pain. Optimal pain control and thus improved quality of life requires combination therapy that includes different pain medications (sustained and immediate release), adjunctive medications, and nonpharmacologic interventions. The precise cause of pain cannot always be identified, but treatment should be based on where the patient says it is. Analgesics work by interfering with the pain transduction, transmission, or modulation in the primary afferent neuronal fibers, the spinothalamic tract, collateral fibers, and high brain centers. Nociception refers to perception of pain.

38. *Answer:* C

Rationale: A breakthrough dose equivalent to 10% to 20% of the 24-hour long-acting dose provides adequate relief to get the pain in control as the episode subsides. Selection of the appropriate analgesia should be based on pharmacokinetic factors and the client's physical needs, age, history of analgesia usage, and organ function. The cause of the pain is not always known. The most appropriate dose of pain medication is the one that controls pain throughout a 24 hour period, including breakthrough pain. Tolerance and physical dependence occur in clients who take opioids regularly (withdrawal syndrome will occur if abruptly stopped); psychological dependence occurs when clients crave the opioid, use the drug compulsively, and continue use despite harm.

39. *Answer:* B

Rationale: Hepatic insufficiency increases the amount of fentanyl, morphine, tramadol, and oxycodone available.

40. *Answer:* D

Rationale: The altered transit time and absorption caused by the tube feedings and the metoclopramide are decreasing the effectiveness of the pain management; this would be the primary indication for pain management adjustment.

41. *Answer:* D

Rationale: Morphine is the most potent and central nervous system–depressing of the agents listed and thus has the potential of causing the most respiratory depression.

42. *Answer:* C

Rationale: Finding an alternative route is the best solution. Sustained-release tablets cannot be crushed; doing so presents a safety risk for the client. Other options involving tube feeding can compromise pain relief by increasing transit time and decreasing gastrointestinal absorption of the tablets.

43. *Answer:* B

Rationale: Aspirin competes with methotrexate for protein-binding sites and kidney excretion, thus liberating more methotrexate into the circulation. This can result in increased blood levels of methotrexate and enhanced toxicity, especially to the bone marrow. Other drugs that compete with methotrexate include sulfonamides, penicillins, nonsteroidal antiinflammatory drugs, and probenecid. These drugs should not be given concurrently with methotrexate; to do so is a safety risk for the client.

44. *Answer:* C

Rationale: Sustained-release morphine has too slow an onset of action to be useful for breakthrough pain. Immediate-release opioids such as morphine solution and hydromorphone are preferred. Around-the-clock dosing on analgesics is recommended in patients with chronic pain. Increased fluid and fiber intake are useful adjuncts to prevent narcotic-induced constipation.

45. *Answer:* B

Rationale: When a client receives meperidine and phenytoin, it can lead to reduced meperidine levels, which may alter pain management. The interaction does not commonly lead to the other identified effects.

46. *Answer:* A

Rationale: Respiratory suppression secondary to central nervous system (CNS)–related sedation requires early recognition to avoid further complications. Gastric upset, orthostatic hypotension, and constipation are not related to CNS suppression.

47. *Answer:* B

Rationale: The main goal during the first round of treatment (other than safety) should be prevention of nausea and vomiting because this will decrease the likelihood of anticipated problems during future rounds. Some medications such as lorazepam may contribute to sedation and amnesia, but this is not the main principle for their use. Delayed nausea and vomiting may occur if agents with this potential are administered. Clients receiving agents such as the platinums require a multiday antiemetic protocol to avoid this problem. Breakthrough nausea and vomiting is often an indication of inadequate antiemetic doses or frequency.

48. *Answer:* C

Rationale: Although pain relief is a respectable goal, family members do need to be cautioned regarding the risk of overmedication related to the risk of respiratory suppression and risk of falls. Constipation and nausea or vomiting as side effects are not safety concerns. Option B indicates a need for teaching regarding pain assessment, which is not as directly focused on safety.

49. *Answer:* B

Rationale: The pharmacokinetics of fentanyl support B as the correct answer. Fentanyl patch onset is 18 to 24 hours and buccal administration is 5 to 15 minutes.

50. *Answer:* A

Rationale: Anxiety is estimated to be present in approximately one third or more of clients with cancer. C is incorrect because the risk factors include all of those provided, including ongoing treatment, which can become draining for clients in terms of coping ability. Other risk factors for anxiety include cancer-related fears (situational anxiety, fear of death) and comorbidities like pain or fatigue.

51. *Answer:* C

Rationale: Anxiolytics serve multiple roles in clients with cancer; however, they are not used for food aversion.

52. *Answer:* A

Rationale: Triazolam is a short-acting sedative–hypnotic agent with minimal daytime hangover effect. Chlordiazepoxide and diazepam are indicated more for anxiety, seizure control, and alcohol withdrawal. Phenobarbital is a long-acting sedative.

53. *Answer:* C

Rationale: Tolerance to the sedating properties of barbiturates occurs rapidly and allows for rapid titration of the drug. Stevens-Johnson syndrome does occur, but it is rare. Rebound anxiety and loss of concentration and depression of affect are not usual side effects of barbiturates.

54. *Answer:* B

Rationale: The use of a phenothiazine (prochlorperazine) or high-dose meperidine in a client with brain metastases might lower the seizure threshold. Thus, phenytoin might be used as a prophylactic anticonvulsant in a client with brain metastases. Neither granisetron and dexamethasone nor naproxen and dexamethasone lower the seizure threshold. Although codeine may lower the seizure threshold, option B is the best answer because prochlorperazine lowers the seizure threshold, and normeperidine (the metabolite of meperidine) may also lower the seizure threshold.

55. *Answer:* B

Abrupt withdrawal can lead to an increased likelihood of psychosis, seizures, and coma. Although anxiolytics can be used for anticipatory nausea, this is not a major indication to avoid abrupt discontinuation. In addition, they can enhance pain control, but this also is not an indication against abrupt discontinuation.

56. *Answer:* C

Rationale: Benzodiazepines can cause sedation, cognitive impairment, dizziness, and lightheadedness, which increase the risk of falls. Fall precautions should be used, and this client may not be safe left home alone. In addition, these medications may cause respiratory depression, especially in individuals with lung cancer and a history of chronic obstructive pulmonary disease or if the patient's respiratory status has been compromised. Options B and D are important questions that need to be addressed, but they are not as critical as option C.

57. *Answer:* B

Rationale: Buspirone has similar mechanism of action, but the different structure leads to reduced incidence and severity of side effects compared with chlordiazepoxide, which is an intermediate-acting benzodiazepine.

The remaining options are not relevant for this comparison. Another concern for chlordiazepoxide would be it uses the CYP 3A4 pathway, which could cause potential problems if the client was receiving a medication that is metabolized by one or multiple CYP enzymes. We do not have that information in this scenario.

58. *Answer:* C

Rationale: The majority of the serotonin reuptake agents can contribute to sexual dysfunction. The other options are not expected side effects.

59. *Answer:* D

Rationale: Ifosfamide, high-dose methotrexate, and busulfan have the potential to cause seizures in individuals receiving these agents as part of their cancer therapy. Bleomycin, carmustine, gemcitabine, cyclophosphamide, and dacarbazine do not have this as a common potential risk factor.

60. *Answer:* A

Rationale: These agents have a greater potential to cause drug interactions without great likelihood of effective seizure prevention. Non–enzyme-inducing medications such as valproic acid, levetiracetam, and lamotrigine are more commonly used and well tolerated with limited drug interactions.

61. *Answer:* D

Rationale: Lowering the seizure threshold can cause seizures in an individual whose seizures were previously well controlled. The seizure threshold can be lowered by bupropion, isoniazid, tricyclic antidepressants, meperidine, propoxyphene, and phenothiazines. It can also be lowered by trauma, febrile episodes, and tumor pressure within the brain. Because the seizures have been well controlled, adherence is less likely to be a problem. Sleep disturbances would not affect seizure threshold. Workup may be needed to determine spread of disease, but from a nursing viewpoint, the other options are more appropriate initially.

62. *Answer:* A

Rationale: There can be multiple causes for seizures in an individual experiencing a seizure for the first time. A neurologic consult would provide necessary expertise to be certain the cause has been identified and treatment selected that would maintain optimal quality of life. This may not be caused by spread of the cancer. There is no evidence that dual therapy is more effective than monotherapy. Phenobarbital and phenytoin are no longer the gold standard because they cause drug interactions caused by enzyme induction.

63. *Answer:* A

Rationale: Gabapentin can be effective for neuropathic pain in clients with cancer; do not assume a seizure indication for the medication. It would be important to address the indication for the medication because sedation versus seizure risk have different safety concerns. Drug–drug interactions are always possible but should not be the initial action in this client. Gabapentin can cause sedation and weight gain, but this is not the initial action if it has not been a problem for this client.

64. *Answer:* A

Rationale: Oprelvekin is still being evaluated for use in cancer treatment. The Food and Drug Administration has approved it to reduce platelet transfusions caused by low platelet nadirs. Allergies to the product are not regarded a common problem at this time.

65. *Answer:* D

Rationale: Granulocyte-macrophage colony-stimulating factor (sargramostim) is a multi-lineage growth factor that stimulates production of secondary cytokines such as tumor necrosis factor, interleukin-1, and macrophage colony-stimulating factor. Pegfilgrastim, darbepoetin, and oprelvekin are single-lineage growth factors.

66. *Answer:* C

Rationale: Prevention of febrile neutropenia is more effective than treatment of febrile neutropenia with granulocyte-colony stimulating factor or granulocyte-macrophage colony-stimulating factor. Neutropenia is influenced by the treatment protocol and patient-related factors. Oprelvekin has not been shown to decrease mortality.

67. *Answer:* B

Rationale: The neutropenia level for an indication would be absolute neutrophil count less than $500/mm^3$. The thrombocytopenia level would be platelet count less than 75,000 cells/mm^3. D is not included as an approved indication for growth factors.

68. *Answer:* A

Rationale: Hematopoietic growth factors for the myeloid line enhance the production of granulocytic myeloid cells. It is thought that they do not promote tumor activity by stimulating bone marrow stem cells. They are not used as a primary treatment for breast cancer, and they can shorten the duration of neutropenia.

69. *Answer:* B

Rationale: A nonsteroidal antiinflammatory drug is effective for bone pain. Vials of proteins such as filgrastim (granulocyte-colony stimulating factor) should not be shaken vigorously because doing so will degrade the protein. Hematopoietic growth factors should be given 24 hours after chemotherapy.

70. *Answer:* B

Rationale: Granulocyte-colony stimulating factor increases phagocytic activity and stimulates production of neutrophils. It does not interact with the erythroid or platelet cell lines.

71. *Answer:* D

Rationale: Bone pain is the main side effect of filgrastim. This occurs as a result of expansion of granulocytic precursors in the client's bone marrow. Often, a client's peripheral white blood count will be correspondingly high.

CHAPTER 26

1. *Answer:* B

Rationale: Integrative medicine involves both complementary and alternative medicine and conventional (also called traditional or Western) medicine. Some, but not all, of the alternative therapies are evidence based.

Holistic healthcare refers to modalities that integrate the body, mind, emotion, spirit, and environment of a person; not all of these modalities are outside of conventional medicine. Discouraging the use of all complementary therapies actually encourages the clients to be secretive regarding their use.

2. *Answer:* D

Rationale: Osteopathic medicine focuses on the relationship between the structure and function of the body; it uses physical manipulation, as well as conventional medical therapies, to facilitate self-healing in the individual.

3. *Answer:* C

Rationale: The National Cancer Institute Office of Cancer CAM distinguishes two broad categories of health care practices that fall outside of conventional medical treatments. In addition they lists eight major categories, which are alternative medical systems, energy therapies, exercise therapies, manipulative and body-based methods, mind–body interventions, nutritional therapeutics, pharmacologic and biologic treatments, and spiritual therapies. This, however, is also complex and not universally recognized. Ayurveda is based on the principle that maintaining balance in the body, mind, and consciousness helps to preserve health and treat illness. Ayurveda is regarded a whole medical system of CAM. There is ongoing work to achieve a universally accepted categorization to help people receiving or using complementary therapies understand more about the therapies offered.

4. *Answer:* A

Rationale: There are currently no standards of practice or processing regulations for aromatherapy; essential oils have a wide range of quality levels. Aromatherapy targets physical imbalances, as well as psychological and spiritual issues. Although individuals can develop an allergy to the transporting vehicle, this is not a major safety concern.

5. *Answer:* C

Rationale: Feldenkrais refers to a method that teaches movement and manipulation to increase body awareness. Gentle manipulation of the skull to reestablish natural configuration and movement is cranial osteopathy. Lymphatic therapy is the use of vigorous massage to stimulate flow of lymphatic fluid. The technique that uses movement and touch to restore balance to the body is called the Alexander technique, and it is not part of the Feldenkrais method.

6. *Answer:* B

Rationale: Dance therapy, physical therapy, and Qi Gong are forms of manipulative and body-based complementary and alternative medicine practices. The other choices are not body-based practices.

7. *Answer:* C

Rationale: Studies have shown that achieving a relaxed state of mind can decrease perceived levels of stress, relieve muscle tension, enhance a sense of well-being, and boost the immune response. It is a mindfulness-based form of stress reduction that involves training clients to develop awareness of experiences moment by moment and in the context of all senses. Guided imagery techniques may include the use of a coach (or audio or video recording) who narrates the imagery, but this is not a requirement to practice meditation.

8. *Answer:* C

Rationale: Neurolinguistic programming focuses on changing thought patterns, such as the use of a gratitude journal to focus the mind on the positive. A and D refer to yoga; B refers to T'ai Chi.

9. *Answer:* B

Rationale: Herbal therapy can be taken in a variety of ways and can cause drug interactions. Herbal therapy products are not regulated by the Food and Drug Administration and should always be monitored by a healthcare provider to ensure safety. Hydrotherapy is the use of baths and compresses to enhance absorption. Although herbs may be used in baths, that is not the primary focus of this form of therapy.

10. *Answer:* D

Rationale: In Reiki, the practitioner directs the flow of energy by placement of the hands on the body in specific patterns (without deep pressure) to redirect restore energy flow. Therapeutic touch is described in A, B refers to healing touch, and C describes magnetic therapy.

11. *Answer:* D

Rationale: Psychosocial status and age-related developmental issues can be influenced by the use of complementary therapies. Cultural practices may influence the tendency of the client and family to use complementary therapy with or without healthcare professional knowledge or approval. Although cost may influence a client's decision to forego traditional therapy for less expensive complementary therapies not all complementary therapies are less expensive. Physicians may or may not be supportive of the client's use of complementary therapy; nurses play an important role in maintaining open communication and avoiding safety issues.

12. *Answer:* A

Rationale: Possible improvement in quality of life is a valid reason to use alternative medicine, along with the cost of the medicine being less than conventional medicine. The other answers may be cited by patients but do not accurately represent complementary and alternative medicine (CAM) or conventional medicine. The field of CAM does not have a foundation of evidence-based practice, although the practices are widely accepted in some geographic areas. Claims of cancer remission associated with certain CAM are frequent but are not based on reliable clinical data. CAM should not act as a replacement for conventional medical assessment and treatment.

13. *Answer:* D

Rationale: The volume of information available on any approach, traditional or alternative, should not be interpreted as evidence of clinical effectiveness. Oncology nurses can assist clients in accessing credible information by asking a series of questions about the therapy and about the practitioner who will be administering the therapy. The other answers are valid questions and should be considered before any treatment plan.

14. *Answer:* A

Rationale: Originating in India, Ayurveda is based on the principle of maintaining balance in the body, mind, and consciousness and is used to preserve health and treat illness. Aiming to restore an internal balance, interventions may include proper diet, hydration, and lifestyle alterations. Homeopathy is based on the precept of healing through the administration of specific substances, whereas osteopathic medicine focuses on the relationship between the structure and the function of the body. Combining five elements, fire, earth, metal, water, and word, which correspond to various organs and tissues in the body, is a tenet of traditional Chinese medicine.

15. *Answer:* C

Rationale: Acupuncture needles in one part of the body can affect the pain sensation in another part of the body when impulses stimulate the nerve fibers in the dorsal horn of the spinal cord. Acupuncture treatments could create a placebo effect and could help clients to refocus their concentration, but these are not the main actions of the therapy. Acupressure uses pressure applied to the skin surface with the finger and thumb. It is similar to acupuncture, but needles are not used.

16. *Answer:* A

Rationale: Homeopathy uses substances in hyperdiluted concentrations for symptom management or disease resolution. The other answers are not systems of healing.

CHAPTER 27

1. *Answer:* A

Rationale: Many drugs can alter platelet development; aspirin, clopidogrel (Plavix), and sulfonamides are just a few. Others include digoxin, furosemide, heparin, phenytoin quinidine, and tetracycline.

2. *Answer:* B

Rationale: Infection precautions are important to include in a care plan for a patient with a low absolute neutrophil count. Changing water pitchers frequently is encouraged; removing them is unnecessary. Furthermore, there should not be any fresh flowers or plants in the room or near the vicinity of the patient. Sterile technique for central lines is definitely indicated; clean technique for indwelling urinary catheters and feeding tubes is appropriate.

3. *Answer:* D

Rationale: Patients with tumor invasion of the bone marrow are at a higher risk for neutropenia because of a smaller reserve of normal cells. Patients who are malnourished are at a high risk for neutropenia because of poor nutritional status. Patients who receive radiation to a major bone marrow production site such as the sternum, skull, pelvis, or long bones are at a risk for becoming neutropenic. A patient with hypoalbuminemia, not hyperalbuminemia, is at risk for neutropenia.

4. *Answer:* D

Rationale: D is the only correct answer. If the chemotherapy dose is reduced and will not compromise the goal of cancer treatment, growth factor is not recommended. However, if the chemotherapy dose cannot be reduced, growth factor may be prescribed. Colony-stimulating growth factors for neutrophils are not prescribed for anemia or clients undergoing radiation.

5. *Answer:* C

Rationale: Patients who have a hypercoagulation state from a paraneoplastic syndrome are at risk for thrombocytopenia. Although biotherapy agents modulate the immune system, the potential for alteration of the blood cells remains unknown. The occurrence of thrombocytopenia after high doses of interferon has not been evident in clinical studies. Normal bone marrow function and growth factors do not place patients at risk for thrombocytopenia.

6. *Answer:* A

Rationale: Altered mucosal barriers such as mucositis increase the client's risk for infection. The other options describe nursing interventions to assist in infection prevention.

7. *Answer:* D

Rationale: Hemorrhage in cancer patients occurs because of alterations in hemostasis or coagulation mechanisms, such as disseminated intravascular coagulation. Hemorrhage does not occur from chemotherapy administration, platelet count greater than $100,000/mm^3$, or hematocrit above 30%.

8. *Answer:* D

Rationale: Patients with liver metastasis are at risk for tumor-induced fever. Patients with an absolute neutrophil count of $2000/mm^3$ or greater are not at high risk for a fever. Platelet counts do not contribute to a fever. Patients who are 3 weeks from an operative procedure are unlikely to experience a fever.

9. *Answer:* A

Rationale: Febrile neutropenia in a cancer patient is defined as having an absolute neutrophil count $<1000/mm^3$ and a single temperature of higher than 38.3° C (101° F) or a sustained temperature of 38° C (100.4° F) or higher for more than 1 hour.

10. *Answer:* B

Rationale: Lymphopenia, a reduction in the number of B or T lymphocytes, places the patient at risk for opportunistic infections.

11. *Answer:* C

Rationale: Fever can be a side effect of bleomycin, biotherapy (including interferon), and vancomycin administration. Acetaminophen is often given to reduce headache or tumor-induced fever.

12. *Answer:* C

Rationale: Circulating neutrophils are comprised of segmented neutrophils (segs) and bands and are important to fighting infection. If a patient has a decreased number of circulating neutrophils in the blood, the risk of infection is increased. It is important for nurses to know how to calculate an absolute neutrophil count. The ANC is calculated by taking the % neutrophils (segs 1 bands) multiplied by WBC.

13. *Answer:* C

Rationale: Platelets arise from the myeloid stem cells. Lymphoid stem cells produce lymphocytes. Megakaryocyte is an immature platelet. Epithelial stem cells produce skin cells.

14. *Answer:* D

Rationale: Prolonged neutropenia can result in sepsis and septic shock. The other options do not result from prolonged neutropenia.

15. *Answer:* B

Rationale: It is important for the nurse to understand the risk for developing myelosuppression before administering a chemotherapy regimen. Intermediate risk is defined as 10% to 20%; high risk is defined as greater than 20%. The other options are not chemotherapy regimens associated with an intermediate risk of myelotoxicity. The other options are chemotherapy regimens associated with a high risk of myelotoxicity.

16. *Answer:* D

Rationale: The normal life span of red blood cells is 120 days. The normal life span of neutrophils is 1 to 3 days, and the normal life span of platelets is 10 to 12 days.

17. *Answer:* B

Rationale: Invasive procedures such as rectal medications should be avoided in patients with thrombocytopenia. The other options are all appropriate precautions used to prevent or minimize bleeding.

18. *Answer:* B

Rationale: The most important physical barriers against invasion of organisms are the skin and intestinal mucosal barrier. From the mouth to the anus, there is a mucosal barrier, which serves as the first line of defense against pathogens. A venous access device and an indwelling urinary catheter are not barriers to infection but may actually be sources of infection. The immune system is not a physical barrier.

19. *Answer:* C

Rationale: The absolute neutrophil count is calculated by multiplying the % of neutrophils (Segs [22] + Bands [4]) by the actual white blood cell count. In this case, 22 + 4 = 26%. 0.26 × 1700 = 442.

20. *Answer:* C

Rationale: Implementation of an institutional standard of care for febrile neutropenia includes obtaining cultures (blood and urine), chest radiography (posteroanterior and lateral), viral and vancomycin-resistant enterococcus swabs if indicated, and prompt administration of intravenous antibiotics within 1 hour of evaluation. Computed tomography is not indicated and the abdomen was already found to be normal on assessment.

21. *Answer:* A

Rationale: One of the potential sequelae of prolonged hemorrhage is shock. Because of numerous blood transfusions caused by hemorrhage, patients with cancer are at risk for the development of viral disease such as human immunodeficiency virus, hepatitis C, and hepatitis B and unfortunately may experience transfusion reactions. Blood clots are not associated with hemorrhage.

22. *Answer:* A

Rationale: Granulocytes include basophils, eosinophils, monocytes, and neutrophils.

23. *Answer:* D

Rationale: It is important for the nurse to teach S.L. about appropriate measures to take to prevent infection and when and whom to call for medical assistance. Although a white blood cell (WBC) count may indicate S.L.'s immune system's ability to fight infection, an absolute neutrophil count (ANC) is more reflective because the neutrophils can be low when the WBC count is normal. Chemotherapy is typically not ordered and administered if the ANC is less than 1500/ mm³ or the WBC count is less than 1000/mm³. The patient does not have signs of dehydration or a fever.

24. *Answer:* C

Rationale: Neutrophils and lymphocytes are part of the white blood cell components and infection. Erythrocytes are red blood cell components. Levels of platelets below 20,000/mm³ increase the patient's risk for severe bleeding.

25. *Answer:* B

Rationale: The client is also at risk for spontaneous bleeding and should follow bleeding precautions. Unless the client is actively bleeding, platelets are usually administered for platelet levels of 20,000/mm³ or lower. Chemotherapy is usually held if the platelet count is less than 100,000/mm³. There is no indication that the patient is terminally ill; thus, hospice would not be the next step.

26. *Answer:* C

Rationale: Nadir refers to the lowest point blood cells reach after a cancer treatment. Nadir occasionally happens after biotherapy administration but this is not a regular occurrence.

27. *Answer:* A

Rationale: A nosebleed that is difficult to control should alert the nurse that the patient may have a low platelet count. A temperature of 100° F (37.7° C) is not indicative of infection. Nausea and excessive fatigue are unfortunate, but not life threatening, occurrences that may occur after chemotherapy administration.

28. *Answer:* B

Rationale: Interferon, interleukin-2, and vancomycin can all induce fever.

29. *Answer:* A

Rationale: Radiation of 20 Gy or more to the major bone marrow production sites (pelvis, ribs, sternum, skull, metaphyses of the long bones) will result in myelosuppression and may cause prolonged cytopenias.

30. *Answer:* A

Rationale: This information would provide the nurse with the approximate time to expect the patient's nadir and to suspect an infection with the presentation of fever.

31. *Answer:* B

Rationale: Red blood cells, white blood cells, and platelets are mature cells that are released into the peripheral circulation from the bone marrow.

32. *Answer:* D

Rationale: Chemotherapy-induced myelosuppression is the most common dose-limiting adverse event for patients receiving cancer treatment. Although uncomfortable, constipation and nausea and vomiting are side effects that can be managed with aggressive antiemetic therapy and stool management protocols. Severe diarrhea can certainly be a reason to stop chemotherapy or reduce dose but is not the most common dose-limiting adverse event.

33. *Answer:* C

Rationale: Filgrastim (Neupogen) is administered at a dose of 5 mcg/kg/day (rounding to the nearest vial size by institution-defined weight limits). It is typically given 24 hours or up to 4 days after treatment until the postnadir absolute neutrophil count recovers to normal or near normal levels by laboratory standards. It should never be administered before chemotherapy is given. Pegfilgrastim (Neulasta) is administered as a single dose of 6 mg per cycle on the day after treatment.

34. *Answer:* C

Rationale: Neutrophils provide the first line of the body's defense against bacterial infection by localizing and neutralizing bacteria.

35. *Answer:* D

Rationale: Prophylactic antibiotics are only used in patients with hematologic malignancies or in those patients who are at very high risk for febrile neutropenia. The regimen used is typically institution or region specific based on common infectious agents.

36. *Answer:* A

Rationale: Erythropoiesis-stimulating agents (ESAs) do not prevent anemia but stimulate the production of cells in patients with anemia. ESA administration is associated with inferior survival. Unfortunately, there is a risk of thrombosis, hypertension, and seizures with ESA administration. Patients need to be warned of these risks; informed consent with administration is indicated.

37. *Answer:* A

Rationale: When the platelet levels drop below 100,000/mm³, the client has thrombocytopenia.

38. *Answer:* A

Rationale: When a patient has febrile neutropenia, vital signs indicative of clinical deterioration are decreased blood pressure and increased respiratory and pulse rates.

39. *Answer:* D

Rationale: D is correct. The risk for infection is higher when the absolute neutrophil count (ANC) is below 1000/mm³. A refers to anemia; B refers to thrombocytopenia; in C, the ANC is not low.

40. *Answer:* B

Rationale: Folate deficiency, not excess, is a contributing factor for anemia.

41. *Answer:* D

Rationale: Prolonged fever and chills can result in increased metabolic activity and oxygen consumption, which lead to an increase of fatigue, muscle weakness, myalgias, and dyspnea. Fever and chills for a lengthy period of time is not associated with a decrease in circulating cancer cells or an increase in activity.

CHAPTER 28

1. *Answer:* B

   Rationale: Xerostomia is a drying of the oral mucosa, resulting in loss of saliva caused by damage that occurs to the salivary glands subsequent to radiation therapy. Dysphagia, mucositis, and trismus do not result in dry mouth. Dysphagia is an inability to swallow or difficulty in swallowing. Mucositis is inflammatory lesions of the mucous membranes and may include the intestine. Trismus is contraction of the muscles of mastication.

2. *Answer:* A

   Rationale: Large bowel obstructions occur less frequently than small bowel obstructions and commonly occur in the sigmoid colon. Causes of large bowel obstructions are cancer, volvulus, and diverticulitis.

3. *Answer:* B

   Rationale: Absence of bowel sounds may be a sign of obstruction, which is a potentially life-threatening complication. Although increasing fluid intake is recommended, inadequate fluid intake is not a life-threatening complication. Some patients may require laxatives and experience abdominal cramping; some may only have bowel movements every other day. These are not life-threatening complications.

4. *Answer:* C

   Rationale: Xerostomia is definitely related both to the cumulative radiotherapy dose and the volume of salivary gland tissue included in the treatment portals. Young adults are more likely to recover salivary flow than older patients. Management of xerostomia consists of both salivary substitutes and salivary stimulation; the latter is more beneficial in patients with residual salivary function. Of the salivary substitutes, mucin-based products are better tolerated and have a longer duration of action than methylcellulose-based products.

5. *Answer:* B

   Rationale: Because esophageal cancer can invade surrounding structures, symptoms may occur that are related to compressive effects of the enlarging mass on adjacent structures. Dysphagia is one of the classic symptoms of esophageal carcinoma. Infection, anxiety, and anorexia are symptoms that may occur with a cancer diagnosis and accompanying treatment but are not the likely cause of dyspnea and dysphagia.

6. *Answer:* B

   Rationale: Eating popsicles wets the mouth and numbs the mucosa and is an intervention that may provide moisture to the oral mucosa. Decreasing intake of liquids will cause less moisture to be present. The other two answers may irritate the mouth and cause excessive burning.

7. *Answer:* D

   Rationale: Antiemetics should be administered around the clock to prevent nausea. Medicating after vomiting does little to relieve nausea that preceded the emesis. Intake of fatty or fried food may contribute to nausea, and caffeine does not affect nausea. Modifying the diet to include bland, chilled foods with liquids served separately and replacing fluids with popsicles or sports drinks is recommended.

8. *Answer:* C

   Rationale: The early symptoms of esophagitis include difficulty and pain on swallowing and epigastric pain. Esophageal pain that worsens indicates progressing esophagitis. The other answers involve inflammation in various other parts of the body.

9. *Answer:* A

   Rationale: Papain (found in papaya) and amylase (found in pineapple) are enzymatic agents that break down saliva. The other agents act as stimulants to increase the saliva or may be too drying.

10. *Answer:* B

    Rationale: Ascites is associated with various tumors, mainly intra-abdominal malignancies. Ovarian cancer accounts for 38% of ascites.

11. *Answer:* C

    Rationale: The location of the colostomy is the main determining factor. A cecostomy or ascending colostomy produces semifluid or mushy stool. A transverse ostomy drains mushy stool at irregular intervals, usually after meals. A descending or sigmoid colostomy produces soft to formed stool and can be regulated by irrigation. The amount and type of food eaten and fluid intake are not the most important factors in determining the consistency and volume of colostomy output.

12. *Answer:* D

    Rationale: Patients with a history of rheumatoid disorders, diabetes, and HIV are at risk for xerostomia.

13. *Answer:* A

    Rationale: Diarrhea results in electrolyte imbalances, including potassium loss and low sodium. Hypercalcemia is often seen in clients with breast cancer or multiple myeloma with bone metastases, and hypophosphatemia is typically seen in clients treated for diabetic ketoacidosis. Hyperkalemia occurs when the kidney is unable to excrete potassium, often seen in patients with renal failure.

14. *Answer:* D

    Rationale: High-fiber and roughage-based diets stimulate peristalsis and prevent constipation. Milk can be constipating. Fluid intake should be 3000 mL/day.

15. *Answer:* B

    Rationale: Corticosteroids, such as dexamethasone (Decadron), are most effective when combined with serotonin antagonists to prevent and relieve nausea and vomiting. Classic steroid side effects are not seen when steroids are used for the short term to manage nausea and vomiting. They increase appetite and do not cause dysphagia.

16. *Answer:* A

    Rationale: Some salivary function can return after the cessation of treatment, but the patient should understand that xerostomia may be permanent. A decrease in salivary flow occurs within the first week of treatment, and medication is not always indicated and often does not totally prevent or eliminate this side effect. Chemotherapy does not usually affect xerostomia.

17. *Answer:* B

Rationale: Dysphagia is usually insidious and slowly progressive. It is usually associated with head and neck, esophageal, and lung cancers with lymph node involvement. Dysphagia may be caused by anticholinergic drugs and psychotropic medications that impair the gag reflex and swallowing.

18. *Answer:* B

Rationale: Ovarian and colorectal cancers most commonly cause distal bowel obstruction. Cholangiocarcinoma, gallbladder, and pancreatic cancers are the most common tumors causing duodenal obstruction.

19. *Answer:* A

Rationale: Although all of these may be appropriate to institute in patients with ascites, providing pain medications and nonpharmacologic pain strategies, such as relaxation, imagery, music, distraction, and healing touch, is the most important.

20. *Answer:* A

Rationale: The head of the bed should be elevated 45 to 90 degrees, with head slightly forward while eating, but this position should only be maintained for 45 to 60 minutes after oral intake. Explore the need for alternative methods for providing nutrition, such as total parenteral nutrition (TPN), only if intake is not possible via oral route. Other actions can be tried before suggesting TPN. It is important to minimize swallowing difficulty by avoiding milk products, alternating solids with liquids, and encouraging chewing thoroughly on the strongest side of the mouth.

21. *Answer:* A

Rationale: Mucositis and esophagitis are related to 5-fluorouracil, cytosine arabinoside, and etoposide. Of the chemotherapeutic agents listed, busulfan, docetaxel, and carboplatin are not implicated.

22. *Answer:* C

Rationale: Antiemetics such as 5-HT3 antagonists, opioids, and chemotherapeutic agents in the vinca alkaloid class can cause constipation. Side effects of 5-fluorouracil are nausea, mucositis, and diarrhea.

23. *Answer:* D

Rationale: Women and those younger than 50 years of age have increased incidence of nausea and vomiting. Patients with delayed gastric emptying have an increased risk of nausea and vomiting. Hypercalcemia, tumors of the central nervous system, and bowel obstruction are all risk factors.

24. *Answer:* B

Rationale: Stomatitis is mucositis or ulcerative reaction of the oral cavity. Gingivitis is inflammation of the gum tissues, usually of dental origin. Dysphagia is difficulty swallowing, and xerostomia is a dry mouth.

25. *Answer:* D

Rationale: Combined 5-fluorouracil and abdominal radiotherapy have a synergistic effect to cause diarrhea. Peripheral neuropathy typically occurs with vincristine or vinblastine. Constipation is not a side effect of radiation and 5-fluorouracil. Although thrombocytopenia and low blood counts may occur with radiation, diarrhea is a side effect with life-threatening implications.

26. *Answer:* B

Rationale: The location of the stoma is the most important factor to consider in determining the best type of ostomy appliance for the patient. Pouch selection is based on the consistency of effluent, stoma size, abdominal contour, and the degree of stomal protrusion.

27. *Answer:* C

Rationale: Patients younger than 20 years old have a higher risk for developing mucositis than elderly patients. The severity of mucositis is associated with daily radiotherapy dose, total cumulative dose, and volume of irradiated tissue. The small intestine exhibits injury within a few days of cytotoxic exposure and large intestine a short while later.

28. *Answer:* A

Rationale: Her symptoms indicate a partial bowel obstruction. Gastric outlet obstruction causes pain higher in the abdomen and exhibits sour emesis that is not bile colored and often contains undigested food. Frequent symptoms associated with proximal small intestine obstruction is rapid-onset, bitter, bile-stained emesis that may be projectile. The characteristics of the client's pain are not consistent with bowel perforation and peritonitis, which exhibits a boardlike abdomen and increased pain on movement.

29. *Answer:* C

Rationale: Younger clients are more sensitive to the effects of the prochlorperazine. The combination of prochlorperazine and diphenhydramine can help decrease these effects.

30. *Answer:* B

Rationale: Orabase gel is a topical agent used to treat radiation- and chemotherapy-induced mucositis and esophagitis by protecting, coating, and soothing the oral mucosa. It is not intended to reduce infection or decrease chemotherapy drug exposure to the oral mucosa.

31. *Answer:* D

Rationale: Mucositis is two to three times more likely to occur in hematologic malignancies than in solid tumors such as melanoma, bladder, and breast cancer.

32. *Answer:* C

Rationale: Constipation of 3 days or more is unusual in this client and suggests a need for immediate relief. At 10 days after chemotherapy, patients are at nadir and are susceptible to infection. Rectal medications or treatments should be avoided. Opioids can increase the risk of constipation. Bulk-forming laxatives can take longer to provide relief than oral stimulant laxatives.

33. *Answer:* D

Rationale: Irrigation is appropriate for clients with sigmoid colostomies who are producing formed stool. The patient must have a strong desire to learn the technique. Irrigating is contraindicated if a client is receiving pelvic or abdominal radiation because of the risk of bowel perforation. Irrigating a temporary colostomy can create bowel dependence, and it may take a long time for the client to master the procedure.

Cecostomies are not irrigated because they produce semifluid to mushy stools throughout the day and cannot be regulated.

34. *Answer:* D

Rationale: Oral mucositis is graded as follows: grade 1, mild symptoms; grade 2, moderate pain not interfering with oral intake; grade 3, severe pain interfering with oral intake; grade 4, life threatening with urgent intervention and hospitalization needed; and grade 5, death.

35. *Answer:* B

Rationale: Appropriate management of irinotecan-induced late diarrhea (occurring more than 24 hours after treatment) is loperamide. Patients should be monitored closely for dehydration and fluid–electrolyte imbalances. Atropine is used to treat cramping, spasms, and early diarrhea (occurring during the first 24 hours after treatment). Dexamethasone as a premedication is used to prevent nausea and vomiting. The diet should be modified for all patients who are expected to have diarrhea; management of diarrhea consists of keeping skin clean, dry, and protected with a skin barrier. Both of these nursing measures should be implemented at all times but will not decrease late diarrhea.

36. *Answer:* A

Rationale: Ginger has been found to be useful in treating motion sickness. Its antiemetic properties are due to the local action on the stomach, not on the central nervous system. Its effectiveness has not been established, but some evidence exists to support its usefulness.

37. *Answer:* D

Rationale: Bowel perforation and peritonitis are potential complications of bowel obstruction. Hypokalemia can occur if there is a large loss of gastric secretions either through vomiting or nasogastric intubation. Dyspepsia is not a symptom of bowel obstruction. Fluid overload is not a possible complication to bowel obstruction; dehydration is more of a potential sequela of bowel obstruction.

38. *Answer:* A

Rationale: Palifermin (Kepivance) for prevention of severe mucositis is used in transplant settings and is typically administered intravenously before stem cell infusion. Amifostine (Ethyol) acts as a radioprotector and is administered when radiotherapy is used and mucositis is possible. In addition to pharmacology interventions, a dental examination and cleaning may be necessary before treatment. Initiation of a standardized oral hygiene program is key; this includes using normal saline or salt and baking soda rinses (1/2 teaspoon each in 1 cup of warm water) regularly.

39. *Answer:* A

Rationale: Ondansetron is in a class of medications called serotonin 5-HT3 receptor antagonists. It works by blocking the action of serotonin, a natural substance that may cause nausea and vomiting.

40. *Answer:* B

Rationale: Symptoms are consistent with a bowel obstruction, most likely recurrent colon cancer. A is incorrect because constipation is not a side effect of FOLFOX (folinic acid [leucovorin], 5-fluorouracil, and oxaliplatin) therapy. Diarrhea is the more likely effect of 5-fluorouracil and oxaliplatin. A change in dietary fiber intake and exercise generally do not cause rectal bleeding. Onset of rectal bleeding is not associated with chronic use of laxatives.

41. *Answer:* A

Rationale: A low-residue diet will decrease irritation of the gastrointestinal tract. In addition, decreasing spicy, fried, and fatty foods may help. Diet can affect radiation-induced diarrhea; a high-fiber diet will increase irritation of the gastrointestinal tract. The patient should consume solid foods that contain low residue and high protein and avoid lactose if lactose intolerance has been a problem.

42. *Answer:* B

Rationale: The appliance should be changed every 5 days or as needed for leakage or complaint for peristomal discomfort. Changing it more often will only cause skin irritation. Additional information about colostomy care includes the fact that the opening of the pouch should be cut by ⅛ inch so that skin is protected and not exposed to ostomy contents. The peristomal skin should be cleaned with water, not chlorhexidine (which is very irritating).

43. *Answer:* D

Rationale: Magnesium citrate is of little to no use in prevention of constipation. It is primarily used in the acute evacuation of the bowel. Placing M.H. on a stimulant laxative and stool softener may be more appropriate. A total of 3000 mL/day of fluid intake is recommended every day to decrease the incidence of constipation. A diet that is high in fiber and roughage is recommended. Exercise can help stimulate peristalsis.

44. *Answer:* A

Rationale: Nonsurgical and postoperative intra-abdominal adhesions can cause small bowel obstruction. Nonsurgical adhesions can occur at any time after an infection or completion of radiation therapy. Hernias also can cause small intestine obstruction. Volvulus and diverticulitis cause large bowel obstruction. Gastrointestinal bleeding is not identified as a risk for small bowel obstruction.

45. *Answer:* A

Rationale: The client with HIV is at greatest risk because his immune system is compromised. He also recently took antibiotics, which places him at risk for overgrowth of *Clostridium difficile* or other organisms. For the client with acute myelogenous leukemia in remission, the client is not at increased risk for infectious diarrhea. It is more likely to occur in those traveling outside the United States. The young rhabdomyosarcoma survivor is in remission and not at increased risk for infectious diarrhea. Infectious diarrhea is not a toxicity associated with prostate cancer treatment comprising leuprolide.

46. *Answer:* A

Rationale: Senna is a laxative that chemically stimulates smooth muscles of the bowel and increases contractions. It is often ordered for patients receiving opioids. Methyl-cellulose is a bulk-forming laxative. Docusate is an emollient and lubricant laxative that softens hardened stool and facilitates passage through the lower intestine. Sodium phosphate does not stimulate smooth muscle; it increases the bulk of the stool by causing water retention.

47. *Answer:* C

Rationale: Grade 3 is defined by experiencing more than seven stools per day or a need for parenteral support for dehydration. Grade 1 is fewer than four stools per day over pretreatment level. Grade 2 is four to six stools per day. Grade 4 has physiologic, life-threatening consequences that require urgent care. Grade 5 is death.

48. *Answer:* C

Rationale: Lack of privacy and decreased physical activity are primary mechanisms. Anticonvulsant medications are considered an iatrogenic mechanism for intestinal mobility slowing. Spinal cord compression is a secondary mechanism.

49. *Answer:* D

Rationale: Bacteria such as *Escherichia coli* and *Clostridium difficile* are causes of secretory diarrhea. Enteral tube feedings are unabsorbable substances in the intestine, which can cause diarrhea by drawing water into the intestinal lumen by osmosis. Diarrhea caused by graft-versus-host and inflammatory bowel disease is a result of hypermobility (limited absorption caused by increased motility of the intestines).

). *Answer:* A

Rationale: Obstruction of bowel by tumor can cause constipation, but it is not likely in this case because her surgery showed no evidence of further disease. Bodily wastes need to be eliminated each day, regardless of amount of food ingested. Bowel manipulation during abdominal surgery can decrease peristalsis and motility, resulting in constipation. Opioids and immobility can decrease bowel motility.

CHAPTER 29

1. *Answer:* B

Rationale: There are multiple types of urinary incontinence, all of which involve an involuntary loss of urine. Stress incontinence occurs during laughing, coughing, sneezing, and other physical activities that increase abdominal pressure. Reflex incontinence is characterized by a lack of urge to void or sensation of bladder fullness. Functional incontinence is experienced because of difficulty in reaching or an inability to reach the toilet before urination. Total incontinence is the continuous loss of urine without distention or awareness of bladder fullness.

2. *Answer:* C

Rationale: Urinary incontinence can be attributed to storage or emptying problems (or both). A urethral or prostatic obstruction can prevent urine from exiting the bladder.

3. *Answer:* C

Rationale: Incompetence of the rhabdosphincter is the primary cause of incontinence and may result from a variety of factors, including shortening, not lengthening, the urethra. Unintentional pudendal nerve injury is another factor that may be implicated in postprostatectomy incontinence. This is something that can occur and is a risk associated with surgery that would have been outlined during the consent process.

4. *Answer:* C

Rationale: For the patients described, a loss (not an excess) of bladder, bowel, and rectal reflex contractions can occur. Loss or absence of contractions can lead to urinary incontinence.

5. *Answer:* D

Rationale: Antiemetics and nonopioids have not been associated with urinary incontinence. Sedatives and hypnotics relax smooth muscles and are medication risk factors for incontinence. Chemotherapy agents causing neurotoxic side effects, such as vincristine, oxaliplatin, and ifosfamide, have been associated with urinary incontinence; doxorubicin is not one of those drugs.

6. *Answer:* D

Rationale: Fluid intake should be monitored and limited several hours before bedtime. Excessive alcohol and caffeine intake is associated with urinary incontinence and should be limited or curtailed. Bladder training programs may be advantageous. Although exercise may add to stress incontinence, exercise and mobility are important for all patients with cancer and should not be eliminated.

7. *Answer:* B

Rationale: The risk of catheter-associated urinary tract infections is increased when an indwelling urinary catheter (IUC) is used. An IUC should be a last resort. Instead, instituting nonpharmacologic and supportive techniques to promote urinary continence and prevent skin breakdown is recommended. Lotion should not be applied; instead, a moisture barrier ointment or skin barrier is necessary after each incontinent episode. The perineal areas should be cleansed with a soft washcloth, soap, and water after every voiding. Chlorhexidine may be irritating to the skin and is not recommended.

8. *Answer:* A

Rationale: A neobladder is a urinary reconstructive procedure in which a surgically constructed bladder is created from intestine and attached to the urethra. Thus, patients with any intestinal or urethral issues are not appropriate candidates for the surgery. Factors that exclude creation of a neobladder include cancer extending into the urethra, a past history of inflammatory bowel disease, radiation, or short gut syndrome from previous bowel resection. Patients with a history of benign prostatic hypertrophy and urinary incontinence may be appropriate candidates for the surgery.

9. *Answer:* A

Rationale: An ileal conduit is the only urinary diversion requiring an external collection device. Patients with a continent diversion only need to catheterize through the stoma to drain urine from the reservoir every 4 to 6 hours, not every 3 hours.

10. *Answer:* C

Rationale: The pouch opening should be cut by ⅛ inch so that the barrier clears the stoma and does not allow urine to come in contact with skin surrounding the stoma. Excessive urine contact with skin around the stoma may lead to skin excoriation. The opening of the pouch should be as close as possible to the size of the stoma. The appliance should only be changed every 5 days and as needed for leakage or complaint of peristomal skin discomfort. More frequent changes are unnecessary and costly and may cause skin breakdown. Keeping the appliance clean will decrease odor buildup. Emptying the pouch when it is one-third to half full and before chemotherapy treatment will decrease odor. A full pouch may promote leakage and discomfort.

11. *Answer:* A

Rationale: 5-Fluorouracil is not a nephrotoxic chemotherapeutic agent. Gemcitabine is nephrotoxic; radiation therapy to renal structures may cause atrophy of normal tissue and permanent fibrosis. Many chemotherapeutic agents can cause rapid cell destruction, increasing uric acid formation and development of obstructive stones. Hemolytic-uremic syndrome (consists of concomitant anemia, thrombocytopenia, and acute renal failure) can be induced by mitomycin C administration, other drugs such as cyclosporine, bone marrow transplant, or radiation therapy. This syndrome can lead to renal impairment.

12. *Answer:* D

Rationale: Hypercalcemia of malignancy is a common occurrence in certain cancers, such as breast cancer with metastases, multiple myeloma, squamous cell cancer of the lung and head and neck, renal cell cancer, lymphomas, and leukemia. Cervical cancer renal problems are often related to post renal obstructive uropathy. Pancreatic cancer usually does not cause renal dysfunction.

13. *Answer:* B

Rationale: Patients with renal dysfunction typically have an elevated serum creatinine and blood urea nitrogen, an increase in uric acid and calcium phosphate formation caused by excessive tumor cell destruction, and a decreased creatinine clearance. Fluid and electrolyte imbalances caused by chemotherapy agents can have an indirect effect on kidney function and can lead to renal failure. A positive urine culture is not indicative of renal impairment but may suggest infection.

14. *Answer:* C

Rationale: Closely monitoring intake and output during and immediately after chemotherapy administration is crucial for patient safety. If the urinary output is less than 30 mL/hr, renal impairment is indicated. Aggressive hydration during cisplatin administration includes administering fluids before, during, and after chemotherapy infusion. Sodium bicarbonate administration is used to maintain urine alkalinity.

15. *Answer:* C

Rationale: The nurse is in a key position to talk about emotional and sexual health concerns with patients. It is important to take time to actively listen to the patient's concerns and assist in problem-solving ways to incorporate lifestyle changes. This includes talking about sexual health issues. If the nurse does not feel comfortable or does not have the information the patient needs, referral to a sexual health counselor is appropriate. Although talking with a physician is important, acknowledging that it is normal to have these concerns, and referral to an ostomy support group can provide additional support, parts of each of these answers are incorrect. The nurse should take responsibility to find the best evidence so the patient has correct and useful information as he tries to improve his quality of life.

16. *Answer:* D

Rationale: Electromyography is used to evaluate micturition, bladder filling, and storing function, and cystoscopy is used to identify the site of obstruction. Bladder scanning is used to determine the presence and amount of postvoiding residual urine. Other urodynamic and imaging studies include a cystometrogram and voiding cystourethrogram. A cough stress test may also be used to determine urinary incontinence.

17. *Answer:* C

Rationale: Pelvic exercises and a scheduled voiding program are interventions frequently used for initial treatment of urinary incontinence. Urinary incontinence is common after a radical prostatectomy and can last for several months. An indwelling catheter is usually left in place for a few weeks, and then bladder retraining is started. Incontinence is primarily caused by incompetence of the rhabdosphincter. Some incontinence may persist for several months. Interventions may include establishing a schedule for voiding, gradually increasing the intervals between voiding, and pelvic muscle exercises.

18. *Answer:* C

Rationale: Cisplatin requires aggressive hydration before, during, and after therapy. The other agents do not require aggressive hydration. Daunorubicin can cause the client to experience red urine. 5-Fluorouracil is not associated with renal toxicity but can cause diarrhea and stomatitis. Flutamide is more commonly associated with side effects of hepatoxicity and gynecomastia.

19. *Answer:* D

Rationale: Hypercalcemia commonly occurs with metastatic breast cancer, multiple myeloma, squamous cell cancer of the lung and head and neck, renal cell cancer, lymphomas, and leukemia. Hypercalcemia interferes with the kidneys' ability to concentrate urine. Hyperkalemia, hypocalcemia, and hyponatremia do not commonly occur with breast cancer with bone metastases and cannot cause the kidneys to lose the ability to concentrate urine.

20. *Answer:* C

Rationale: Adult briefs would create difficulty in providing accurate measurement of urine output. B is incorrect; toilet training is preferable to a catheter. If no special measures are taken, the client could be at risk for falling, and accurate measurement of urine output would be difficult. The client should be near a commode for easy access and for measurement of urine output.

21. *Answer:* B

Rationale: Fluid and electrolyte imbalances from some chemotherapy agents can have an indirect effect on kidney function and can lead to renal failure. Radiation therapy may cause permanent fibrosis and atrophy. Hypercalcemia of malignancy causes loss of concentration by the kidneys. Renal hypoperfusion promotes renal damage. Diuretics are not a direct cause of renal failure.

CHAPTER 30

1. *Answer:* D

Rationale: An examination of joint structure and alignment will assist in evaluating the integrity of bones structure and function and potentially uncover any underlying root causes. Assessment of deep tendon reflexes in both legs and arms would assist in determining the level of functional reflex and provide a baseline by which to measure improvement. The evaluation of the patient's mobility and sensory function is helpful in determining damage to sensory nerves and again gives a baseline from which to improve. The patient should inspect herself for cuts, burns, and bruises, but this measure is not part of a physical assessment; instead it is an intervention.

2. *Answer:* B

Rationale: Skin folds are dark, moist areas that retain wetness. Drying will decrease the risk of fungal infection. Applying povidone-iodine (Betadine) will cause the skin to dry out and may increase the risk of breaks in the skin. Bathing the patient daily may be necessary but also increases the risk of the patient not drying carefully and therefore increases the risk of fungal infections. Keeping the room at a cool temperature would reduce perspiration but not impact the risk for fungal infection.

3. *Answer:* C

Rationale: Pain; paresthesia (the sensation of tingling, pricking, prickling, or numbness); and formication (the sensation of worms or insects being under the skin) are the usual sensations patients with perineural tumor spread experience. Patients with diabetic neuropathy experience a reduction in their ability to feel pain or changes in temperature in their hands and feet. Horner's syndrome causes drooping of the upper eyelid and a consistently small pupil on the affected side. The symptoms of pain in or behind the ear, drooling, and an increased sensitivity to sound are associated with Bell's palsy.

4. *Answer:* B

Rationale: With leukopenia, there is an increased risk for infection. A patient with impaired skin integrity is at greater risk because of the break in the first line of defense, the skin. Diarrhea may occur as a side effect of the antineoplastic medication. Constipation is not associated with most antineoplastic medications. Some

antineoplastic agents can cause cardiotoxicity but not dysrhythmias.

5. *Answer:* D

Rationale: A neurologic examination will determine motor, sensory, and reflex loss caused by a spinal cord compression resulting from the prostate cancer metastasis to the spine. Immobilizing the body and instructing the patient not to flex his head, as well as turning the patient every 2 hours and doing skin checks, may be very important after a cause for the numbness and tingling is determined. To give false reassurance before determining the cause of the numbness and tingling is inappropriate.

6. *Answer:* C

Rationale: Changing position decreases the pressure in the area and decreases the risk of skin breakdown. The logroll technique will prevent further injury. The other interventions help to decrease risk of circulatory complications or autonomic dysreflexia but are not related to skin integrity.

7. *Answer:* A

Rationale: Platinum derivatives, such as cisplatin and carboplatin, can cause itching, redness, and swelling within 1 hour after beginning infusion. If this condition is life threatening, it is termed *anaphylaxis* and includes decreased blood pressure, decreased level of consciousness, and airway and breathing compromise. Rituximab can cause a reaction with flulike symptoms, also described as serum sickness. Patients on EGFR inhibitors (cetuximab, gefitinib) can develop acneiform rash, with papules and pustules similar to acne, although this rash contains no comedones and commonly involves the face, back, and upper chest.

8. *Answer:* B

Rationale: A patient with ataxia has a compromised ability to walk or impaired mobility status. Although safety issues regarding mobility, falls, and accessory devices are very important aspects of care, these are considered preventive measures and interventions rather than assessment. Skin integrity, dehydration, electrolyte imbalance, and renal compromise are all issues of concern throughout oncology care but are not specifically related to ataxia.

9. *Answer:* B

Rationale: Generalized exfoliative, ulcerative, or blistering skin toxicity presents as a grade 4 skin rash. Pruritus is a symptom of a grade 2 rash. Severe generalized erythroderma, along with macular, papular, or vesicular eruption, can be found in a grade 3 skin rash.

10. *Answer:* D

Rationale: Rehabilitation activities that help maintain and restore function are tertiary prevention activities. Education is provided at all levels of prevention for informed decision making. Promoting and immunizing are related to primary prevention, which includes preventing and protecting persons from disease.

11. *Answer:* C

Rationale: Cognitive distraction—the use of guided imagery or music therapy—is a common nonpharmacologic intervention used for patients presenting with anxiety and depressive symptoms. Counseling, psychotherapy, and behavioral therapies are psychoeducational interventions with any patients having issues with alterations in mental status. Requesting a sitter for a patient considered unsafe is an intervention to ensure a safe environment for patients in both inpatient and outpatient settings.

12. *Answer:* B

Rationale: In addition to calcium's benefits to bones and teeth, it acts as a catalyst in initiating and controlling muscular contractions and relaxation. Calcium is not involved in creating stomach acidity and does not prevent blood clotting. Calcium is not involved in the production of insulin.

13. *Answer:* A

Rationale: Erythema multiforme is usually a self-limiting hypersensitivity condition of the skin. It can be related to certain infective agents (herpetic viruses) or drugs (phenytoin, nonsteroidal antiinflammatory drugs, penicillins). It has also been known to occur with paclitaxel or radiotherapy. Candidiasis can occur anywhere but is usually found where the skin is folded, such as the armpits. It can appear moist and white or red. Erythema nodosum is a condition that causes rounded lumps or nodules just below the surface of the skin. Rosacea is a chronic skin condition in which tiny blood vessels enlarge and dilate over the face and nose.

14. *Answer:* C

Rationale: The use of assistive devices such as glasses and hearing aids will decrease the distortion of sights and sounds and decrease the client's anxiety, which reduces delirium. The remaining choices may maintain or increase the patient's delirium.

15. *Answer:* B

Rationale: A nursing intervention to protect skin integrity is to adopt and use sterile techniques for invasive procedures such as the insertion of tubing and other venous access devices. Moisturizing and lubricating skin and gentle skin cleansing with mild, pH-balanced skin cleansers are interventions nurses can provide to patients to teach self-care techniques and prevent complications. The use of medications to manage rash is considered a pharmacologic intervention.

16. *Answer:* B

Rationale: Muscle atrophy can occur when a patient has a painful joint condition. The remaining choices—curvature of the spine, generalized decreased upper muscle mass, and bilateral hypertrophy of paired muscle groups—are not related to physical mobility.

17. *Answer:* C

Rationale: When working with cognitively impaired patients, it is important for the nurse to reorient the patient to person, place, and time. Calling the patient by a term of endearment is inappropriate and is not best practice. Confirming identification by checking an identification wristband is standard procedure and is important, but it does not contribute to reorienting or maintaining cognitive function in the client. Neglecting to touch the patient may increase his or her anxiety.

18. *Answer:* B

Rationale: Changing a patient's position every 2 hours is an intervention to increase physical functioning, especially for a patient who is physically impaired or incapacitated. Placing a call light within reach when the patient is left alone is an intervention designed to decrease risk of further complications of immobility, allowing the patient an opportunity to reach out to the health care team when in distress. Placing the bed in a low position and raising the two side rails at the HOB is an intervention meant to maximize safety for the patient, whereas discussing risk factors for impaired mobility incorporates the family into the patient's care and provides necessary education.

CHAPTER 31

1. *Answer:* B

Rationale: A pneumothorax is caused by air in the pleural space. An empyema is an abnormal accumulation of infected fluid or pus in the pleural space. Diffuse parenchymal lung disease is a general term for a lung disorder that affects the deeper aspects of the lung tissue. A pleural effusion is a collection of abnormal amounts of fluid in the pleural space.

2. *Answer:* D

Rationale: A pneumonectomy is removal of the entire lung. Individuals can usually learn to adapt to the change. However, it will be important to avoid additional respiratory risk factors such as smoking. Preventive care such as vaccination to prevent pneumonia or the flu and early treatment of infections will also be important.

3. *Answer:* B

Rationale: A history of lung cancer, surgery, chronic obstructive pulmonary disease, heart disease, cardiac stents, and asthma are all risk factors for alterations in ventilation. Receiving treatment for tuberculosis, diabetes, and latex allergies are not significant risk factors. Cholecystectomy would impact respiration initially; however, the surgery was three months ago in this scenario.

4. *Answer:* B

Rationale: An empyema is an abnormal accumulation of infected fluid or pus in the pleural space and is treated with systemic antibiotics. Radiation therapy is done to reduce obstructions caused by lung tumors. Epinephrine is used to treat anaphylaxis. Oxygen is used to treat anaphylaxis or the hypoxemic client.

5. *Answer:* B

Rationale: All of these considerations are important, but medication management and the availability of emergency care are the priorities. Mismanagement of medications could result in significant problems that would require emergency care. The availability and location of such care are important to discuss in advance. This also influences the reporting of changes to the local healthcare provider, depending on availability versus having to contact the cancer treatment center that might be coordinating the treatment plan. Rural access to services can be a challenge and should be anticipated with initial planning of care. Awareness of cognitive function will help caregivers know when the patient can be left unattended. Activity prioritization and energy conservation strategies allow the client to be able to have some choice in activities.

6. *Answer:* C

Rationale: Bleomycin and radiation therapy place a client at high-risk for pneumonitis. The other options are not associated with this client's therapy regimen.

7. *Answer:* D

Rationale: Tapering of glucocorticoids rather than "stopping" them abruptly is necessary to avoid a flare-up of the pneumonitis. The nurse should have a baseline assessment of the lungs, but a complete blood count is not needed at this time unless there are other clinical indications for it. Cough suppressants and antipyretics are part of management for radiation-induced pneumonitis.

8. *Answer:* B

Rationale: Dyspnea, a nonproductive cough, and a fever during the infusion are the cardinal signs of pulmonary toxicity of drug-induced pneumonitis, and the nurse needs to stop the chemotherapy immediately. A crash cart may become necessary but is not the immediate intervention. Chest radiography is also not an immediate need, but arterial blood gas evaluation would be included in near immediate care. Oxygen may be required, but stopping the chemotherapy is the primary and immediate intervention. Epinephrine is helpful in treating anaphylaxis

9. *Answer:* C

Rationale: It is anticipated that the arterial blood gas evaluation to show decreased oxygenation and respiratory alkalosis. Hypoxia and hypocapnia are expected. Metabolic acidosis would present with a decreased not increased pH.

10. *Answer:* B

Rationale: Cetuximab is an example of a targeted therapy agent with a number of potential pulmonary abnormalities, including acute pneumonitis, bronchiolitis, and hypersensitivity reactions. It also can increase the risk of radiation pneumonitis. Clients with radiation-induced pulmonary toxicity are more likely to experience pleuritic chest pain. Clients with pulmonary toxicity are likely to have diminished diffusion capacity of the lungs for carbon monoxide, which measures the ability of the lungs to transfer gas from inhaled air to the red blood cells in pulmonary capillaries.

11. *Answer:* B

Rationale: Glucocorticoids decrease local inflammation. Bronchodilators relax airway constriction thus increasing airflow to the lungs. Antibiotics are used to treat sensitive infections, which may have a component of pulmonary inflammation. However, the target of the antibiotic treatment is the bacterial infection. Diuretics decrease fluid overload.

12. *Answer:* [?]

Rationale: Pulse oximetry provides a noninvasive estimate of blood oxygen levels by measuring the percentage of hemoglobin that is saturated with oxygen. Lung diffusion testing measures how well the lungs exchange gases; although it is an important part of testing for lung function, it is not a STAT procedure. Chest radiography detects structural abnormalities but does not provide information about oxygen level. A sputum culture detects infectious organisms, and results take several days.

13. *Answer:* D

Rationale: Sitting upright and leaning forward with the elbows on a table will increase the ease of respiration and reduce the work of breathing. Lying down, lying in a semi-Fowler position, or sitting with the legs crossed increases respiratory effort.

14. *Answer:* B

Rationale: Prayer and meditation have been shown to be effective in decreasing the sense of dyspnea. There is not sufficient evidence to support the use of grape seed extract. Morphine and incentive spirometry are not complementary therapies. Incentive spirometry would transiently increase respiratory effort.

15. *Answer:* A

Rationale: Dyspnea is a subjective experience that can best be evaluated from the client perspective. includes difficulty breathing, the feeling of an inability to get enough air, and the emotional reaction to those sensations. Clients usually can describe it in their own terms and are in the best position to determine symptom worsening or improvement. The clinician may not have the same sense of severity as the client. Dyspnea can indeed be present with many different conditions but must be rated by the client if they are able to do so.

16. *Answer:* A

Rationale: Hypoproteinemia decreases oncotic pressure in the microvasculature. Heart failure increases hydrostatic pressure. Atelectasis increases negative pressure in the pleural space. Acute pain increases blood pressure and respirations. These other options do not decrease the oncotic pressure in the microvasculature.

17. *Answer:* D

Rationale: Tachypnea, dullness to percussion, absent breath sounds, egophony, and a slight fever are classic symptoms of a pleural effusion. Symptoms associated with lung metastasis would depend on size, number, and location. Signs of anemia include dyspnea on exertion, fatigue, weakness, headache, decreased blood pressure, tachypnea, and tachycardia. Signs of pulmonary fibrosis include moist rales, tachypnea, and dyspnea.

18. *Answer:* A

Rationale: The speed of accumulation is the best predictor of symptoms of a pleural effusion. If it develops gradually over time, clients tend to tolerate larger volumes of fluid. Transudative fluid is related to system factors such as hypoalbuminemia, cirrhosis, congestive heart failure, and nephrotic syndrome, causing an effusion. Exudative fluid is usually related to local factors such as metastatic tumor or infections, causing an effusion. Although talc pleurodesis may be indicated, it will partially depend on the severity of symptoms and goals of treatment.

19. *Answer:* A

Rationale: The presence of air in the pleural space is a pneumothorax, which causes a loss in the vacuum normally present and eventual lung collapse. Although radiation therapy to the lung and bleomycin can cause respiratory side effects, pneumothorax is not usually one of them. The treatment will depend on the size of the collapse; if small, it may resolve on its own, a larger one may require the placement of a chest tube to evacuate the air. Surgery is not usually indicated unless the client develops additional complications such as a fistula.

CHAPTER 32

1. *Answer:* A

Rationale: An obstruction of the lymphatic system interferes with movement of lymph fluid into the circulatory system and leads to lymphedema with an overload of lymph fluid in the interstitial spaces. Edema is an accumulation of fluids in the interstitial space. Lymphedema is secondary to obstruction of the lymphatics, not the presence of fluid in the peritoneal cavity. Swelling, pain, and erythema of an extremity most likely indicate a potential infection.

2. *Answer:* D

Rationale: Regular measurement of extremities facilitates early recognition of changes. Another nursing action for treatment and prevention was the use of elastic sleeves and graded wraps serve to facilitate movement of lymph out of the arm. Sterile technique with chemotherapy is always indicated and is not specific to lymphedema. It is also important to avoid use of a limb that is at-risk for lymphedema as a site for venous access. Use of electronic or automated pressure cuffs on a sustained basis is not indicated on an arm at-risk for lymphedema. Carefully applied massage therapy has been shown to be beneficial, but vigorous weight lifting with the affected limb is not indicated. Moderate use limits risk while allowing lymphatic fluid to drain normally.

3. *Answer:* B

Rationale: Lymphedema may occur initially years after the surgical procedure even if there were no previous problems. Less invasive breast surgery still requires lymph node dissection for staging. Sentinel node mapping does not eliminate the need for node dissection for biopsy, which can contribute to future lymphedema. Although less extensive node disruption with breast conservation and radiation therapy may well decrease the risk of lymphedema, it does not eliminate that risk.

4. *Answer:* A

Rationale: Increased pigmentation, prominent superficial veins, and the presence of thickening, pitting, and erythema of the skin are indications of changes consistent with lymphedema and should be addressed early. Deep venous thrombosis would result in dull aching pain and potentially extremity swelling, warmth, and erythema.

Edema is accumulation of fluid in the interstitial space. Arterial emboli would result in a cool extremity with pallor.

5. *Answer:* B

Rationale: An infection of the affected limb increases risk of lymphedema. High-dose radiation therapy to the nodes draining the extremity affected by the cancer is more likely to result in lymphedema. Overuse of a limb is a greater risk factor than immobility. There does not appear to be a relationship between deep venous thrombosis and lymphedema.

6. *Answer:* C

Rationale: Redness may indicate infection and requires prompt intervention. The other options result in delay of treatment of the underlying problem.

7. *Answer:* A

Rationale: A client should expect a reasonable degree of comfort after treatment for lymphedema. Weight, vital signs, and dyspnea are not important factors related to lymphedema.

8. *Answer:* D

Rationale: Seeking information to plan for a plane trip indicates awareness of a potential concern. Sentinel node biopsy does not eliminate the risk of lymphedema. Although the acute postoperative concerns are most likely past, lymphedema may occur at any time in the future. Lymphedema is not related to medications for breast cancer.

9. *Answer:* C

Rationale: Decreased plasma oncotic pressure from processes such as liver failure and malnutrition results in increased fluid in the tissues. Raised hydrostatic pressure causes fluid to be driven from the capillaries into the interstitial spaces. Increased capillary permeability from vascular injury such as burns, radiation, drug reactions, and infection contributes to the accumulation of fluid in interstitial spaces. Increased capillary pressure, when the volume of blood is expanded or with obstruction, will also contribute to the accumulation of fluid in interstitial spaces.

10. *Answer:* D

Rationale: Hypothyroidism, hypoproteinemia, hypoalbuminemia, poor nutrition, and sepsis are associated with edema in clients with cancer, as are antiangiogenesis chemotherapy agents.

11. *Answer:* B

Rationale: Although deep venous thrombosis can contribute to edema, hypotension is not a risk factor. The client with pain and stiffness may decrease use of an extremity, which could increase edema, but these are not direct risk factors for edema. Paroxysmal nocturnal dyspnea is not a risk factor for edema unless it is associated with other factors such as heart failure.

12. *Answer:* B

Rationale: Hypoproteinemia contributes to edema by shifting fluids into the interstitial space. An S2 heart sound is normal; blood pressure and pulse usually increase with edema; peripheral pulses usually diminish as a result of poor cardiac output.

13. **Answer:** B

Rationale: Skin breakdown on the extremity is of particular concern for clients with cancer who also have lymphedema. Fluid retention and edema may actually occur after prolonged standing; the safety concern is the risk of infection with the breakdown. Bed rest does not facilitate diuresis; avoiding a dependent state in the extremities is important. Sepsis is a risk for all clients with cancer who have central lines; it is not unique to those with edema.

14. **Answer:** A

Rationale: Metastatic disease that has moved into the cardiac space through local advancement, spread by blood or lymph systems, or obstruction from adenopathy can cause clients to develop pericardial effusions. The likelihood of symptoms with a malignant pericardial effusion is related to how rapidly the fluid accumulated. Radiation-related immune suppression does not cause pericardial effusions. Cardiotoxic agents usually have an effect on the musculature or cardiac conduction system. Cardiac tamponade resulting from the accumulation of excess fluid in the pericardium may result from pericarditis or injuries to the heart.

15. **Answer:** A

Rationale: Tachycardia, jugular vein distention, and decreased peripheral pulses are seen if the effusion has accumulated rapidly. Dyspnea (both at rest and with exertion) may also be reported by the client with a pericardial effusion. Chest radiography showing an enlarged heart accompanied by a wide mediastinum would be indicative of a potential malignant pericardial effusion. Chest pain is usually dull, jugular venous distention is unlikely, and cough is usually nonproductive. Echocardiography, not electrocardiography, allows measurement of volume of an effusion.

16. **Answer:** D

Rationale: Preexisting heart disease increases the risk because of a compromised cardiac status. Systemic lupus erythematosus and bacterial endocarditis are also risk factors. High fractions of radiation therapy that include significant portions of the heart are more likely to cause effusions. Diabetes and deep venous thrombosis do not increase the risk.

17. **Answer:** D

Rationale: High-dose cyclophosphamide damages the cardiac endothelium, which can lead to myocardial necrosis and death. High-dose cyclophosphamide is also associated with atrial fibrillation, atrial flutter, and AV block, but not with bradycardia. Paclitaxel may cause asymptomatic bradycardia. 5-Fluorouracil can cause coronary artery spasm. Anthracyclines cause cardiomyopathy.

18. **Answer:** D

Rationale: Many clients do not have symptoms, and no intervention may be chosen depending on performance status. The head of bed should be elevated, diuretics are not helpful, and clients should be taught energy-conserving measures.

19. **Answer:** D

Rationale: Techniques to improve relaxation, strategies to conserve energy, and modifications to activity designed to conserve energy are all aspects of patient education interventions to relieve symptoms and improve quality of life in patients with malignant pericardial effusion. Oxygen therapy is a pharmacologic intervention recommended for this patient population but is not part of any patient education initiatives.

20. **Answer:** A

Rationale: Cancer therapies affect both cardiac function and conduction. Individuals with abnormal potassium and chloride levels are at increased risk of showing symptoms of these changes. Anthracycline-related cardiotoxicity in the form of cardiomyopathy occurs in up to 40% of clients depending on the cumulative dose administered.

21. **Answer:** C

Rationale: When administered with taxanes (paclitaxel and docetaxel), doxorubicin has been shown to be more toxic, leading to early heart failure or left ventricular dysfunction (LDV). Cremophor EL, found in paclitaxel, contributes to the problem. Daunorubicin causes cardiomyopathy, methotrexate has no cardiac toxicities, and high-dose 5-fluorouracil can cause coronary artery spasm.

22. **Answer:** C

Rationale: Subacute cardiac toxicities occur within 4 to 5 weeks after therapy and are often reversible. Acute changes occur within 24 hours of drug administration and are usually self-limiting, stopping when the drug is stopped. Chronic changes are not typically reversible though they can often be effectively managed with good supportive care.

23. **Answer:** D

Rationale: Although history of smoking and advanced age are associated with an increased risk of cardiotoxicity, standard-dose cyclophosphamide, the presence of bone metastases, and a primary diagnosis of lung cancer are not. High doses of cardiotoxic chemotherapeutic agents administered over shorter periods of time create higher dose exposures to sensitive tissues, thus increasing the risk of toxicity.

24. **Answer:** C

Rationale: Exercise strengthens cardiac muscle, thus increasing function. Dexrazoxane protects cardiac muscle against the effects of doxorubicin. Dexamethasone does not have a role in prevention of cardiotoxicity. Smoking cessation, lipid-lowering drugs, and a low-fat diet do have a role in cardiac health in general but are not specifically preventive strategies for doxorubicin-related cardiomyopathy. Oxygen therapy is not a preventive against cardiotoxicity.

25. **Answer:** B

Rationale: A normal ejection fraction is more than 60%. A decrease of more than 5% over baseline or an ejection fraction of less than 45% requires dose reduction. The dexrazoxane dose should be continued as recommended for the cardioprotectant effect. The client is already demonstrating changes in the ejection fraction—the ejection fraction should be followed closely.

26. *Answer:* B

Rationale: Alkylating agents associated with acute myopericarditis, pericardial effusions, and heart failure are cyclophosphamide and ifosfamide. Proteasome inhibitors may cause cardiotoxicity. Antimetabolites can cause coronary artery spasm. Monoclonal antibodies inhibit certain pathways critical to cardiac function, which may increase the risk for cardiac toxicity. Tyrosine kinase inhibitors may cause cardiotoxicities through the inhibition of various target pathways, although cardiac adverse events are rare. Anthracyclines may cause free-radical–mediated cardiac tissue injury.

27. *Answer:* C

Rationale: Most treatment regimens for breast cancer include an anthracycline, which is a risk factor for cardiomyopathy.

28. *Answer:* C

Rationale: Disseminated intravascular coagulation is an abnormality of the clotting cascade that causes coagulopathies. Thrombocytopenia is a decrease in the number of thrombocytes or platelets. Anemia and neutropenia indicate decreased hemoglobin and neutrophils, respectively.

29. *Answer:* C

Rationale: A pulmonary embolism usually causes a sharp, stabbing chest pain. Other findings include dyspnea, shallow respirations, tachypnea, and a sudden onset of anxiety. This may progress to cardiopulmonary arrest. Paroxysmal nocturnal dyspnea is defined as acute dyspnea occurring at night, waking the client after 1 to 2 hours of sleep, and is associated with pulmonary congestion caused by congestive heart failure.

30. *Answer:* A

Rationale: An arterial embolus obstructs arterial flow, causing cool or cold extremities and pallor. Other findings include severe pain and an absent or decreased pulse. A dull ache in the calf and a feeling of tightness are more characteristic of deep venous thrombosis. Unilateral edema of the involved extremity is also indicative of a potential venous occlusion.

31. *Answer:* B

Rationale: Tamoxifen is associated with clot formation. Monoclonal antibodies are not a risk factor. Family history does not factor unless there is a history of Factor V leiden or other coagulopathy, nor does administration of monoclonal antibodies.

32. *Answer:* B

Rationale: Intact skin integrity indicates adequate perfusion. Clients should have warm extremities; blood pressure and fatigue are not associated with deep venous thrombosis.

CHAPTER 33

1. *Answer:* C

Rationale: Cancer cell division and growth are associated with increased protein metabolism and hyperglycemia, presumably to meet the energy demands of malignant tumors. Carbohydrate metabolism is altered in malignant states, leading to hyperglycemia. Vitamin and mineral deficiencies are not associated with malignancies, although individual clients may develop deficiencies or require additional amounts. If liver function is adequate, medications are metabolized normally by liver enzymes. Malignant tumor metabolism is not associated with increased fat metabolism.

2. *Answer:* C

Rationale: There are many sequelae of prolonged anorexia. Long-term anorexia contributes to decreased calorie and protein intake with subsequent loss of fat and muscle mass, muscle and visceral organ (not bone) atrophy, weight loss, and weakness. Cancer patients experience hypoalbuminemia, anemia, and decreased bone marrow production, including compromised humoral and cellular immune function, e.g., impaired neutrophil function.

3. *Answer:* A

Rationale: The syndrome described is cachexia. Anorexia is defined as a loss of appetite accompanied by decreased oral intake. Secondary cachexia is manifested by involuntary weight loss and lethargy based on mechanical factors, such as obstruction, malabsorption, or treatment-induced toxicities, such as nausea or vomiting or alterations in taste. Failure to thrive is a global decline with weight loss and accompanying functional decline.

4. *Answer:* B

Rationale: Corticosteroids and megestrol acetate may stimulate appetite. Metoclopramide (Reglan) at low doses may stimulate gastrointestinal motility and decrease early satiety and nausea, thus stimulating appetite. Muscle relaxants and opioids are used to decrease pain. Methylphenidate is a stimulant that may curb appetite.

5. *Answer:* C

Rationale: Using the gastrointestinal (GI) tract maintains the integrity and functioning of the bowel wall and helps maintain normal GI flora. A healthy bowel provides the benefits of regulated absorption of nutrients and stimulation of the immune system, which protects the blood from contaminants in food, thus reducing the risk of infection. Total parenteral nutrition (TPN) is far more costly than oral or enteral nutrition. Parenterally infused nutrients are introduced directly into the circulation, making that route the quickest method for speedy delivery. A potential drawback to the constant level of nutrients infused may be an alteration in the normally intermittent hormone release and may provoke a higher metabolic rate. TPN, oral, and enteral nutrition all provide the same benefit of supporting adequate vascular fluid volume.

6. *Answer:* B

Rationale: Any of the answers could contribute to weight loss, but B is the most likely reason because gastric resection is associated with postprandial dumping syndrome, which may lead to significant weight loss. Surgical procedures may cause alterations in ability to eat and patients are often NPO immediately before and after surgery, but this does not explain a loss of 20 lb in a short period of time. Cachexia is a progressive deterioration associated with muscle wasting when protein or calorie requirements are not met and usually occurs over a lengthy period of time. Depression may decrease the patient's ability to eat, affecting quality of life, but probably is not associated with this significant weight loss.

7. **Answer:** A

Rationale: Lung, pancreatic, and gastric carcinomas are those most often associated with cachexia. Other disease-related risk factors include acquired immunodeficiency syndrome, infections, septic states, and inflammatory diseases.

8. **Answer:** C

Rationale: Metabolic disturbances, treatment side effects, and a proinflammatory cytokine environment are physiologic factors associated with anorexia. Depression and anxiety are psychological factors.

9. **Answer:** D

Rationale: Serum albumin and transferrin reflect protein stores in the body. Erythrocyte sedimentation rate is a measure of sedimentation of red blood cells that accelerates with inflammation and infection. Creatinine is an indicator of kidney function, and bicarbonate is an indicator of serum pH, an important buffer of acidity. Activated partial thromboplastin time is indirectly related to nutrition. The liver manufactures these components of the anticoagulation process. Without adequate amino acids, synthesis of these proteins may lag, especially in liver disease.

10. **Answer:** D

Rationale: Patients and their family members should be taught to monitor for signs and symptoms of dehydration. These include dry skin and mucous membranes, poor skin turgor, and decreased urinary output. Dehydration can occur in patients with severe nausea and vomiting. Decreased energy is a symptom of malnutrition.

11. **Answer:** B

Rationale: Cachexia is a complex process involving anorexia, metabolic alterations, release of cytokines, and other catabolic factors that lead to skeletal muscle wasting. Primary cachexia appears to be mediated by a number of proinflammatory cytokines, including tumor necrosis factor. Some of the metabolic alterations that occur with cachexia include decreased gluconeogenesis, alterations in glucose metabolism, and increased metabolic rate. Cachexia is present in 80% of patients at death.

12. **Answer:** C

Rationale: Malnutrition deprives the body of the components for wound healing and can lengthen hospital stays. Malnutrition associated with malignancy results in a loss of lean muscle mass rather than a reduction of fat stores. Adequate nutrition is needed for the patient to tolerate the side effects and adverse reactions associated with cancer treatment.

13. **Answer:** A

Rationale: Patients should have access to favorite foods (within dietary restrictions). Cold or room temperature foods should be encouraged, as should soft foods and those that are nutritionally dense. Hot or spicy foods should be discouraged. Liquids should be limited at mealtimes; they may cause early satiety and nausea. B is incorrect because maximizing food preferences and access to favorite foods within dietary restrictions is encouraged. Instant breakfast powder can be added to other foods to increase caloric intake, and review of food options is helpful to find new ways to ensure adequate nutrition.

14. **Answer:** D

Rationale: Measurements of height, weight, mid-arm circumference, skinfold thickness, and calculation of ideal body weight should be done. Body mass index should be calculated before, at intervals during, and after therapy.

15. **Answer:** D

Rationale: Tumors have an altered protein and carbohydrate metabolism, use anaerobic glycolysis, and have an increased rate of gluconeogenesis. There is an increased uptake of amino acids by tumor.

16. **Answer:** D

Rationale: Cancer typically causes loss of appetite, anorexia, and cachexia. Weight loss may result from acute or chronic diarrhea caused by radiation therapy and other chemotherapy drugs and because of protein-calorie malnutrition caused by the metabolic effects of the tumor. Weight gain is typically caused by inactivity, effusions, and steroid use.

17. **Answer:** B

Rationale: Dysgeusia is an unusual, often unpleasant, taste perception. Hypogeusesthesia describes a decrease in the acuity of the taste sensation. Ageusia is an absence of the taste sensation or "mouth blindness." Cachexia refers to progressive deterioration with muscle wasting that occurs when protein or calorie requirements are not met.

18. **Answer:** A

Rationale: The feeding bag and tube must be changed daily to avoid contamination. Before each use, the tube placement must be checked by aspirating gastric contents, observing for air bubbles by placing distal end of tube in water, and injecting air (not water) and listening with stethoscope over stomach. After each feeding, the nasogastric tube must be flushed with 30 mL of water. Keep the head of the bed elevated 30 degrees during and for 1 hour after infusion.

19. **Answer:** A

Rationale: Patients who complain about taste alterations typically experience the following: a constant or intermittent metallic and bitter taste, increased or decreased threshold for sweets, increased threshold for salty and sour tastes, and decreased threshold for bitter taste. Patients also have meat, coffee, and chocolate aversions.

20. **Answer:** A

Rationale: Total parenteral nutrition (TPN) should not be unrefrigerated for more than 4 hours prior to administration. Hyperkalemia is not a usual electrolyte disturbance that occurs with TPN administration; hyperglycemia or hypoglycemia is more likely. If a sudden cessation of TPN occurs, 10% dextrose in water solution should be infused peripherally at same rate as TPN. A dextrose solution of 50% is too high and can cause venous irritation if administered peripherally at a fast rate. Although verification of blood return before connecting the intravenous tubing to the central venous catheter is indicated, a blood return does not need to be continuously monitored every 2 hours. Checking for blood return at the start of every infusion and every shift is recommended.

21. *Answer:* B
    Rationale: The serum albumin level (half-life, 20 days) reflects the availability of protein within the past month. Hypoalbuminemia is common in patients with cancer. A normal albumin level is 4 g/dL; in a patient with cancer, the average albumin level is 2.9 g/dL. Cholesterol levels decrease when caloric intake is low; a low cholesterol level may detect inadequate intake but not malnutrition. Red and white blood cell counts are not indicative of malnutrition.

22. *Answer:* B
    Rationale: Spices and herbs can enhance taste and increase appetite. Fluid intake should be increased, not decreased, at mealtimes. The aroma of foods may actually stimulate taste. Amifostine (Ethyol) is only used when the patient is receiving radiotherapy (RT) to possibly prevent tissue damage and subsequent taste loss caused by RT.

23. *Answer:* B
    Rationale: Any weight loss can adversely affect nutritional reserves. However, weight loss of greater than 5% of body weight indicates that the patient may require the professional assistance of a dietician or nutritional intervention. Development or worsening of symptoms such as dehydration, fatigue, early satiety, constipation, mucositis, or nausea, which inhibit their ability to eat or drink, may require nutritional support. Fever increases the need for additional calories. Mouth soreness and sensitivity and queasiness may be medically managed with oral soothing agents and antiemetics that enable the patient to eat.

24. *Answer:* A
    Rationale: Taste alterations can lead to a decrease in food intake and anorexia. This can result in a negative, not positive, nitrogen balance from decreased protein intake.

25. *Answer:* B
    Rationale: The hyperosmolar enteral feedings are introduced slowly to promote tolerance and absorption of the formula, avoiding diarrhea. Aspiration caused by reflux of the liquid formula is a potential risk that is decreased by elevating the head of the bed 30 degrees or higher as tolerated. *Euthyroid* means normal thyroid hormone levels and is unrelated to enteral feedings. Dehydration is a condition corrected by enteral feedings, and unless there is congestive heart failure, the fluid provided in the enteral feeding remains in the vascular system, not causing dyspnea. If the patient develops hypoglycemia, it is related to excessive insulin, either endogenous or exogenous. Edema is not a side effect of enteral feeding.

26. *Answer:* C
    Rationale: A predigested formula is indicated when a patient has malabsorption.

27. *Answer:* C
    Rationale: Sugar-free lemon drops or smooth, flat, tart candies stimulate production of saliva, which can improve taste. Commercial mouthwashes contain alcohol, which dries the mucosa and may lead to further taste changes and mucosal damage. Meat served hot would not affect the taste changes; cold foods are usually better tolerated. Oral care should be done before and after meals.

28. *Answer:* D
    Rationale: Treatment-induced nutritional problems are often handled successfully by medication and self-care actions. Cancer-associated nutritional problems are best resolved by successful treatment of the malignancy. Extended nutritional counseling may or may not be beneficial based on individual compliance.

29. *Answer:* A
    Rationale: Early nutritional intervention, while the tumor is still small, has the best chance to alter client outcomes.

CHAPTER 34

1. *Answer:* B
   Rationale: The International Association for the Study of Pain (IASP) identifies pain as a sensory and emotional experience associated with actual or potential tissue damage or described in terms of such damage. The damage may not have occurred yet and may not be apparent on tests. The client's report of pain is seen as the most important for describing the experience. Although involving the family will most likely be beneficial, it is not as critical as the client's report. In addition, collaborative care is important but not part of the IASP definition.

2. *Answer:* C
   Rationale: Individuals with peripheral neuropathy are especially at risk of falls when walking on uneven surfaces. Although pain or discomfort related to pressure or temperature is a concern, it is not a safety-specific concern. Similarly, the impact on quality of life is a concern but is not a safety factor.

3. *Answer:* C
   Rationale: Clients with cancer have pain related to multiple causes that are likely to require different treatments. Not all problems are related to the cancer diagnosis, and focusing too narrowly on that relationship can lead to inferior care. There are adequate numbers of pain medications and treatments that do not interfere with chemotherapy. Although addiction is a fear, this attitude should not be allowed to interfere with willingness to treat the pain adequately.

4. *Answer:* A
   Rationale: The patient is describing neuropathic pain, which usually results from compression, inflammation, infiltration, ischemia, or injury to the peripheral, sympathetic, or central nervous system. Centrally mediated pain

is characterized by radiating and shooting sensations with a background of burning and aching. Sympathetically maintained pain is caused by autonomic dysregulation. Peripheral neuropathic pain is characterized by a numbness and tingling sensation.

5. *Answer:* C
Rationale: Nociceptive pain can include somatic pain from bone, joint, or connective tissue, and poorly localized visceral pain. In addition, visceral pain results from nociceptor activation secondary to distention, compression, or infiltration of the thoracic or abdominal tissue. Nociceptive pain is caused when special nerve endings—called nociceptors—are irritated; it produces a dull or sharp aching pain that can be mild to severe. Neuropathic, not nociceptive, pain includes pain caused by autonomic dysregulation and pain radiating down the arm.

6. *Answer:* C
Rationale: Perception is accurately described. B describes transduction, not transmission. The definitions for option A and option B are transposed. An action potential is generated, and the pain message begins its way to the central nervous system. During transmission, the action potential continues to the dorsal horn. Modulation is described correctly except that the neuromediators inhibit the transmission of the pain impulses at the dorsal horn.

7. *Answer:* A
Rationale: Bone metastasis leading to destruction or compression of the bone on nerves and soft tissue is the most common source of cancer pain. Bone metastases are common in the following malignancies: breast, prostate, lung, and multiple myeloma.

8. *Answer:* D
Rationale: These complaints are indicative of peripheral neuropathy. Platinum compounds, vinca alkaloids, taxanes, thalidomide, interferon, cytosine arabinoside, and bortezomib have the highest incidence of peripheral neuropathy.

9. *Answer:* A
Rationale: Withdrawal occurs in clients who are physically dependent on an opioid when abrupt cessation occurs. The administration of an opioid antagonist can also precipitate withdrawal. This is a physiologic phenomenon that the client cannot control. Tolerance means that after repeated administration of an opioid, a given dosage begins to lose its effectiveness; it begins to have a shorter duration of action and then less analgesic action. Addiction is a psychological occurrence when clients have an overwhelming need to obtain and use a drug for a nonmedical purpose.

10. *Answer:* D
Rationale: Biologic age cannot be used when choosing a pain assessment tool for the pediatric population; rather to improve interpretation of the assessment findings, the clinician should select a measure appropriate to the development stage of the child.

11. *Answer:* B
Rationale: The client is experiencing incident pain, which is increased pain with movement or activity. It is important to address pain preemptively, before anticipated activity, so the best response is to increase the dose of the breakthrough opioid analgesic medication. The client should also take the breakthrough medication approximately 30 minutes before activity so that the medication will be most effective while the client is moving and hence the client can move and complete activities of daily living more easily and comfortably.

12. *Answer:* C
Rationale: Pentazocine is not an optimal drug of choice for any type of pain because of the psychomimetic effects. When agonist–antagonists are added to pure agonists, the combination can also prevent full receptor binding of the agonist and can precipitate withdrawal in some clients.

13. *Answer:* C
Rationale: Bisphosphonates are used for the relief of pain in osteolytic bone metastases such as metastatic breast and prostate cancer.

14. *Answer:* B
Rationale: The celiac plexus block is a surgical intervention for pain related to pancreatic cancer. The other options are not autonomic nervous system blocks.

15. *Answer:* B
Rationale: This individual is describing peripheral neuropathic pain. The tricyclic antidepressants (TCAs) can be effective for this pain. The TCAs block the reuptake of serotonin, norepinephrine, and dopamine in the central nervous system. Anticonvulsants such as gabapentin may also be helpful. No research suggests that the serotonin-specific antidepressants are as effective for pain. Analeptics are used to counteract sedation, and benzodiazepines are used for pruritic pain and anxiety associated with pain.

16. *Answer:* C
Rationale: Analeptics such as Ritalin may counteract sedation and may improve quality of life. Another commonly used analeptic is dextroamphetamine.

17. *Answer:* D
Rationale: In addition to physical stimuli, pruritus is mediated by histamine release from mast cells, prostaglandins E2 and H2, substance P synthesized in C fibers, cytokines, serotonin, neuropeptides, and opioids along the afferent pathway. However, epinephrine does not mediate pruritus.

18. *Answer:* B
Rationale: Cisplatin, cytarabine, taxanes, epidermal growth factor receptor inhibitors, mammalian target of rapamycin inhibitors, interferon, and interleukin-2 are antineoplastic therapy agents that increase the risk of pruritus. Erythromycin is an antibiotic. Mycosis fungoides and renal disease do increase the risk of pruritus, but they are not antineoplastic agents.

19. *Answer:* C
Rationale: The patient description is accurate, and occurrence generally increases at night. Laboratory findings generally include hypoactive or hyperactive thyroid, elevated blood urea nitrogen and creatinine, abnormal liver function test results, and hyperglycemia. It is also important to minimize vasodilation.

20. *Answer:* D
   Rationale: Pharmacologic interventions include diphenhydramine, cimetidine, corticosteroids, naloxone, methylnaltrexone, butorphanol, and capsaicin.

21. *Answer:* A
   Rationale: Pruritus transmission is closely linked to the transmission of pain and is conducted along polymodal C-nociceptors. The stimuli can originate anywhere along the afferent pathway, and is often linked to an internal cause.

22. *Answer:* B
   Rationale: Risk factors include melanoma, hematologic malignancies including leukemia and lymphoma, diabetes, polycythemia vera, age older than 70 years, and dehydration.

23. *Answer:* B
   Rationale: H1-receptor antagonists are the first drugs of choice for pruritus. Small doses of opioid antagonists are sometimes used for pruritus caused by intraspinal analgesia but would not be the first choice. Rotating opioids takes time and interrupts the pain management plan, and meperidine is not a drug of choice. Placing a fan in the room does not manage the underlying cause of the pruritus.

24. *Answer:* D
   Rationale: Scratching should be avoided because it can disrupt the skin integrity and lead to significant infections. Medicated baths can help with pruritus, but the temperature should be cool to minimize vasodilation. Alcohol consumption can cause vasodilation and contribute to pruritus. Distraction methods such as television and other activities may be helpful because pruritus is often exacerbated with stress and anxiety. The most important action is to ensure that the client and family understand safety risks associated with pruritus.

25. *Answer:* C
   Rationale: Symptoms that cluster with fatigue include pain, depression, and sleep disturbances. One theory of fatigue is that vascular endothelial growth factor levels have been associated with fatigue, causing impaired thyroid blood flow, leading to hypothyroidism.

26. *Answer:* A
   Rationale: Cancer related fatigue occurs in 70% to 80% of clients with cancer, can be a chronic condition after treatment, and is more common in individuals with comorbidities and underlying diseases.

27. *Answer:* B
   Rationale: Fatigue is a common dose-limiting side effect in up to 70% of individuals undergoing immunotherapy or biotherapy. Although it occurs in up to 80% of individuals receiving radiation, because the duration of the treatment is shorter, it is less likely to be identified as a dose-limiting side effect.

28. *Answer:* B
   Rationale: Darbepoetin alfa and erythropoietin are both growth factors that stimulate the production of red blood cells in the bone marrow. Oprelvekin is a platelet growth factor, and sargramostim and pegfilgrastim are white blood cell growth factors.

29. *Answer:* C
   Rationale: It is important to take part in some type of activity or exercise as tolerated. Studies show that clients who exercise have decreased levels of fatigue. Putting Evidence into Practice (PEP) guidelines from the Oncology Nursing Society recommend exercise as an intervention for fatigue. Too much sleep will not assist with the fatigue and may lead to nighttime sleep disruptions. A diet should be balanced with adequate amounts of protein, and schedule adjustments with prioritizing needs are important to manage the overwhelming fatigue.

30. *Answer:* B
   Rationale: Depression and fatigue often have overlapping features: therefore a differential diagnosis is important. Although hemoglobin levels should be examined, platelet counts are not reliable indicators in the assessment of fatigue. Although fatigue can only be measured by asking the client, the family can indicate the impact it has on the client's quality of life.

31. *Answer:* A
   Rationale: Eighty percent of those surveyed assumed sleep problems were caused by the treatment. Sixty percent assumed the problems would be short lived, and almost 50% assumed physicians could do nothing to alleviate their sleep problems. Sleep disturbance does have a significant impact on quality of life and can often occur in patients with no history of sleep problems.

32. *Answer:* C
   Rationale: Melatonin and circadian rhythm are believed to be the primary regulatory processes influencing sleep. There are four stages of sleep from the lightest (stage 1) progressing to stage 4, which is the deepest part of the sleep cycle. Adults' sleep patterns are typically 4 to 6 cycles of REM and NREM sleep. Older individuals have decreasing levels of melatonin, which can change sleep patterns.

33. *Answer:* A
   Rationale: Melatonin mediates or regulates the day and night rhythms; normally, the levels increase at night during sleep and decrease during the daylight hours. Melatonin decreases with menopause and age, and this is reflective of the fact that as people age, they experience sleep disturbances more often.

34. *Answer:* B
   Rationale: Arising at the same time each morning facilitates a routine that enhances sleep. It may not be helpful to go to bed when not tired. Routine exercise is helpful, but exercise should be avoided 2 to 3 hours before bedtime. Exercise can stimulate the client and lead to insomnia right before bedtime. If clients awaken at night, it may be helpful to leave the bed and return when sleepy.

35. *Answer:* C
   Rationale: Individuals who are sleep deprived are at significant risk for falling asleep when driving or operating equipment. Benzodiazepines carry a higher risk of tolerance and dependence, and withdrawal has

been associated with risk of seizures. Sleep disturbance greatly impacts quality of life but there is no available evidence that sleep disturbances directly impact treatment tolerability.

36. **Answer:** D

Rationale: Factors that negatively influence sleep include female gender, advanced age, physical inactivity, and alcohol intake.

37. **Answer:** A

Rationale: Dark circles under the eyes, nystagmus, incorrect word use, slurred speech, frequent yawning, and ptosis of the eyelids are all physical signs of sleep deprivation. Stuttering and a loud voice are not usually associated with sleep disorders.

CHAPTER 35

1. **Answer:** C

Rationale: The definitions of *culture* and *religion* are fairly uniform throughout current professional literature, but *spirituality* is more elusive and defined in different ways depending on the group or individual involved. Spirituality refers to how a person perceives his or her place in the world and determines how a person relates to and interacts with other people, animals, nature, and the world. Culture is a world view of a set of traditions, attitudes, and practices that are transmitted from generation to generation by a particular society, group of people, or institution or organization. Religion is an organized system of worship. Diversity is the condition of being composed of differing elements, including different races or cultures.

2. **Answer:** B

Rationale: Race is based on appearance and is a social definition; ethnicity is defined by a common heritage and culture. Asian American and Pacific Islanders are racial groups that include more than one ethnic subgroup. Cubans are an ethnic group that includes multiple racial groups. Culture, not ethnicity, encompasses a group's world view, religion, economy, language, environment, uses of technology, and social structure.

3. **Answer:** B

Rationale: Poverty is defined based on annual household income; guidelines vary in different states. Individuals who have lived in poverty may have been exposed to factors such as low nutritional quality, stress, or comorbidities that influence health outcomes. Those under the poverty line may have had less access to health services including screenings and health information, which also affects prognosis. Therefore the same treatment may not have the same effect for those living in poverty. People may be reluctant to self-identify as qualifying for sliding scale services because of their personal or family pride. People may regard "free" services as substandard and potentially an invasion of their privacy.

4. **Answer:** B

Rationale: For some cultures, avoiding direct eye contact is a way of showing respect. Although eye contact can be seen by some cultures as a source of comfort and support, in others it may be seen as intrusive. The potential relationship to depression cannot be determined without further interaction.

5. **Answer:** D

Rationale: Unfortunately, personal knowledge of other cultures is often based primarily on our exposure and assumptions. Cultural awareness is not necessarily aligned with professional education. Self-proclaimed knowledge does not automatically qualify an individual for the taskforce, and everyone benefits from more awareness of cultural differences.

6. **Answer:** D

Rationale: Scientists believe that more than half of the difference in survival can be attributed to later stage at detection and tumors that are more aggressive and less responsive to treatment. Additional factors include the presence of multiple chronic conditions, and various sociodemographic factors. While lower adherence may affect outcomes, there is no evidence that race moderates the relationship between adherence and outcomes. Decreased adherence is a biased assumption.

7. **Answer:** C

Rationale: American Indians may carry objects believed to guard against witchcraft or have objects that are considered curative; they are given to the client by the native healers. The latter may be considered sacred. As long as the object does not interfere with the client's care, there is no harm in leaving it on. If for some reason it needs to be removed, consult with the family if the client is comatose.

8. **Answer:** D

Rationale: Japanese culture often expects a wife to be a primary caregiver. Other family members may also share the duties. Insisting, or having the patient insist, that the wife go home is insensitive to the cultural values and beliefs that may shape this family's behavior. Doing nothing ignores the possibility of caregiver burnout. The best course of action is to discuss with the family a schedule whereby other family members may assist in caring for the client and allow the patient's wife time to rest.

9. **Answer:** B

Rationale: Becoming culturally competent requires an ongoing process that begins with self-awareness. Ideally, one should begin to assess his or her personal cultural beliefs and professional values and identify how these help to shape personal behaviors and attitudes. The process of cultural awareness includes the recognition of one's biases, prejudices, and assumptions about individuals who are different. Without an awareness of the influence of one's own cultural or professional values, the healthcare provider runs the risk of engaging in cultural imposition, which is imposing one's beliefs and values on another culture.

10. **Answer:** A

Rationale: Cultural desire is characterized by a desire to learn and become culturally aware, knowledgeable, and skillful. This is a self-imposed learning that is distinct from cultural knowledge required by clinical standards.

11. *Answer:* D

Rationale: Program success is greatly enhanced when respected leaders are involved in all phases of a project. In this instance, the healthcare team can work with a respected American Indian leader to address the low participation. If recommended, a respected Indian healer might perform a cleansing ceremony and blessing of the mammography machine. This may help the women to feel more comfortable and be more willing to participate in mammography screening.

12. *Answer:* D

Rationale: The community should be involved in all phases of the project, beginning with the needs assessment to the final completion and dissemination of results. The most important aspect of program development is the involvement of those affected by the issue being discussed. Nurses in the same clinic may not have an adequate awareness of the community.

13. *Answer:* D

Rationale: The meaning of and reaction to a life-threatening diagnosis is largely influenced by culture. Cultural or religious factors may affect interest in clinical trial participation, coping throughout the disease progression, and end-of-life issues.

14. *Answer:* A

Rationale: One's spirituality and religiosity may manifest differently at different stages. Religion describes organized systems of faith that follow regulated (individual or group) practices intended to enhance spirituality. Fatalistic views can occur in deeply religious individuals. Conversely, those who believe they have accepted the will of a higher being may exhibit behaviors that seem fatalistic to others but can still be spiritually meaningful. Each patient's relationship with these concepts is different.

15. *Answer:* A

Rationale: Spiritual distress may be experienced by many patients, resulting from a sense of abandonment by their greater power; inability to find meaning in their cancer diagnosis; or a sense that they are being punished, justly or unjustly. It would be important to listen to the client's situation before offering approaches to address the distress. It may be important to learn if the client has been able to participate in religious services, but this may not be the underlying cause of spiritual distress.

16. *Answer:* C

Rationale: The oncology nurse must first recognize his or her own culture, spirituality, or religiosity and how this may impact the perception of others. Education regarding practices and belief systems and attendance at other services can be beneficial, but the personal assessment is the core to an expanded understanding and acceptance of others. Although it would be beneficial to know what other co-workers think, it should follow a self-assessment.

17. *Answer:* C

Rationale: Complementary modalities that have the potential to enhance spiritual well-being include mindfulness meditation; yoga; prayer; and expressive therapies such as art therapy, music therapy, and journaling. Although herbal drinks may be recommended and used by certain cultural groups, further research is needed to support their use from an evidence-based perspective.

CHAPTER 36

1. *Answer:* C

Rationale: The protocols for estrogen receptor–negative breast cancer contain agents that commonly cause alopecia. She may have noticed some change after her first round, but it may be more extensive now. Although the goal of treatment is for her to be cancer free, that is not influencing how she feels about going out. Her feelings about hair loss need to be addressed because these changes may be the most obvious in public. A referral to Look Good Feel Better is an important resource, but it should not be a substitute for an honest discussion about her feelings and her body image.

2. *Answer:* A

Rationale: Greater than 40 Gy usually causes permanent damage to the hair follicles in the treated field, 30 to 35 Gy may cause temporary hair loss, and 20 to 25 Gy may cause shedding of some hair. If feasible, a maximum dose of less than 16 Gy at less than 5 mm under the surface of the skin is preferred to minimize damage to hair follicles.

3. *Answer:* A

Rationale: The core content of B, C, and D are factual, but they do not demonstrate sensitivity to the client's concerns. If hair loss is inevitable with the planned treatment, it is important for the nurse to listen and be sensitive to the client's concerns, keeping communication open and respectful.

4. *Answer:* C

Rationale: The safety concerns are sun damage and heat loss, both of which can be significant. Pushing the client to deal differently is not appropriate, nor is focusing on resources that do not support the apparent plan to use no covering. At this time, the client is not voicing negative emotions that may lead to self-destructive behaviors.

5. *Answer:* B

Rationale: The adverse effects of body image disturbances have implications for client safety and should be given priority. Clients may experience significant emotional problems that could lead to potentially life threatening actions. A focus on adverse effects is the nurse's responsibility and does not (initially) require referral. The other responses are information-seeking interventions not necessarily within the scope of the nursing role and may require the expertise of other healthcare professionals.

6. *Answer:* C

Rationale: Serving as a volunteer represents actions and reintegration, with constructive channeling of energies. Action is a higher level of adaptation than planning and displays of knowledge.

7. *Answer:* D

Rationale: Various cultures place different values on body image and the significance of certain body organs and other changes. If a client is already struggling to cope with the disease, treatment side effects, and quality of life issues, body image changes may be more challenging. Studies have shown that most clients want to be asked about body image, but they may not know how to initiate the conversation without sounding overly concerned. The impact of body image changes can last for years and actually change over time depending on other events and developmental stages in the client's life.

8. *Answer:* C

Rationale: Patient concerns tend to be related to function (speech and exercise tolerance); but health professionals' concerns for the patient were anatomic defects and the patient's body image.

9. *Answer:* A

Rationale: Hormone therapy can cause significant changes in appearance that impact body image. The weight changes may be more difficult to counteract than in those patients who have had a sex organ removed. Healthcare professionals must evaluate possible outcomes of both treatments and chances of adverse effects that accompany both options. Doses can be adjusted as necessary, but some side effects of hormone therapy may be unavoidable.

10. *Answer:* D

Rationale: Nurses often find it more difficult to allow clients to share negative emotions, but it may be the most supportive role of a nurse. In addition the nurse can begin to provide the client with helpful information regarding how to cope with the changes experienced. Grief has no time frame; there is not a defined time for moving on. Conversations with family may be helpful, but they do not address changing body image. Education may be part of a nurse's tasks, but it is not directly related to the patients' acceptance of body image changes.

11. *Answer:* D

Rationale: Active listening, education about body image changes, and stressing the temporary nature of side effects are all positive coping strategies. Avoiding a discussion with the patient may worsen adverse effects after body image changes occur.

12. *Answer:* A

Rationale: Art therapy can assist clients to integrate body image and to develop insight regarding recovery and survival. Strength training and physical exercise can assist with maintenance of function, socialization, and a sense of normalcy. A focus on mindfulness can decrease perceived stress and anxiety. Support from family and friends is important, but it cannot be implemented by the healthcare professional.

CHAPTER 37

1. *Answer:* D

Rationale: All individuals experience some level of distress related to their diagnosis and treatment. Thus, all are faced with coping challenges.

2. *Answer:* C

Rationale: The patient is attempting to derive meaning from the stressful experience of cancer. Problem-focused coping is directed toward reducing or eliminating a stressor; emotion-focused coping is directed toward changing one's own emotional reaction. These are types of behavior seen as individuals attempt to cope with a stress in their lives.

3. *Answer:* C

Rationale: Distress is multifactorial in nature and may be psychological (cognitive, behavior, emotional), social, or spiritual in nature. It may interfere with effective coping related to diagnoses, physical symptoms, and treatment. Avoidance is considered an ineffective coping process.

4. *Answer:* D

Rationale: The trauma of the cancer experience can cause posttraumatic stress disorder (PTSD), a delayed clinical response. PTSD can manifest in many ways, including altered cognitive, behavioral, emotional, and physiologic responses. Individuals may self-medicate with alcohol or drugs to assist with coping. Although this is a known phenomenon related to a cancer experience, it is not a "normal" phase or a long-term effect. A.D. should receive counseling.

5. *Answer:* A

Rationale: Ineffective coping can occur in a crisis situation and lead to suicidal thoughts and actual attempts. The priority should be to address coping with each visit to determine the need for intervention. Similar-sounding and -looking medications, drug-to-drug interactions, and family abuse of the client's medications are always important to address but are not the major concern for this situation.

6. *Answer:* B

Rationale: Factors that influence coping are related to diagnosis, treatment, psychological comorbidities, social situation, cultural practices and beliefs, and gender. B is the only answer that describes a coping response.

7. *Answer:* C

Rationale: J.P. is demonstrating signs of anxiety that may include agitation, restlessness, sleep disturbances, sweating, shortness of breath, lightheadedness, and palpitations. There may also be manifestations of increased autonomic activity, weight gain or loss, and mood changes. There is no indication this individual is post-treatment, so this would not be considered posttraumatic stress disorder. Nor is there any evidence of a history of manic-depressive disorder. It is more likely that this is an acute anxiety reaction. Distress with this diagnosis would be anticipated; however, the intensity of the symptoms should be addressed to decrease the stress for the client.

8. *Answer:* C

Rationale: These options articulate common risk factors for depression at the time of a cancer diagnosis. Depression can occur in anyone with a new cancer diagnosis. Evidence indicates it to be most prevalent for pancreatic and head and neck cancer. Advanced stage of cancer is also a contributing factor. Long wait times in the clinic are frustrating but not necessarily a major cause of depression.

9. *Answer:* B

Rationale: Sodium or potassium imbalance, both hyper- and hypothyroidism, and adrenal insufficiency have been identified as potential factors for depression with a cancer diagnosis. Although anemia may be a factor, hypercalcemia is seen as a significant causative factor. Fever is a potential factor, but the more common vitamin deficiency is vitamin B12 or folate deficiency.

10. *Answer:* C

Rationale: Denial may be a conscious or unconscious attempt to deny the knowledge or meaning of the diagnosis. It can lead to adverse effects if the relevance of symptoms or need for treatment is denied. As a coping mechanism, it should not be considered dysfunctional; it may be unconscious. It should not delay the response of a healthcare team.

11. *Answer:* C

Rationale: The National Comprehensive Cancer Network's Distress Thermometer is a linear scale of measuring distress. Ten is the highest score and represents severe distress. A score of 4 or greater triggers further evaluation or referral to psychosocial services.

12. *Answer:* A

Rationale: The goal is to decrease caregiver signs of stress and anxiety. Expected outcomes would include the caregiver expressing increased feeling of support and lower feelings or no feelings of burden, maintaining his or her own physical and psychological health, identifying resources available to help giving care and verbalize mastery of the care situation, and feeling confident and competent to provide care. It is desirable for the patient to exhibit enhanced social interactions, but this does not focus on the caregiver. It is important for caregivers to master coping skills, but this would not be an expected initial outcome.

13. *Answer:* D

Rationale: A collaboration to identify strengths and resources would enhance the ability of the patient and caregiver(s) to understand factors that can be modified, recognize the sources of stress, and expand personal skills and knowledge. Active listening is important; responses may include confrontation, and this should not be avoided when it is indicated. Establishing stretching goals is not indicated until they feel confident with their ability to deal appropriately with the stress of the disease and its treatment; goals should be realistic. Evidence indicates that both sexuality and spirituality issues can contribute significantly to distress and should be actively addressed, not avoided.

14. *Answer:* D

Rationale: Education programs can often lead to improved outcomes. Knowledge of stressors helps to prevent increased stress, and individual preferences should always be considered in care plans. Alternative approaches may actually serve to improve the effectiveness of pharmacologic interventions rather than vice versa.

15. *Answer:* D

Rationale: An initial screening provides a baseline to allow monitoring for change over time. It is important to have this baseline on all patients. Changes in disease status (remission, recurrence, and progression) tend to increase distress. The National Comprehensive Cancer Network recommends that standards should be implemented toward individual treatment plans and include the involvement of multiple disciplines, especially licensed mental health professionals, to enhance outcomes.

16. *Answer:* C

Rationale: Indicators of depression include changes in appetite and sleeping patterns, fatigue, poor concentration, and recurrent thoughts of death or suicide. Patients may also exhibit diminished pleasure or interest in most activities; psychomotor agitation or slowing; feelings of worthlessness; or excessive, inappropriate guilt. When symptoms persist for more than 2 weeks, depression is indicated. The other three options are actually indicators that support more focused or involved interventions because of the enhanced potential for distress.

17. *Answer:* B

Rationale: Paroxetine (Paxil) and sertraline (Zoloft) are selective serotonin reuptake inhibitors. Venlafaxine, trazodone, and bupropion are atypical antidepressants. Tranylcypromine and phenelzine are monoamine oxidase inhibitors. Amitriptyline is a tricyclic antidepressant, not an atypical antidepressant.

CHAPTER 38

1. *Answer:* C

Rationale: The emotional distress response is seen as a normal response to cancer, different from clinical depression, posttraumatic stress disorder, or anxiety disorder, and should be addressed. Professional intervention will enhance the ability of the client and family to cope and manage self-care responsibilities. Emotional distress is a combination of social, spiritual, physical, financial, and psychological (not psychiatric) stressors. Psychiatric responses are seen as uniquely different. It is seen as existential and psychological (not psychiatric) concerns that are common in clients with cancer.

2. *Answer:* C

Rationale: Client teaching will help with anxiety and fears. Client teaching is a nursing intervention. Nurses are not able to alter the age-specific developmental tasks that are important at a given age. Although they do not want to hear about a very poor prognosis, clients often struggle with the uncertainty of their prognosis. Their previous life experiences and related learned coping patterns are history that cannot be altered.

3. *Answer:* A

Rationale: Psychological needs vary depending on the individual, his or her developmental stage, phase of disease trajectory, past coping skills, and available emotional and practical resources. All clients should be routinely screened for distress with at least a general screening checklist to identify the level and source of their distress so that further evaluation can be completed. Many institutions use the Distress Thermometer, which is a unidimensional screening tool.

4. *Answer:* D

Rationale: Although the nurse may help the client to identify the current social support system, only the client can determine the need to, or ways in which to, strengthen it. Evaluation of the effectiveness of current coping strategies can be initiated by the nurse based on demonstrated behaviors and awareness of usual reaction in other clients. Instruction in relaxation, imagery, and other holistic stress reduction techniques is an intervention the nurse can offer to the client. Learning takes participation and practice, but the instruction is a nursing action. Providing referrals as needed to the psychiatric liaison nurse, psychologist, or social worker also is a nursing function. Cooperation is important for maximum benefit, but the referral can be initiated by the nurse.

5. *Answer:* B

Rationale: Self-negation and self-blame are the defining characteristics that differentiate between low self-esteem and the other mood states. Fear of death is not necessarily related to feelings about self. Neurotic anxiety is a mental disorder in which particular situations cause irrational anxiety and distress; thus, the individual avoids those situations. Although Mrs. R has withdrawn, the greater change is related to her sense of self-worth and self-esteem; no mention is made of role abandonment.

6. *Answer:* C

Rationale: Reinforcement of her approaches to self-care is a behavioral approach that reinforces the desired behavior and is therefore the best response. A referral for rehabilitative counseling is premature at this time. Avoiding all demands on C.D. for her care does not facilitate adaptive behavior. Having the family assume responsibility for her wound care fosters dependency, not self-care.

7. *Answer:* D

Rationale: Assisting the client to explore his/her personal value system and sense of purpose and meaning in life will facilitate the setting of meaningful personal goals. Identifying perceived threats and providing accurate information on risks is more applicable for individuals with posttraumatic stress disorder. Assisting the individual to list priorities within his or her personal, professional, and social responsibilities will facilitate addressing ineffective role performance.

8. *Answer:* A

Rationale: Anxiety is correct, and these are classic signs of anxiety. The stimulus is diffuse, thereby ruling out fear and phobias. The presenting physical symptoms are not typical of delirium.

9. *Answer:* A

Rationale: Hyperthyroidism, hormone-secreting tumors, hypoglycemia, and sepsis are abnormal metabolic states seen in clients with cancer that can increase the risk for anxiety as a psychological state requiring intervention. Hormone-secreting tumors,

hypoxia, delirium, and hypoglycemia are risk factors, as are electrolyte imbalances, sepsis, and paraneoplastic syndromes.

10. *Answer:* B

Rationale: Pharmacology management for anxiety includes anxiolytics, azapirones, antihistamines, antidepressants, and atypical neuroleptics. Medications that can contribute to the risk for anxiety include corticosteroids, neuroleptics (especially those causing akathisia), thyroxine, bronchodilators, antihistamines, decongestants, and opioid-induced hallucination.

11. *Answer:* B

Rationale: First it would be important to know the client's concerns and fears. This will help to facilitate better coping. Privacy, meditation, spiritual rituals, and the intervention of clergy may be helpful, but their efficacy cannot be determined without first discussing fears and coping strategies with the patient.

12. *Answer:* D

Rationale: Potential somatic symptoms that can occur as sequelae of anxiety include nausea, vomiting, headaches, and a change in bowel habits. Contact with reality is intact, there has been no indication of flashbacks, and there is no record of previous psychological disorders. Posttraumatic stress disorder, bipolar disorder, and psychotic stress disorder are not indicated in this scenario.

13. *Answer:* C

Rationale: Contact with reality is intact, so psychotic disorder is not true. No history of mood swings is given, thus eliminating bipolar disorder as a possibility. Although generalized anxiety stress may be present, the experience of flashbacks may be indicative of posttraumatic stress disorder.

14. *Answer:* D

Rationale: It is important to assess for delirium with this client, who may be experiencing behavioral changes related to metastatic disease. The other options are valid considerations, but organic causes of behavior must be ruled out first.

15. *Answer:* A

Rationale: Although all of those factors are important to consider, only the chemotherapeutic agents represent a treatment-related risk factor.

16. *Answer:* C

Rationale: Crises and social support can be affected by interventions, but the nurse has limited control of these. Although a history of suicidal thoughts is important to consider, interventions to enhance symptom control, particularly pain, may have a more direct effect on depressive symptoms.

17. *Answer:* B

Rationale: Low positive affect, with symptoms of anhedonia and cognitive and motor slowing, are all associated with physiologic signs of depression. Symptoms of fatigue, change in appetite, and psychomotor agitation or slowing lasting 2 or more weeks are clinical assessment findings associated with depression that should be further evaluated. Depression is a state of feeling sad or discouraged. Anxiety is a state of feeling uneasy and apprehensive in response to a vague, nonspecific threat; findings include facial pallor, tense posturing, vocal tremors, and diaphoresis. Psychosis refers to disintegration of personality and loss of contact with reality; findings include inappropriate affect, disheveled dress, sweaty hands, and tremors. Panic is acute anxiety, terror, or fright; findings include labile emotions, hyperactivity, sighing respirations, and over talkativeness.

18. *Answer:* C

Rationale: Listening nonjudgmentally and trying diversional techniques as a possible method of alleviation are indeed important nursing interventions. This would be a priority to allow more thorough assessment. When there is no physiologic basis for the symptoms, treatment of somatic complaints that are aspects of depression is contraindicated because such actions reinforce these maladaptive behaviors and symptoms. It is, however, important to do a thorough assessment because many clients with cancer have physical symptoms and anxiety. Referral to a psychologist may be required. To ask the client to "buck up" is asking the impossible and instilling guilt. The symptoms are real to the client, and diversion may help.

19. *Answer:* D

Rationale: At one time, it was thought that clients with cancer did not attempt suicide. However, with cancer now being a chronic disease, suicidal thoughts and attempts are more common. Therefore, this is the most important concern to address to prevent a negative outcome. Although the remaining options are important to address, the safety priority issue is suicide. Certainly, interference with social roles and lack of compliance with medical treatment may likely contribute to the depressed mood. Similarly, individuals may regress psychologically with loss of function secondary to cancer and cancer treatment.

20. *Answer:* D

Rationale: Loss of purpose, beliefs, and trust is indicative of spiritual distress. Anxiety symptoms are not present, ineffective coping is not specific enough, and the client is not exhibiting any self-negating behavior indicative of self-esteem problems.

21. *Answer:* B

Rationale: Offering to listen is a therapeutic response and acknowledges the client's discomfort. The other reactions do not facilitate open communication and can damage rapport.

22. *Answer:* C

Rationale: Symptoms presented are indicative of powerlessness. Anxiety and spiritual distress are not represented by these symptoms. Ineffective coping is not specific enough.

23. *Answer:* B

Rationale: Loss of personal control is just that, personal; therefore, an individual's pattern of coping is the primary influencing factor. The duration of time since the diagnosis may be a factor, especially during the initial trauma and if the course has been extensive, but it is not as strong as the individual patterns of coping. Similarly, response of family and friends may be influenced, but

these also are evaluated by the client. Assessment of the personal meaning of the loss is important to know, but again, the individual pattern of coping will influence the response.

24. *Answer:* C

Rationale: "Let's spend some time talking a little more about your feelings" is an open-ended statement to elicit individual perceptions of the response without jumping to conclusions of a diagnosis of loss of personal control. Referring to the doctor does not help the client process his feelings. Having his wife do more things for him may not address the real issue. Similarly, developing a routine schedule may not address the issue if it is lack of personal control.

25. *Answer:* D

Rationale: Management of symptoms is a basic nursing intervention in facilitating a client's sense of personal control. Optimal nursing management of symptoms will decrease the client's sense of things being out of control. Having family make decisions for the client will most likely increase the problem. The remaining options would be additional potential interventions after symptom control is accomplished.

26. *Answer:* D

Rationale: Seeking the opinions of both the client and family about his care is most facilitative of his sense of control. Although the other options represent doing something that may well be beneficial for the client, they are not directly facilitating his sense of control.

27. *Answer:* D

Rationale: Statements of suicidal intentions require immediate response for further assessment by a healthcare professional and probably referral to a mental health professional. Inability to perform activities of daily living and noncompliance with treatment regimen require problem solving by care providers to avoid other problems. Refusal to discuss personal feelings may be a pattern of coping and the client's choice.

28. *Answer:* D

Rationale: The client is most likely experiencing grief. Grief is defined as changes in thinking, feeling, and behaving that occur in response to loss of a valued object or person, including personal goals, plans, or abilities. It would be beneficial to facilitate the understanding that the identified feelings are most likely related to losses secondary to the cancer diagnosis and treatment. Focusing on the parent's death may take the focus off the perceived personal losses and the appropriateness of that as a cause of grief. Labeling this as depression and offering medications does not facilitate verbalization of concerns. Countering the statement with information regarding an excellent prognosis does not facilitate discussion regarding the client's perception of changes and potential threats. Grief may be related to the uncertainty experienced regarding prognosis.

29. *Answer:* A

Rationale: Cancer as a disease and many of the current treatments frequently cause changes in body structure and function. The other options identify factors that all people may experience. Changes in body structure and function are more specific to the experiences of cancer diagnosis and treatment.

30. **Answer:** A

Rationale: Risks for complicated grief include perception of death as preventable, ambivalent relation to the deceased; coexisting medical conditions; and coexisting financial or legal problems. Although we should not neglect the care of the client, the daughter is at risk of complicated grief because of what is likely an ambivalent relationship with her father. Optimal pain control is always important, and the patient is your first concern. But as a nurse, you have responsibilities and resources to support the family as well. Reprimanding the daughter for blaming her father will not serve any meaningful purpose at this time.

31. **Answer:** A

Rationale: One's past experiences are basic to one's grief responses throughout life; therefore, this response is the most basic point. The other options are also applicable as well, but it will be important not to mask somatic symptoms with sedative medications and thus interfere with coming to terms with feelings of grief.

32. **Answer:** A

Rationale: Encouraging discussion of the feelings related to the loss will facilitate expression and resolution. The remaining responses represent strategies that will most likely block grief work and resolution of the loss.

33. **Answer:** D

Rationale: A 35-year-old widower who prides himself on keeping all of his wife's possessions and visiting her grave daily for the 5 years since her death while neglecting his other responsibilities is the best answer because of the evidence of a prolonged and unresolved grief process. The other responses represent normal grief responses.

34. **Answer:** D

Rationale: Withdrawal or social isolation could be a symptom of clinical depression and deserves further evaluation. The other options represent normal grief responses, especially this early in the grief experience.

CHAPTER 39

1. **Answer:** D

Rationale: Approximately 66% of patients across all cancer types reported that discussion about sexuality during cancer care was important. Sexuality issues are a significant long-term effect of cancer treatment and should be discussed to allow early interventions.

2. **Answer:** B

Rationale: When nurses do not discuss sexuality, the patient may infer that changes in sexuality are to be expected, that there are no effective treatments, or that the subject is not an important one. Patients are often more comfortable discussing sexuality issues with nurses; if the nurse does not initiate the topic, patients are not likely to assume the physician will discuss it.

3. **Answer:** D

Rationale: Chemotherapy treatments can produce harmful effects in a fetus. Birth control is critical during chemotherapy even if the patient has decreased fertility. Although pain with intercourse can occur with drying or breakdown of membranes, that is not the major safety concern. Not all chemotherapy agents cause vaginal mucositis; the specific agents are not listed here, so D is the best answer.

4. **Answer:** C

Rationale: Sexuality-related effects of hormone therapy for men include gynecomastia, feminization, erection dysfunction, decreased fertility, penile or testicular atrophy, and a decrease or loss of libido. Women may experience decreased vaginal lubrication, vaginal atrophy, change in libido, masculinization, and amenorrhea, as well as temporary or permanent menopause, which may include menopausal symptoms of mood swings, hot flashes, sleep disturbance, and dyspareunia. Sexuality-focused concerns are usually related to these treatment effects.

5. **Answer:** A

Rationale: Unfortunately, professionals not practicing in radiotherapy lack adequate knowledge to discuss side effects; ongoing education is important. It is inappropriate to assume sexuality is not a concern for those older than 70 years of age. Pelvic radiation in women may cause decreased vaginal lubrication, a hardened clitoris, dyspareunia, a change in vaginal sensation, risk of infection because of decreased vaginal lubrication, a change in usual sexual expression, shortening of the vaginal vault, decreased elasticity of the vagina or vaginal stenosis, increased vaginal irritation, urinary incontinence, or bowel changes. Prostate brachytherapy causes erectile dysfunction in 6% to 61% of men.

6. **Answer:** C

Rationale: Although antimetabolites and antitumor antibiotics as single agents do not directly cause sexual dysfunction, they can potentiate dysfunction when given with alkylating agents. Chemotherapy side effects of oral stomatitis, dry mouth, nausea, fluid retention, fatigue, pain, and others may affect sexual functioning or libido. Infection is a concern during neutropenia, but sexuality concerns also need to be addressed.

7. **Answer:** C

Rationale: Numbness and other sensation changes after lumpectomy or mastectomy can affect sexual pleasure for a woman, which can then have an impact on her partner. Individuals with mastectomies can have phantom breast and nipple sensations. Postlumpectomy changes can include "electricity-like" shock sensations. A postmastectomy implant does not result in a normal-appearing breast. C indicates that she and her husband are attempting to address concerns related to their decision.

8. **Answer:** C

Rationale: Individuals are rarely aware of the potential for retrograde ejaculation and the impact it may have on a partner. Hormone therapy may be indicated for further therapy, but it is not due to the surgical changes per se. Testicular shrinkage is not related to prostatectomy. Sleep disturbances and fatigue are not sexual changes directly related to the surgery.

9. *Answer:* A

Rationale: Changes in speech and the ability to whisper may have an impact on the spouse. The sensations of respirations from the stoma may be unexpected. Drooling may be considered unattractive. Although providing nutrition may be seen as caring, it does not address the issue expressed by the spouse.

10. *Answer:* C

Rationale: This model allows healthcare providers to obtain the information to plan interventions at the appropriate level based on their ability and identified client needs. Referrals to individuals with advanced degrees are appropriate, but all nurses should have a basic understanding about the implications for concerns related to sexuality. The PLISSIT model is appropriate to guide care planning throughout the disease and treatment course.

11. *Answer:* B

Rationale: Introducing the subject of sexuality to clients and their partners conveys acceptability that discussing sexuality is appropriate. It is not a blanket permission for all sexual behaviors. It should also include permission not to engage in sexual activity. All nurses are able to provide sexuality information at this level.

12. *Answer:* C

Rationale: Age and total amount of radiation dosage affect risk of sterility in females. Age does not affect risk of sterility for males. However greater than 5 Gy radiation will cause permanent sterility in males. For females, 95% of individuals receiving 20 Gy fractionated over 5 to 6 weeks before the age of 40 years will experience sterility.

13. *Answer:* B

Rationale: A comprehensive proposed model for sexual assessment is ALARM (activity, libido, arousal and orgasm, resolution, and medical history relevant to sexuality), BETTER (bringing up the topic, explaining that sexuality is part of quality of life and nursing care, telling the patient about resources, timing the discussion to the patient's preference, educating the patient about the side effects of treatment that have an impact on sexuality, and recording should be made in the patient notes that the topic has been discussed), and PLEASURE (partner, lovemaking, emotions, attitudes, symptoms, understanding, reproduction, and energy).

14. *Answer:* C

Rationale: The majority of patients do not recall a fertility risk discussion at time of diagnosis. 80% of men and women treated with mechlorethamine, Oncovin (vincristine), procarbazine, or prednisone (MOPP) have their fertility affected. A total of 35% of men treated with Adriamycin (doxorubicin), bleomycin, vinblastine, or dacarbazine (ABVD) have their fertility affected, and it is usually recovered. Fertility in males may reverse (improve) as late as 4 years after treatment; thus, serial measurements are important for planning birth control.

15. *Answer:* B

Rationale: The couple's beliefs and values regarding therapeutic abortion and consequences of potential risk to the fetus must be addressed. Anesthesia risk is similar for pregnant women regardless of the diagnosis. Careful planning is necessary for diagnostic procedures, but not all need to be avoided. Chemotherapy can be delivered after the first trimester under the supervision of a high-risk obstetrician.

16. *Answer:* B

Rationale: Although providing information is important, it must be done without imposing personal values into the conversation. Body image is one component of sexuality that can be affected by cancer and its treatment. The nurse often must initiate these discussions to communicate to the patient that this topic is open and that the nurse is available to listen or advise. Suggesting the need for referral may imply to the client that there are significant problems. Providing resources for erotic stimulation implies an expectation that may not be appropriate for every client.

17. *Answer:* A

Rationale: Preservation of fertility in both male and female clients should be the initial priority; options later may be more restricted. First of all the nurse should be focused on listening to the client, not providing details regarding impact of the treatment and options available. It is important to address the patient's survival concerns but also to have frank discussions about future fertility. This includes preservation before treatment and discussions of adoption and other options as needed.

18. *Answer:* A

Rationale: Premature menopause caused by chemotherapy can affect libido, body image, and the ability to engage in sexual intercourse. Libido will be decreased, intercourse is possible with use of vaginal lubricants, and side effects of chemotherapy such as fatigue and vaginal changes affect sexual functioning.

19. *Answer:* C

Rationale: Myths or misconceptions can escalate anxiety and interfere with sexual functioning. Discussing how is not as important now as knowing misunderstandings.

20. *Answer:* B

Rationale: Clients and significant others should be informed of the possibility of erectile dysfunction after surgery. The degree of erectile dysfunction is related to the extent of the surgery and success of nerve-sparing procedures. After the degree of dysfunction is established, a variety of means of achieving sexual pleasure can be discussed. Retrograde ejaculation is a side effect of an abdominoperineal resection but is a moot point if he cannot achieve an erection. He will probably not internalize the effect of these changes on his self-concept of masculinity before leaving the hospital. The discussion should start with communication about the risk for erectile dysfunction.

21. *Answer:* B

Rationale: By using the phrase "some women," the nurse communicates a common response and provides an opportunity for the patient to express her concerns. Asking about appearance changes is important for body image problems but may not necessarily affect sexuality.

22. *Answer:* A

Rationale: Often the partner is reluctant to initiate sexual activities for fear of hurting the client or because the partner assumes that the client does not want to have sex. Communication of desire between the patient and her partner can address these concerns.

23. *Answer:* B

Rationale: Management of ostomy appliances by securing the bag or changing position will help prevent accidental spilling of contents. Discuss anal intercourse at a later time unless they specifically introduce the subject. A folded towel placed above the ostomy acts as a bridge over the ostomy site. There are no restrictions to sexual positions.

24. *Answer:* B

Rationale: Loss of ovarian function results in vaginal changes of decreased elasticity and lubrication, which may make sexual intercourse painful. A hysterectomy does not cause a total loss of sexual desire, and although fear of sexual intimacy and changes in self-concept may occur, they are psychological responses and are not present in every woman having a hysterectomy.

25. *Answer:* B

Rationale: Most chemotherapy is excreted from the body in the first 72 hours. During this time, they should use condoms. Oral sex should be avoided unless they are using condoms. Although his physician should know about the activity so that he can reinforce safety issues, and although the activity may be inappropriate in a hospital setting, it is not a primary focus if it is done in a private setting.

CHAPTER 40

1. *Answer:* A

Rationale: Disseminated intravascular coagulation (DIC) is a life-threatening metabolic emergency that is usually seen in critically ill patients. It is also considered an oncologic emergency. Cancer treatment can also increase the risk of DIC, which is cumulative with the more treatment the patient receives. For example, immunosuppressive chemotherapy can leave the patient susceptible to severe infections or sepsis, which increases the risk of DIC.

2. *Answer:* D

Rationale: The pathophysiology of disseminated intravascular coagulation involves extensive rapid triggering of the coagulation system, which results in abnormal activation of thrombin formation. Clotting factors are depleted. Fibrinolysis and the clotting pathways continue at a rapid rate.

3. *Answer:* C

Rationale: Exercise and weight bearing are essential to maintaining bone mass; thus, immobility contributes to the development of hypercalcemia. The other factors listed have not been found to be contributing factors for the development of hypercalcemia.

4. *Answer:* A

Rationale: The four main metabolic changes associated with tumor lysis syndrome (TLS) are hyperkalemia, hyperphosphatemia, hypocalcemia, and hyperuricemia. Hyperkalemia can cause cardiac conduction abnormalities, muscle weakness, or paralysis. Hyperphosphatemia can cause a deposit of calcium phosphate in the renal parenchyma, leading to hypocalcemia. This can lead to changes in mental status, parkinsonian movements, and papilledema. Hyperuricemia is caused by massive cell death in TLS and can lead to acute renal failure.

5. *Answer:* B

Rationale: Disseminated intravascular coagulation (DIC) is characterized by the initiation of the coagulation cascade. The platelet count will be decreased or low, not elevated. DIC also leads to decreased fibrinogen levels, a prolonged prothrombin time, elevated blood urea nitrogen, and can cause renal failure. Coagulation, clotting, and platelet destruction are the main features in DIC; although anemia and changes in iron levels can occur, they are not the primary findings in this condition. In DIC, the activated partial thromboplastin time is prolonged because of the rapid consumption of clotting factors. Protein C is initially overactive in DIC but eventually becomes overwhelmed, and levels decrease. Schistocytes are often present in peripheral smears in patients with DIC. Their presence is not diagnostic but indicates underlying abnormal coagulopathy.

6. *Answer:* D

Rationale: Of all the available, heparin therapy interferes with thrombin production and is often given for the management of intravascular clotting. The goal of heparin therapy is to maintain a partial thromboplastin time at one to two times the normal levels. Low-dose heparin would minimize the risk of bleeding. Vasopressors may be used to treat an associated hypotension, which the patient is not experiencing. Fibrinolytic therapy may be given after the heparin therapy. The patient may require mechanical ventilation at some point; however, not based on the current status of the client.

7. *Answer:* B

Rationale: Intravenous administration of drugs increases the risk for anaphylaxis because of the rapid systemic effect. Other factors associated with an increased risk of anaphylaxis are high dosages, naturally occurring agents, and intermittent administration.

8. *Answer:* B

Rationale: Local osteolytic hypercalcemia (LOH) accounts for approximately 20% of hypercalcemia in patients with malignancy. In LOH, the bone provides a place for tumor growth, and tumor cells produce various cytokines, which lead to calcium reabsorption from the bones. Osteoclasts are active at the site of the tumor cells.

resulting in breakdown of bone and an increase in calcium levels which accounts for nausea, loss of appetite, and confusion. William syndrome is a genetic condition present at birth that can affect young children and causes elevations in blood calcium levels. Humoral hypercalcemia of malignancy accounts for approximately 80% of hypercalcemia of malignancy cases. It is most often found in patients with little or no bone metastases. A total of 1% to 20% of patients with sarcoidosis have renal involvement, which affects the renal tubules and increases bone reabsorption of calcium, causing hypercalcemia.

9. *Answer:* B

Rationale: Acral cyanosis, or mottled extremities, is a hallmark of disseminated intravascular coagulation (DIC). Heart rate is usually increased, not decreased. Bowel sounds may be decreased but are not a specific sign of DIC. Specific gravity is not applicable in this condition.

10. *Answer:* A

Rationale: Hypercalcemia is defined as abnormally high levels of calcium (>10.5 mg/dL) and is the most common oncologic emergency, occurring in 10% to 20% of all patients with cancer. Tumor lysis syndrome is estimated to occur in approximately 2% of oncology patients. The syndrome of inappropriate antidiuretic hormone secretion is characterized by hypo-osmotic hyponatremia and affects 1% to 2% of all patients with cancer, small cell lung cancer in particular. Disseminated intravascular coagulation is estimated to occur in 1% of hospitalized oncology patients.

11. *Answer:* D

Rationale: Platelet transfusions are helpful in the treatment of disseminated intravascular coagulation because platelets contain platelet factor III, a substance that strengthens the endothelium; prevents petechial hemorrhage; and aids in the conversion of prothrombin to thrombin, acting as a "mechanical plug" by adhering to the vessel wall. Additional treatment options include fresh-frozen plasma, and, less commonly, packed red blood cells.

12. *Answer:* B

Rationale: When a hypersensitivity reaction is suspected while infusing a medication, the first intervention is to stop the infusion of the offending agent. There is no indication in this scenario that any of the other actions—calling a code, intubating the patient, or initiating cardiopulmonary resuscitation—are necessary at this time.

13. *Answer:* B

Rationale: The pulmonary system could be severely compromised in patients with disseminated intravascular coagulation (DIC) because of inadequate exchange of oxygen and CO2, possible pulmonary edema, and pulmonary emboli. Pulmonary status assessment can be determined through auscultation for wheezes, crackles, and stridor. Obtaining a sputum for cytology is not useful in DIC. Providing adequate hydration and measurement of intake and output pertain most closely to the renal system rather than the pulmonary system.

14. *Answer:* A

Rationale: Hypercalcemia is demonstrated by an elevated calcium level. Patients with a diagnosis of lung cancer and breast cancer comprise about 80% of all patients in whom hypercalcemia develops. Mental status changes are one of the signs and symptoms of hypercalcemia.

15. *Answer:* C

Rationale: Patients with moderate hypercalcemia would likely experience constipation, bloating, increasing abdominal pain, and dehydration. Mild hypercalcemia would illicit symptoms of nausea or vomiting, loss of appetite, generalized weakness, and dehydration. Ileus, seizures, coma, ataxia or pathologic fractures, renal failure, and abnormal electrocardiographic changes are seen in patients who have severe hypercalcemia. Dysuria, flank pain, hematuria, paralysis, weakness, and spasms of the extremities are associated with tumor lysis syndrome.

16. *Answer:* C

Rationale: This particular patient has several risk factors for systemic inflammatory response syndrome, including recent antineoplastic treatment resulting in neutropenia, implanted medical device (port-a-cath), age older than 65 years, poor nutritional status, and hospitalization. Tumor lysis syndrome is most closely associated with large bulky tumors. Disseminated intravascular coagulation is usually related to leukemias and solid tumors. Although hypersensitivity reactions can occur with a variety of antineoplastic agents, they are most commonly experienced with platinums, taxanes, L-asparaginase, procarbazine, etoposide, and monoclonal antibodies.

17. *Answer:* A

Rationale: In treating patients with hypercalcemia, the aim is to reduce serum calcium absorption, increase urinary calcium excretion, and decrease intestinal calcium absorption. Initially, the patient is given 0.9% saline intravenously to increase circulating volume. Calcitonin then works to reduce the serum calcium level. A loop diuretic is often instituted to reduce fluid overload, but it does not reduce serum calcium. After rehydrating the patient, bisphosphonates are administered. Vasopressor drugs are not normally used in the treatment of hypercalcemia.

18. *Answer:* A

Rationale: Clinical criteria associated with systemic inflammatory response syndrome include temperature higher than $100.4°$ F ($38°$ C) or below $96.8°$ F ($36°$ C), heart rate greater than 90 beats/min, respiratory rate greater than 20 breaths/min, and white blood cell count greater than 12,000 cells/mm^3.

19. *Answer:* B

Rationale: Signs and symptoms of anaphylaxis include urticaria and angioedema. Pain or itching around intravenous insertion sites describe a localized hypersensitivity reaction. Feelings of fatigue are common in patients with cancer but are not indicative of anaphylaxis.

20. *Answer:* B

Rationale: Sepsis usually presents with two or more of the following manifestations: temperature greater than $100.4°$ F ($37.9°$ C), heart rate greater than 90 beats/min, respiratory rate greater than 20 breaths/min, and white blood cell count greater than 12,000 mm^3 or less than 4000/mm^3. No mention is made of serum calcium or symptoms of hypocalcemia. Also, no mention is made of signs or symptoms of bleeding as seen in disseminated intravascular coagulation. The client's blood sugar is not significantly elevated as in diabetic shock.

21. *Answer:* D

Rationale: Because an anaphylactic reaction may be a life-threatening emergency, appropriate emergency equipment and drugs should be readily available. Diazepam is not a normal premedication for preventing hypersensitivity reactions. Because every agent has the potential to cause anaphylaxis, patients are not rejected from studies for this reason alone. Premedications may be given as a precautionary measure. Vital signs usually are taken more often for a drug with anaphylactic potential, especially during the first hour.

22. *Answer:* A

Rationale: Factors that can increase a patient's risk for tumor lysis syndrome (TLS) include a large bulky tumor mass, chronic renal insufficiency, oliguria, dehydration, acidic urine, exposure to nephrotoxins, splenomegaly, extensive lymphadenopathy, and ascites. Treatment risk factors include cisplatinum, etoposide, cytarabine, immunotherapy, monoclonal antibodies, radiation therapy and hormone therapy. Tetany is not a risk factor for TLS but can result from the processes of TLS.

23. *Answer:* B

Rationale: This patient has risk factors for the development of syndrome of inappropriate antidiuretic hormone secretion (SIADH). Small cell lung cancer accounts for more than 75% of all tumors associated with SIADH. Patients receiving platinum products are also at higher risk of SIADH. SIADH is not usually seen in patients with colon cancer.

24. *Answer:* B

Rationale: The patient is experiencing moderate hyponatremia with neurologic changes, which should alert the nurse to implement seizure precautions immediately to ensure safety for the patient. There is no indication that the client has complaints of pain. Encouraging good mouth care is essential for any patient on a fluid restriction but is not an immediate nursing action in this case. The patient would be placed on a fluid restriction based on his serum sodium level.

25. *Answer:* D

Rationale: Emergency treatment of the syndrome of inappropriate antidiuretic hormone secretion may be required if the client experiences significant neurologic changes because this can lead to an irreversible neurodegenerative disorder called central pontine myelinolysis.

CHAPTER 41

1. *Answer:* C

Rationale: The leptomeninges are the two innermost layers of the meninges. Cerebrospinal fluid (CSF) circulates between these layers. Leptomeningeal metastases are often seen in acute leukemias. It is metastatic spread of malignant cells through the CSF spaces. Lymph node metastases are also seen with leukemias. The spleen and the liver can be involved, but this is less common.

2. *Answer:* A

Rationale: Patients with increased intracranial pressure (ICP) can display a variety of neurologic symptoms, including headaches, blurred vision, lethargy, and changes in level of consciousness. Some of the most emergent late signs and symptoms comprise Cushing's triad and include bradycardia, respiratory depression, and hypertension. B and C describe digestive and neurologic symptoms. A variety of urinary symptoms are related to ICP depending on the cause. Urinary frequency is more often found than decreased urination.

3. *Answer:* B

Rationale: Intracranial pressure (ICP) is normally between 7 and 15 mm Hg in a supine adult. A "high normal" level of 20 to 25 mm Hg may require treatment; the goal is ICP less than 20 mm Hg. A Romberg test is a test of the ability to sense stimuli within the body regarding position, movement, and equilibrium. The cerebral perfusion pressure is a measurement of the pressure gradient driving the cerebral blood flow and the availability of oxygen and the metabolites to the brain.

4. *Answer:* C

Rationale: The most common presenting symptom of spinal cord compression (SCC) is neck and back pain. Pain can occur before the actual compression of the spinal cord and before the development of any neurologic symptoms. The common progression of symptoms in SCC is pain, motor weakness, sensory loss, motor loss, and autonomic dysfunction.

5. *Answer:* D

Rationale: Hyperventilation is the quickest short-term method to decrease intracranial pressure (ICP). Vasoconstriction decreases cerebral blood volume and ICP. It requires the patient to be sedated, intubated, and ventilated to a PCO2 between 26 and 30 mm Hg. The other options can be used to decrease inflammation, shrink radiosensitive tumors, or debulk or resect tumors but are not the fastest method to decrease dangerously high ICP.

6. *Answer:* B

Rationale: The administration of stool softeners to prevent constipation and antiemetics to prevent vomiting is appropriate to prevent an increase in the intracranial pressure (ICP). ICP may also increase as the patient's activity increases. Nursing measures to prevent increases in ICP include minimizing environmental stimuli and maintaining bed rest with the head of the bed elevated 15 to 30 degrees to promote venous drainage. The Valsalva maneuver should be avoided in clients with ICP, and they should avoid lifting or turning in bed. Range of motion exercises with 5-lb weights are not related to increased ICP.

7. *Answer:* D

Rationale: The most common cause of spinal cord compression (SCC) in patients with cancer is metastatic tumor invasion. The thoracic area of the spinal column is the most frequent site of metastasis that causes SCC.

8. *Answer:* A

Rationale: Pain caused by spinal cord compression may actually increase in the supine recumbent position and is usually relieved in the sitting position. Pain caused by a herniated disc often decreases in a supine position.

9. *Answer:* B

Rationale: Physical examination should include vertebral palpation and percussion, which can elicit tenderness at the area of the spinal cord compression (SCC). Physical examination of patients with SCC does not usually include lumbar puncture or digital rectal examination. Although not diagnostic of SCC, physical examination of patients with cancer includes chest auscultation.

10. *Answer:* C

Rationale: Although all of these choices could possibly cause cardiac tamponade, the most common cause is malignant disease that causes a pericardial effusion. The severity of the cardiac tamponade depends on the amount of fluid in the pericardium, rate of accumulation, and degree of compromise.

11. *Answer:* A

Rationale: Plain spine radiographs are usually obtained and can identify up to 85% of vertebral lesions. Bone scans are more sensitive than radiography in detecting vertebral abnormalities. Magnetic resonance imaging (MRI), computed tomography, and myelography are used as definitive diagnostic tests for spinal cord compression (SCC). Because an MRI is noninvasive, it has commonly replaced myelography. Lumbar puncture may be completed to assess cerebrospinal fluid but is not a diagnostic for SCC.

12. *Answer:* D

Rationale: The neurologic status of patients with spinal cord compression (SCC) is the most important prognostic indicator. Neurologic status includes ambulatory status. Weight loss, although an important general prognostic indicator, is not the most important prognostic indicator in SCC.

13. *Answer:* C

Rationale: Obstruction of the superior vena cava can occur as the results of extrinsic compression by tumor or enlarged lymph nodes or as a result of intrinsic obstruction by thrombosis or tumor.

14. *Answer:* C

Rationale: Corticosteroids, which reduce spinal cord edema and pain, are usually the initial treatment to address the neurologic deficits seen with spinal cord compression (SCC). A high dose is usually given initially via intravenous bolus as soon as SCC is suspected, followed by subsequent regular dosing as treatment continues; then a gradual tapering of the dose is done. Radiation therapy is used in radiosensitive tumors. Surgery can be used to decompress a vertebral body or in recurring tumors previously treated with radiation. Chemotherapy generally has a limited role; it may be used as an adjuvant with radiation therapy.

15. *Answer:* A

Rationale: Non-Hodgkin lymphoma and advanced lung cancer most commonly cause superior vena cava syndrome. As the lymph nodes and superior vena cava become squeezed and compromised, the blood flow slows, and a complete blockage can occur.

16. *Answer:* B

Rationale: The best diagnostic studies to detect structural abnormalities are computed tomography and magnetic resonance imaging studies. An electrocardiogram and an echocardiogram can detect cardiac abnormalities that result from obstruction of the superior vena cava but not the obstruction itself. A barium swallow may detect an esophageal obstruction but not superior vena cava obstruction. Cervical spine radiography and myelography would not detect obstruction of the superior vena cava.

17. *Answer:* C

Rationale: Obstruction of the superior vena cava causes jugular vein distention and edema of the face, neck, upper thorax, breasts, and upper extremities. Abdominal distention and fever are not associated with superior vena cava syndrome (SVCS). Tachycardia, not bradycardia, usually occurs with SVCS. Cheyne Stokes respirations are not indicative of SVCS.

18. *Answer:* C

Rationale: Although patients with cerebrovascular accidents may have increased intracranial pressure (ICP), the principal cause in clients with cancer is a space-occupying lesion. Metabolic complications, chemotherapy, and radiation therapy do not tend to cause ICP. Other potential causes of ICP in patients with cancer include hemorrhage, venous sinus thrombosis, meningitis, head trauma, infarction, and abscess.

19. *Answer:* B

Rationale: Treatment of superior vena cava syndrome (SVCS) includes treatment of the underlying causative disease. Administration of chemotherapy is the preferred treatment for clients with malignancy-related SVCS. Tissue plasminogen activator is not instilled into a patent central catheter. Heparin use is controversial for patients with SVCS. Chemotherapy is not usually administered until a histologic diagnosis is obtained.

20. *Answer:* C

Rationale: The immediate treatment of intracranial pressure (ICP) includes administration of corticosteroids and osmotic diuretics to decrease cerebral edema. Calcium channel blockers, β-blockers, nitroglycerin, and cardiac glycosides are not given to decrease ICP.

21. *Answer:* A

Rationale: Close attention to subtle early symptoms is important in the early diagnosis of superior vena cava syndrome (SVCS). The inability to complete usual activities may be a sign of progressive dyspnea. Patients with obstruction of the superior vena cava usually have dyspnea in the supine position. Although fever is not diagnostic of SVCS, patients should be instructed to call physicians with a fever over 100.5° F (38° C). Patients with obstruction of the superior vena cava should avoid measurement of blood pressure in the affected extremity.

22. Answer: C

Rationale: Treatment of superior vena cava syndrome (SVCS) includes treatment of the underlying disease, which can include chemotherapy or radiation therapy. Assessment for pancytopenia is necessary. Although corticosteroids may be used, a side effect of corticosteroids is hyperglycemia, not hypoglycemia. Use of diuretics may cause hypotension because of volume depletion, not hypervolemia. Antibiotics are not used to treat SVCS.

CHAPTER 42

1. Answer: D

Rationale: Rarely does cancer affect only an individual. Family units, social acquaintances, coworkers, and even healthcare professionals are affected in multiple ways by someone else's cancer diagnosis. Their issues must also be addressed with appropriate support and resources.

2. Answer: C

Rationale: Although use of sentinel node technology and lumpectomy has decreased the disruption of lymphatic drainage, these individuals who have nodes resected and receive radiation are still at risk for lymphedema and must be instructed that it is actually a risk for the remainder of their lives. The term *survivor* was appropriate from the time of her diagnosis. Although 5 years disease free is a significant milestone, it is not a guarantee for freedom from concerns related to her breast cancer.

3. Answer: C

Rationale: The number of survivors continues to rise steadily; 59% of cancer survivors are 65 years of age or older, and 64% of cancer survivors have survived 5 years or more. Although the number of cancer survivors continues to increase, even individuals greater than 5 years out continue to be at risk for late effects. The most common cancer sites in the survivor population are breast (22%), prostate (20%), colorectal (9%), and gynecologic (8%).

4. Answer: B

Rationale: Late effects can manifest years later, which is part of why there is a need for an evidence-based approach to survivorship after treatment has completed. All survivors are at risk for late effects. Long-term side effects may continue after treatment is completed. It is important to focus on optimal treatment of short-term side effects so that they do not become a recurring pattern for the client. Long-term and late effects vary according to disease, treatment, comorbid conditions, and age of patient. This is an evolving area of cancer treatment.

5. Answer: A

Rationale: Cardiovascular consequences include congestive heart failure, cardiomyopathy, carotid artery disease, valvular heart disease, and electrical or conductive system disease; these can continue to occur as the individual ages. Spiritual concerns are often seen in survivors but are not side effects to cancer treatment. The psychological and cognitive concerns continue through survivorship, especially fear of recurrence and continuing problems with memory, concentration, and expressing thoughts. Unfortunately, even individuals greater than 5 years from their diagnosis continue to experience challenges with insurance, and their treatment may still be affecting their health and well-being.

6. Answer: D

Rationale: Although the overall risk for second malignancies is relatively low, breast cancer is the most frequently seen second malignancy in young women who were treated with mantle radiation for Hodgkin disease. Breast tissue is dense in young women, but mammography remains the best option for screening at this time. Often, tumors occur as late effects and usually occur more than a decade after initial treatment.

7. Answer: B

Rationale: Standardized guidelines for the follow-up care of adult cancer survivors are rare. Transfer back to primary care is decided on a case-by-case basis by either the referring oncologist or the insurance plan. Primary care physicians and other medical specialists see more long-term cancer survivors than oncologists even though there are few guidelines to help with assessing long-term and late effects of cancer therapies.

8. Answer: A

Rationale: B, C, and D are essential for the client to be able to plan for care posttreatment. Information about long-term and late effects are important but should be communicated in writing.

9. Answer: C

Rationale: Although much of the fear associated with cancer gradually subsides over time, an underlying fear can remain permanently. This fear can be triggered at the time of medical follow-up visits, during an anniversary of diagnosis or painful procedures, or at any time a suspicious symptom arises. Although survivors have varying needs for continued psychosocial support after therapy is completed, few are considered to have overt mental illness because of their cancer diagnosis. Family members also usually become less reactive with time, although they may always have some fear. Referrals to counseling are indicated for patients or family members with debilitating fears.

10. Answer: A

Rationale: The average age of cancer survivors continues to rise. This aging population requires providers with knowledge about both the normal aging process and the impact of cancer treatment. We cannot wait until we know all possible side effects; we must act on the knowledge currently available and continue to document new findings. Clients usually want to maintain contact with their oncology provider. D is true of all cancer treatment; it is not unique to survivorship.

11. Answer: D

Rationale: Survivor's guilt is a normal reaction to surviving a life-threatening illness and is often triggered by a return to the clinic, hospital, or support group.

Survivors can compare themselves to others with recurrent disease or to those who have died, and this can provoke mixed reactions and guilty feelings about doing well.

12. **Answer:** D

Rationale: Prevention and detection as part of a survivorship plan includes promotion of healthy behaviors to include physical activity, diet, tobacco cessation, and sun protection as well as regular screenings. Survivorship care should include assessing for late effects. Referral for posttraumatic stress disorder is a treatment intervention, not a prevention care plan.

CHAPTER 43

1. **Answer:** B

Rationale: Palliative care is defined as care that provides symptom management, comfort, and support to clients living with a life-threatening illness. Hospice is a program of care that focuses on comfort (body, mind, and spirit) through the end-of-life; care is initiated when the client has less than 6 months to live.

2. **Answer:** C

Rationale: The client and the family are the focus in palliative care. Symptoms are anticipated, prevented, and treated skillfully rather than waiting for them to occur. The psychosocial, emotional, and spiritual symptoms are regarded as important as the physical symptoms. The intent of palliative care is not to extend life.

3. **Answer:** D

Rationale: Palliative care is indicated when there is advanced disease with prognosis of less than 1 year, debilitating symptom burden from disease or treatments, significant social or psychosocial distress, or a Karnofsky performance status less than 50%. Family members are included in planning, but the care is not indicated only when they are unable to provide the care or when they are not realistic.

4. **Answer:** A

Rationale: With expanded acceptance of palliative care, more facilities are adopting programs, including home-based programs, long-term care and nursing home programs, acute care–based teams, and ambulatory clinics. Certification is already available for physicians, nurses of all levels, social workers, and chaplains through the Center to Advance Palliative Care. Family member acceptance of a referral is important but not necessarily an indicator of the growing acceptance of the specialty. Likewise, developing skill sets in symptom management is important but not an indicator of growing acceptance of the specialty.

5. **Answer:** D

Rationale: Studies show that clients receiving palliative care are experiencing lower symptom intensity, improved quality of life, and longer survival periods. The focus is on quality of life and symptom control, not on more aggressive care. Palliative care accepts death but does not focus on stopping or avoiding other treatment.

6. **Answer:** A

Rationale: Symptoms that cause the greatest client distress should be addressed first by the interdisciplinary team. After symptoms have been assessed and interventions initiated, the next priority is developing a therapeutic relationship with the client and family. This will help in assessment of family coping and discussions about end-of-life planning.

7. **Answer:** C

Rationale: Palliative care continues through hospice and is not distinctly separate. The other options are all correct.

8. **Answer:** C

Rationale: The challenge in hospice tends to be extremely late referrals. Life-prolonging therapies are not usually an integral part of hospice. Hospice care involves an acceptance of death, allowing families to engage in their cultural traditions for the end of life, as long as the traditions are not detrimental to the client.

9. **Answer:** D

Rationale: Prolonged grief is correctly described. Disenfranchised grief is grief that occurs when the loss cannot be openly acknowledged such as a nonsanctioned relationship. Anticipatory grief occurs before the physical death of a loved one. Complicated grief is a disturbance in the normal process of grief.

10. **Answer:** A

Rationale: The dual process model of loss-oriented coping and restoration-oriented coping proposes that both aspects are necessary for adjustment to the loss. Loss-oriented coping concentrates on and works through some aspect of the loss experience itself. Restoration-oriented coping is the mastering of new tasks, reorganizing life, and developing a new identity. The model shows the dynamic nature of grief.

11. **Answer:** A

Rationale: The Joint Commission launched a certification process for hospice inpatient palliative care programs in 2011. Certification programs for the other levels of service are not currently available.

12. **Answer:** C

Rationale: When hospice or palliative care services are not available as an organized program, nurses can facilitate collaboration with other professionals to develop the best plan for the client and family. Receiving supportive services is not contingent on waiving traditional curative care. Assisting with the completion of necessary documentation to document wishes for end-of-life care is not focusing on the services needed. Working with the American Cancer Society is appropriate, but they are not hospice providers.

13. **Answer:** A

Rationale: In contrast to multidisciplinary care, in which each discipline assesses the client and formulates a plan in their specific area of expertise, the interdisciplinary approach requires that the various disciplines collaborate to create a client- or family-directed plan of care. Certification by an individual's professional organization is not a requirement.

14. *Answer:* D

Rationale: During end-of-life care, the priority focus is on addressing the underlying cause rather than just treating the outward symptom. Pain, if a problem, will be addressed, but there is always an attempt to identify the underlying cause. Interventions initially identified as beneficial may no longer be appropriate based on life expectancy. Determining the meaning of quality of life for the client or family will be addressed but is not the initial priority.

15. *Answer:* B

Rationale: It is important to avoid using the term "starvation" and work with the family to understand cancer cachexia. Feeding tubes and calorie counts are not indicated at the end of life. Focusing on the living will does not address their concerns unless it specifically addresses the use of nutritional support.

16. *Answer:* A

Rationale: Frequent oral care will enhance the client's comfort and improve the appearance of the oral cavity for the family. Hydration via intravenous or enteral fluids is not a comfort-focused intervention. Family may provide fluids, but doing so on an hourly basis may induce caregiver strain and increase stress. Complex chemotherapy regimens may no longer be indicated, but that is not addressing the comfort issue.

17. *Answer:* C

Rationale: The intent is to avoid aspiration and yet not have the client experience withdrawal if medications are not continued orally; consider alternative routes for essential medications. Adding hydration is not a comfort measure. Also, having family offer foods may contribute to aspiration.

18. *Answer:* D

Rationale: Causes for fluid loss at the end-of-life may require medical orders to treat nausea, vomiting, diarrhea, diuresis from excessive diuretics, and fevers contributing to diaphoresis. Although pulmonary secretions may seem extreme, they usually are not enough to cause dehydration.

19. *Answer:* D

Rationale: Anticholinergic medications such as scopolamine, atropine, and hyoscyamine can be used to dry secretions. Hormone-induced diuresis, if it is the syndrome of inappropriate antidiuretic hormone secretion, may require demeclocycline or urea. If the diaphoresis is bothersome to the client it can be treated with an antipyretic if a fever is present. Anticholinergics are not indicated for opioid toxicity.

20. *Answer:* C

Rationale: Dehydration symptoms (dry mouth, most commonly) may indicate opioid toxicity because of dehydration, which could be treated with fluids. Myoclonus (quick, involuntary muscle jerk), hyperalgesia (an increased sensitivity to pain), and allodynia (pain due to a stimulus that does not normally provoke pain) are terms used to describe this effect. Oral secretions may be suctioned gently via the oral cavity. It is common for the client to sleep more at the end of life and to not require fluid intake.

21. *Answer:* C

Rationale: There can be multiple causes for altered breathing patterns. Life expectancy and severity will determine the need to intervene.

22. *Answer:* D

Rationale: D describes the position that provides the client with the most support and decreases the work of breathing.

23. *Answer:* B

Rationale: If the client perceives the symptoms as interfering significantly with quality of life and the life expectancy is sufficient, antibiotics may be indicated. It is best to avoid the term "death rattle" with the family and help them to understand that noisy respirations such as snoring are most likely not bothersome to the client.

24. *Answer:* B

Rationale: The client's life expectancy and perceived impact on quality of life should guide the decision to tap a pleural effusion. Many pleural effusions do recur. The benefits and burdens associated with the tap should guide the decision. If the life expectancy is limited, chemotherapy may not be indicated for the underlying disease.

25. *Answer:* D

Rationale: A fan blowing on the face or a cool cloth may actually be sufficient for symptom relief. If the client did not require oxygen therapy earlier, he or she will be less likely to require it at the end of life. If the client required it earlier, the need may persist, but a mask is often bothersome to the client and interferes with family communication.

26. *Answer:* D

Rationale: Effective interventions for dyspnea include cool sensations applied to the face, administrating opioids for comfort, and providing support to lessen anxiety. Benzodiazepines are not indicated unless there is significant anxiety. There is evidence to support that nebulized morphine is not effective. More studies are needed to determine the efficacy of nebulized fentanyl. If the client is not already taking opioids, starting long-acting agents is not indicated at this time. The client may require and benefit from short-acting agents.

27. *Answer:* B

Rationale: Noisy respirations are usually more bothersome to the family than the client. Anticholinergic agents may be beneficial; provide regular mouth care for the drying and accumulated secretions. Help the family to understand the changes in respirations at the end of life but avoid the term "death rattle" because this may be disturbing to the family. Suctioning of the oral cavity may be beneficial, but avoid deep suctioning, which may cause trauma and stimulate additional secretions.

28. *Answer:* C

Rationale: These findings indicate progression; the team will want to prepare the family. The process starts in the periphery, not centrally. Extra blankets and heating are not effective at this time and may actually increase discomfort. Vital signs will not change the plan of care; communicate caring and presence in other tangible ways.

29. *Answer:* C

Rationale: If the client is hypoactive, it may be associated with metabolic abnormalities and dehydration. Delirium is common at the end of life. Toxins would not be a concern unless something indicates otherwise. Sedative medications at night can actually contribute to delirium and are probably not indicated. There is little reason to believe the client will move into a hyperactive state at this time.

30. *Answer:* B

Rationale: The uses of haloperidol and quetiapine are accurately described. Benzodiazepines and opioids can contribute to delirium. A benzodiazepine may not be the drug of choice; providers would also not want to discontinue the opioids abruptly because the client may experience withdrawal. At the end of life, metabolic abnormalities do not necessarily require treatment unless there is an indication it would make the client more comfortable.

31. *Answer:* D

Rationale: For mild delirium at the end of life, avoid overstimulation. Interventions for the problems in the remaining options should be evaluated for appropriateness based on the client's life expectancy.

32. *Answer:* B

Rationale: The diagnostic criteria for delirium include disturbances in attention (reduced ability to direct, focus, sustain, and shift attention) and awareness (reduced orientation to environment). It frequently develops in a short period of time, represents a change from baseline, and tends to fluctuate during the course of the day. If cognitive changes are related to preexisting neurocognitive disorder, this would not be acute confusion or delirium.

33. *Answer:* D

Rationale: Possible causes of delirium may include steroids, infection, opioids, organ failure, metabolic changes, and the effects of disease on the central nervous system.

CHAPTER 44

1. *Answer:* B

Rationale: Further research on these agents is needed. Although the risks and benefits of a central venous catheter should be weighed, that is not the relevant issue in this situation.

2. *Answer:* C

Rationale: Standards of care can be used to identify knowledge gaps and determine the range and level of practice the nurse is prepared to assume. The standards do support the need for patients to be involved in health prevention and promotion. Organizational policies, procedures, and protocols are not an individual nurse's responsibility; standards do guide the organizational development and establishment of these documents. Standards do not provide the specific content for education regarding a given topic.

3. *Answer:* D

Rationale: Oncology Nursing Society standards emphasize collaboration, ethical practice, and diversity to establish universal, high-quality cancer care. Although nursing involvement in evidence-based care is important for quality cancer care, it is not the emphasis of the standard.

4. *Answer:* B

Rationale: Outcomes should result from collaborative diagnoses and be individualized to the patient's needs. Data collection should be systematic, characterized by diversity awareness, continuous (not limited to a brief episode of care), collected from multiple sources, documented, and communicated with members of the multidisciplinary cancer care team. The plan of care should be implemented in concordance with the patient's needs, not just the nurse's identified priorities. Nursing and collaborative diagnoses should be derived from data related to actual and potential health problems.

5. *Answer:* C

Rationale: The standards provide society at large the reassurance that professional nurses have actively worked to define and govern professional cancer nursing practice. The standards do address the 14 high-incidence problem areas common to patients to provide guidance to oncology nurses, not patients. The standards encompass the professional nursing actions, including assessment, diagnosis, outcome identification, planning, implementation, and evaluation as a guide for quality care.

6. *Answer:* D

Rationale: Organizations such as the Centers for Disease Control and Prevention (CDC) have the resources and expertise to promote the establishment of guidelines for common outcomes such as preventing intravascular catheter-related infection. Although CDC guidelines may be used to discuss performance or in orientation for new staff, the most appropriate answer is D.

7. *Answer:* D

Rationale: The quality improvement framework emphasizes using measurable criteria, defining minimum acceptable levels of performance, and collecting data to identify areas for improvement. It is important to address concerns unique to the clinical setting, but the focus of the standards is on the 14 high-incidence problem areas for indicators. The process does not end with implementation of recommendations; it is important to evaluate the effectiveness of the action taken.

8. *Answer:* D

Rationale: The standards provide nursing management and leadership with a recommended format for evaluating performance of staff and resource utilization to accomplish desired outcomes and then justifying current levels or additional levels of resources based on the data. The standards are actually relevant at all levels of generalist staff, advanced-practice specialist, educator, researcher, and nurse managers. The statements about a problem-solving approach and the systematic approach apply more specifically to evidence-based component of the standards.

9. *Answer:* C

Rationale: Evidence-based practice is used to select nursing interventions that create positive outcomes. When patient preferences and cost considerations can be followed, they should be, but the main priority is outcomes.

10. *Answer:* B

Rationale: The standards demonstrate responsiveness to the mandate for the inclusion of evidence-based practice (EBP) by placing it in each of the standards. The use of EBP to guide performance improvement is only one aspect of the mandate. The standards do not integrate nursing practice, research, and education into each aspect of care.

11. *Answer:* C

Rationale: Nurses can contribute in many ways, including identifying study topics, collecting data, and then critiquing and integrating research into practice. Reading published literature is a professional responsibility, but it does not contribute directly to the scientific base of cancer nursing practice.

12. *Answer:* D

Rationale: Generic nursing program graduates should be able to assume nursing care responsibilities to use research evidence to collect and analyze client-related data, develop and evaluate an evidence-based plan of care, participate in oncology nursing research through the identification of research questions, implementation of research findings, or evaluation of outcomes of interventions. Standards do not specifically address staffing levels. Development of a research proposal and seeking funding are skills beyond those of the graduate of a generic program. Although nurses should be able to advocate for patients regarding nonpayment of services, this is not part of the standards or responsibilities of the graduate of the generic nursing program.

13. *Answer:* B

Rationale: Benchmarking data, principles of pathophysiology, and legal data are examples of nonresearch data that can guide evidence-based practice (EBP). Clinical questions should guide the review of literature for EBP but do not contribute to nonresearch evidence. Personal standards guide the performance of the individual nurse. Qualitative patient interviews are usually part of a research study and thus are research evidence to guide practice.

14. *Answer:* A

Rationale: All nurses are expected to be involved in evidence-based practice (EBP). Nursing research is not the only way to be involved and may not be an option for all nurses. Evaluation of clinical quality is an important component of professional nursing as is utilization of EBP, but involvement in EBP is not necessarily an essential component to evaluate quality. Pay-for-performance programs may provide incentives for involvement in EBP, but involvement is not a benefit of pay-for-performance programs.

15. *Answer:* D

Rationale: The integration of the best evidence with professional clinical expertise and patient preferences and values ensures the best patient focused approach for patient safety. Performance improvement and reporting incidents involving patients are components

of evidence-based practice (EBP) and patient safety. Nurses must be aware of look-alike medications for patient safety; however, orientation to these medications is not directly provided by EBP.

16. *Answer:* C

Rationale: Health outcomes may be seriously jeopardized and healthcare costs may soar without evidence-based practice (EBP). The Institute of Medicine has mandated that 90% of all healthcare decisions in the United States will be evidence based by 2020. EBP fosters but does not force comprehensive, outcomes-driven healthcare. Cost-effectiveness analysis is more effective for promoting quality, safe care if it is evidence based but does not require EBP. Using research evidence to collect and analyze data is part of EBP rather than a factor demonstrating the need for EBP.

17. *Answer:* A

Rationale: Research-related roles for oncology nurse generalists focus on identifying problems, collaborating with others to identify potential solutions, participating in research activities, and providing nursing care to clients in the clinical trial setting. However, directing the evaluation of existing research study data analysis is not part of generic preparation for nursing practice.

18. *Answer:* B

Rationale: The entire report, not just the individual components of the study, must be critiqued to determine the appropriate response. Even if it is a high-incidence area, all components of the study must be evaluated for appropriateness. Yes, nurses are interested in the individual's opinion, but that is not the key concern here.

19. *Answer:* A

Rationale: Even though findings may be statically significant, they may not be clinically significant; clinicians must determine that. The nurse's responsibility is to advocate for the improvement of care for your clients, and you are qualified to analyze the feasibility of acceptance of the intervention in the current setting.

20. *Answer:* B

Rationale: The 14 high-incidence priority areas refer to clinical problems that oncology clients most often experience, regardless of setting. They are integrated throughout the standards and are the focus of assessment, intervention, and evaluation.

21. *Answer:* B

Rationale: According to the standards, B supports the outcome standard, A supports implementation, C supports planning, and D supports evaluation.

22. *Answer:* C

Rationale: After the problem of interest has been clearly identified, the next step is to identify the information needed to solve the problem. After the information has been identified, then the literature review is conducted. Getting "buy in" from colleagues and the administration is essential but is not part of the process to use evidence to inform clinical practice.

23. *Answer:* C
    Rationale: The primary goal of a phase IV treatment clinical trial is to evaluate new uses (e.g., different tumor types or settings) after a drug has received Food and Drug Administration approval. Phase I trials evaluate toxicities, phase II trials identify tumor types in which the drug is most likely to be effective, and phase III trials compare the current standard of care with a new drug or combination that is hoped to have better results or have fewer side effects.

CHAPTER 45

1. *Answer:* B
    Rationale: Cognitive and social learning theories are described accurately. Behavioral learning theory purports that learning is based on reinforced observable behaviors. The idea that human behavior is directed by internal or environmental cues is a concept of motivation learning theory. Humanistic learning theory explains that learning is a unique process for each individual, facilitated by a positive environment.

2. *Answer:* C
    Rationale: Questions to answer or discuss include what the client knows or wants to know, cultural or religious beliefs and practice that might impact the process, the language of the client, physical or cognitive impairments that could impact learning, preferred learning style, and educational background. The other concepts listed (e.g., the nurse's knowledge, the budget available) are important, but initial development should be based on answers to the above questions.

3. *Answer:* C
    Rationale: The use of alternative supplements may be a traditional part of the client's cultural or religious beliefs but may also interfere with chemotherapy drugs. Practitioners must be aware of the use of such products and potential interactions. SMART goals facilitate evaluation of the effectiveness of the teaching provided. The ABCD rule promotes the development of clear objectives to guide the content provided. Although the client's family history is important to consider, it is not the priority safety concern initially.

4. *Answer:* D
    Rationale: Consistent use of the acronym SMART in the development of educational programs facilitates the development of appropriate education goals, which can lead to optimal outcomes. Although organization of the educational content and individualization for a specific client are important, they apply to the content more than use of goals to evaluate effectiveness. Clients do need to know what to expect, but they tend not to focus as much on the goals as a description of the program.

5. *Answer:* B
    Rationale: The ABCD rule indicates objectives should include audience (who the learner is), behavior (what the learner is to do), condition (under what circumstances), and degree (how much, to what extent the learner is to perform).

6. *Answer:* C
    Rationale: Preparation for evidence-based teaching will include reviewing practices in the literature, standards of care, and hospital procedure manuals, as well as consulting experts including advanced practice nurses and physicians. These components constitute evidence to guide the development of a teaching plan. Visual aids must support, not drive, the content. Although staffing resources and budget are components to be considered in the next step, starting there will potentially hinder the utilization of the evidence available and thus limit outcomes of teaching. Although there may be literature relevant to cultural concerns, this is not the initial core concern for the development of a program.

7. *Answer:* A
    Rationale: Goal must be SMART—specific, measurable, attainable, realistic, and timely. If they are lacking these characteristics, evaluation of a program will be hindered. Documentation is an integral part of education. Relevancy of the content to the recipients is actually a component of evaluation. Participation in providing the content is not a requirement for evaluation.

8. *Answer:* C
    Rationale: People need information that addresses their immediate concerns. This woman has a new diagnosis of breast cancer, and her immediate need is to learn about breast cancer and its treatment. She does not need education regarding mastectomy because her surgery was lumpectomy. It is too early to begin teaching about continued breast self-examination and follow-up mammography because this would not be a priority for the client at this time.

9. *Answer:* D
    Rationale: The overall purpose of client education is to enable full participation, acceptance of responsibility, and shared decision making. Compliance often implies instructions that the client is expected to obey. Client education focuses on empowering the individual for self-care.

10. *Answer:* B
    Rationale: Learning occurs when a person perceives a need to learn something; therefore, learner-identified needs should receive priority. Learning should be problem centered, is influenced by accumulated life experiences, and may not be accomplished even with instruction.

11. *Answer:* A
    Rationale: Participation in public cancer-related programs is believed to positively affect cancer prevention and detection activities and ultimately cancer morbidity and mortality.

12. *Answer:* D
    Rationale: Multiple factors impact Mr. and Mrs. J. as they deal with the new diagnosis. Theories of adult learning indicate that people have had life experiences that are resources on which to base new learning. These experiences must be acknowledged and dealt with before new learning can take place. Adult learners rarely want an anatomy lesson when what they need are the basics.

The nurse would not want to cause or increase guilt with the implication that D.J. is responsible for causing her cancer, and her consent would be necessary to enroll her in a smoking cessation program.

13. **Answer:** B

Rationale: An organizational framework for health education includes the identification of problems that are of concern to people within a community, specific behaviors that are health related and will address the identified problem, and ways to individualize the program for the target community and evaluate it after presentation to ensure that it meets the needs of the community. Problems identified by the nurse may not be pertinent to the community. Behaviors must be specifically identified; generalizations cannot be measured and will not demonstrate the effectiveness of the program. Programs must be developed specifically for the population targeted, just as all educational efforts are specifically targeted to the person or group being addressed.

14. **Answer:** A

Rationale: Part of the nurse's responsibility is staff education; thus, it would be safe to assume she would have some initial intuition of staff needs (what nurses must know and understand to provide safe care). The self-assessment data by the nurses and performance analysis data will provide additional guidance but do not negate the provider's intuition.

15. **Answer:** D

Rationale: Through Healthy People 2020, the Department of Health and Human Services has established national priorities to improve health and reduce health disparity.

16. **Answer:** D

Rationale: This theory describes how technologic changes are adopted. The stages of change are awareness, interest, trial, decision, and adoption.

17. **Answer:** B

Rationale: This is an example of a conclusion based on analysis of community data. It can lead to potential interventions for testing but is not an intervention. It does not include data and does not discuss a plan for change.

CHAPTER 46

1. **Answer:** C

Rationale: According to meta-analysis of the literature, quality nursing documentation has the following seven characteristics: patient centered; contains the actual work of nurses, including education and psychosocial support; written to reflect the objective clinical judgment of the nurse; presented in logical and sequential manner; written as events occur; reflects variances in the patient's condition; and fulfills legal requirements.

2. **Answer:** C

Rationale: State boards of nursing provide oversight of nursing practice by enforcing the state nurse practice act to protect the health, welfare, and safety of the public. Nurse practice acts define nursing roles, titles, and scopes of practice and define educational program standards,

requirements for licensure, and grounds for disciplinary action. The National Council of State Boards of Nursing develops the NCLEX-RN exam.

3. **Answer:** B

Rationale: The Affordable Care Act provides coverage to Americans with preexisting conditions, protects consumers' choice of doctors, keeps young adults covered (up to age 25 years), ends lifetime limits on coverage, ends preexisting condition exclusions for children, ends arbitrary withdrawals of insurance coverage, reviews premium increases, helps consumers get the most from their premium dollars, restricts annual dollar limits on coverage, and removes insurance company barriers to emergency services. The American Hospital Association in 2003 addressed high-quality hospital care, including a clean and safe environment, protection of privacy, and help when leaving the hospital.

4. **Answer:** A

Rationale: Lifelong learning for professional oncology nurses describes the importance of ongoing formal and informal education for oncology nurses to remain current in knowledge. Oncology certification for nurses is a position statement that describes the contribution of specialized nursing certification to safe and effective cancer care. Cancer pain management addresses the essential nature of pain management, including educational, ethical, legal, socioeconomic components. Survivorship in cancer care is not an Oncology Nursing Society position statement.

5. **Answer:** C

Rationale: Common law is the body of law that is interpreted by the courts and not legislative in nature. A statute is an act of the legislature declaring, commanding, or prohibiting something, a particular law enacted and established by the legislative department of government. Legislation is the act of giving or enacting laws, or the making of laws through the legislation, in contrast to court-made laws. Administrative law is a body of law created by administrative agencies in the form of rules, regulations, orders, and decisions.

6. **Answer:** C

Rationale: Many professional issues can have legal implications, including those stated in A, B, and D. Although professional certification is desirable, certification does not have direct legal implications for the nurse.

7. **Answer:** C

Rationale: State law is the most powerful source of authority for nursing practice and is found in the state-specific nurse practice acts. Licensure is the permission by state authority to practice the act of nursing. Credentialing is the documented evidence of the nurse's authority. Continuing education is a state-specific requirement for nursing education.

8. **Answer:** D

Rationale: Nurse practice acts and professional standards of care are sources used in legal decision making relevant to oncology nursing practice. The other options would increase a nurse's general confidence but are not relevant to her legal standing in this instance.

9. *Answer:* C

Rationale: The durable power of attorney is the designated client advocate to participate in medical decisions if the client becomes incapacitated. An advance directive is a written document from the client that is used to inform healthcare providers of medical management requests in the event they are incapacitated. A legal will is an instrument by a person to dispose of his or her property upon death. An insurance policy does not address a client's medical care. Organ and tissue donation is an election by the client in the event of death.

10. *Answer:* B

Rationale: Malpractice is professional misconduct or unreasonable lack of skill. This nurse was acting outside her professional practice limits. Duty is a legal or moral obligation. Negligence and breach of duty both refer to a lack of action when one is necessary (legally or morally) or when a reasonably prudent and careful nurse would act.

11. *Answer:* C

Rationale: State nurse practice acts and professional standards of care (i.e., American Nurses Association, Oncology Nursing Society) provide sources that can be used in legal decision making. A statute is an act of the legislature declaring, commanding, or prohibiting something, or a particular law enacted and established by the legislative department of government. Licensure is the permission by state authority to practice the act of nursing. State-determined competencies vary from state to state and are not used to discern professional standards of care.

12. *Answer:* D

Rationale: An advance directive is a written document that informs healthcare providers of the medical management requests of patients in the event that they are unable to do so themselves. A living will provides specific instructions about the kinds of healthcare that should be provided or prevented in certain situations; it is not recognized in all states. A do not resuscitate order is used in inpatient settings that support an advance directive. A durable power of attorney is an appointed healthcare advocate or surrogate.

13. *Answer:* A

Rationale: It is the professional nurse's responsibility to know his or her State Practice Act and the fit with job description expectations. This is regulated at the state level and not the federal level. In addition, keeping a list of community service activities will aid the nurse to defend her civic mindedness. Although participation in professional speakers bureaus can assist with enhanced knowledge and networking, it does not directly minimize risk of malpractice. Nurses should be careful to maintain an appropriate relationship with patients and families, one that is caring and professional but not necessarily "close" because such a relationship may decrease professional objectivity.

CHAPTER 47

1. *Answer:* A

Rationale: Although sometimes used interchangeably, morals and ethics have distinct meanings. Morals are personal values or rules based on an individual's upbringing, conscience, cultural, or religious beliefs that serve as a guide to individual moral choice and behavior. Ethics is the study or practice of intentionally and critically analyzing moral choices.

2. *Answer:* A

Rationale: The Code of Ethics for Nurses uses cases to guide the interpretation and application of the code with nine provisions: nurses practice with compassion and respect, are primarily committed to the client, promote health and safety, are responsible for individual nursing practice, owe the same duties to self as to others, establish and maintain healthcare environments (not policies), advance the profession through development, collaborate to meet health needs, and are responsible for maintaining the profession.

3. *Answer:* D

Rationale: Utilitarianism purports that actions are right if they promote happiness and wrong if they promote the opposite. Thus, it judges the appropriateness of an action by the consequence of what will happen if the action is or is not performed rather than judging the action itself.

4. *Answer:* A

Rationale: Deontologic theories are based on the idea of duty. These theories assign a value to the action itself rather than simply judging it by the results it produces. If the nurse wants to know if the proposed action is morally permissible, the right question to ask is not, "What are the likely consequences?" but "Would I expect and wish others to act in the same way, particularly if I am the affected party?" or "Does this action treat those involved as individuals rather than as means to a desired outcome?"

5. *Answer:* A

Rationale: The principle of justice (fairness) is to allocate scarce resources fairly, and abide by institutional or insurance allocation policies.

6. *Answer:* C

Rationale: Veracity is the obligation to tell the truth. Autonomy is respect for persons. Nonmaleficence is not harming or ensuring that the anticipated treatment benefits outweigh anticipated harms. Justice is the fair allocation of resources.

7. *Answer:* B

Rationale: Casuistry is a case-based approach to ethical decision making, focusing on practical decision making in particular cases, and uses paradigm cases for comparison and analysis.

8. *Answer:* D

Rationale: The focus is on emotional commitment and a willingness to act unselfishly for the benefit of others. The approach emphasizes sympathy, compassion, fidelity, discernments, and love. Justice is a core of principle based ethics that promotes fair allocation of scarce resources.

9. *Answer:* A

Rationale: Gadow's narrative-based ethics work puts emphasis on learning the client's story. This approach can increase sensitivity to the details of a case and help the nurse understand the ethical values involved. The focus of this scenario is on teaching nurses an approach to improve care. Obtaining a client's story initially can serve to improve relationships and actually decrease nursing time.

10. *Answer:* B

Rationale: The Joint Commission now includes a standard that requires a mechanism to address ethical issues; an ethics committee is one approach to meeting this requirement. B articulates the three functions of an ethics committee. The American Society for Bioethics and Humanities defines the core competencies for healthcare ethics consultation.

11. *Answer:* D

Rationale: The ethical principle of veracity is the obligation to tell the truth; all communication should be honest. Communication is two way, including sending and receiving messages. Approximately 80% of communication is of a nonverbal nature. Clients should be involved in shared decision making with professionals

12. *Answer:* B

Rationale: Buckman proposes a six-step process. Step 1 sets up the interview, focusing on setting, privacy, and time constraints of those involved. Steps 2 and 3 involve obtaining information from the client, mainly discovering how much the client knows and what he or she wishes to know. Step 4 is giving the patient the bad news. Steps 5 and 6 attempt to address the patient's emotional responses and to strategize and summarize to ensure patient comprehension. Throughout this process, nonverbal communication is important; the nurse should always listen to what the client says but should also observe what is not being said.

13. *Answer:* C

Rationale: Confidentiality and privacy are values related to the ethical principle of autonomy. They both play important roles in providing respect and autonomy for persons. Protected health information is discussed in the Health Insurance Portability and Accountability Act.

14. *Answer:* D

Rationale: The Health Insurance Portability and Accountability Act requires the protection and confidential handling of protected health information (PHI). Although the incarceration record may be public record, the incarceration is PHI and should remain confidential. Nurses have an obligation to protect the clients from this type of violation.

15. *Answer:* A

Rationale: The use of this model will provide the nursing staff with the client's cultural perspective of the illness situation. During illness, culture frequently influences behavior. It would be important to document the information in the medical record and share it with the healthcare team, but it does not require informed consent. Documentation will facilitate the appropriate honoring of traditions and guide necessary teaching regarding potential impact on the cancer treatment. Although family should be included in discussions, it is not appropriate to use them as the interpreter for other than the aspects of day-to-day care.

16. *Answer:* A

Rationale: What constitutes informed consent is open to interpretation by all parties to the situation and varies by individual values, beliefs, and culture. A reasonable person standard supports disclosing what an ordinary person in the client's position would consider significant (subjective) in deciding whether or not to consent to the procedure or treatment. The subject standard supports the inclusion of what a particular client may need or want to know in order to make a decision. Many factors may alter an individual's decision-making capacity, and ability should be reassessed on an ongoing basis as part of the informed consent process. Competency or the lack of competency is a court decision; decision-making capacity is a clinical judgment.

17. *Answer:* A

Rationale: Presence is the expectation that the nurse must be aware of his or her own value system, beliefs, and biases and consider them when working with client decision making and informed consent, including asking to be relieved of care for the clients if personal values, beliefs, or biases impede the provision of quality care.

18. *Answer:* B

Rationale: The nurse's first obligation is to care for the client, but he or she may also have obligations to the research study. These obligations can become a balancing act for the nurse. If the nurse had indicated the client did not understand what he or she signed, a different issue would be involved and the nurse would be obligated to follow-up with the manager and investigatory team. In addition, the nurse who heard the expressed concerns should follow-up in an attempt to clarify the nurse's concern.

19. *Answer:* D

Rationale: Clinical research is conducted to gain new knowledge for the benefit of future clients; the client involved may or may not receive benefit and must understand that fact. Clients who are nearing the end of life and not ready to acknowledge it may have a tendency to agree to greater risks than usual. Nurses must be certain the client is aware of the risks involved and the fact that he or she may not benefit. Nurses must be comfortable enough with the study to answer basic questions and to know when it is important to contact the investigator(s) to address additional questions. In addition the subject always has the option to drop out of the study after signing the informed consent.

20. *Answer:* B

Rationale: Palliative care is specialized medical care for people with serious illnesses. It is focused on providing clients with relief from the symptoms, pain, and stress of a serious illness. The goal is to improve quality of life for both the client and family. Active palliative care can include curative goals with the hope of restoration rather than curing. End-of-life care or comfort care is best delivered through a hospice setting. The primary goal is symptom control or comfort, and the secondary goal is providing a good death for the client and support for the family.

21. *Answer:* B

   Rationale: Healthcare providers are required to give clients written information about their right to participate in their own healthcare decisions and to complete advance directives. Completion of advance directives is not mandatory, and they are not necessarily honored across state lines. Medical power of attorney establishes the individual who will make health decisions for the client if he or she is unable to make them.

22. *Answer:* C

   Rationale: A do not attempt resuscitation (DNAR) is not an advance directive; it is expressed wishes regarding resuscitation. A DNAR can be initiated by a medical power of attorney. Renewal of DNARs and physician orders for life-sustaining treatment is not regulated by state law; it is an institutional policy.

23. *Answer:* A

   Rationale: Early discussions among family members regarding desires and expectations will help to decrease uncertainty under times of stress and facilitate clarification of the client's wishes.

24. *Answer:* D

   Rationale: Healthcare professionals have a responsibility to act to protect the child and promote the child's welfare. Parents have the right to make decisions for their children. This type of action to administer blood in opposition to parents' wishes requires court action, not an ethics committee decision.

25. *Answer:* C

   Rationale: Beneficence is the principle of doing good. In this case, the emergency department physician determined that the client's condition was reversible, that the client could be returned to his/her previous state of health, and that the action of doing good outweighed the "no heroics" advance directive.

CHAPTER 48

1. *Answer:* B

   Rationale: The patient should have been identified as at risk for falls, and precautionary measures should have been initiated. Individuals who have been independent previously do not always realize how chemotherapy will affect their mobility. There is no indication of failure of communication or monitoring. This was a patient safety issue.

2. *Answer:* D

   Rationale: The 1999 Institute of Medicine report "To Err is Human: Building a Safer Health System" provided several strategies for improvement including those articulated in A, B, and C. Continuing education and professional education, although important, has not been mandated.

3. *Answer:* C

   Rationale: Including older adults and those with comorbidities in clinical trials supports evidence-based care. Including patient outcome data in quality monitoring plans facilitates the identification of a plan for improvement. Developing a healthcare information technology system improves documentation and monitoring systems. Although the model addresses accessible, affordable cancer care, it does not mandate free care. In addition, although staff should be adequately trained, it does not address mandatory certification or education.

4. *Answer:* D

   Rationale: Certainly, all of the options articulate components of quality care and important aspects for the nurse to consider when working in cancer care. D is a more specific example of the role of collaboration and coordination of care.

5. *Answer:* C

   Rationale: Although all of the aspects included in the options are important to quality, option C is the key priority. If this step of planning is not accomplished the other aspects are at risk for not being relevant.

6. *Answer:* C

   Rationale: PDSA (plan, do, study, act) is a model for quality improvement developed by the Associates in Process Improvement. The other options pertain more to generic goals.

7. *Answer:* C

   Rationale: Multidisciplinary collaboration involves working together with other disciplines to facilitate optimal outcomes. Knowledge of health literacy of the client and family is important but may not involve collaboration. A standard of care in one institution may not be appropriate in another. Integration of educational materials facilities client care but may not involve multidisciplinary collaboration.

8. *Answer:* C

   Rationale: Mandated, strict oversight by an individual or specific discipline will serve to limit true multidisciplinary collaboration. Individuals with different skill levels have to learn to work together. If an individual identifies more closely with another discipline than his or her own, it may interfere with representation of his or her discipline on the team. Identification of resource options is an important component of care and not a barrier to collaboration.

9. *Answer:* B

   Rationale: B addresses collaboration across educator, administrator, and staff clinician roles; each brings different strengths. D serves to integrate the roles of researcher and clinician. Staff nurses often feel inadequate to review relevant research literature. Focusing only on staff nurses is not addressing collaboration across roles.

10. *Answer:* C

   Rationale: Collaborating with the staff will show that the certified nurse values their views, concerns, and expertise. Therefore, this would build cooperation among the staff members. Conducting an educational program will only provide the staff with information. Evaluating the care of their clients is giving their personal opinion. Having a way to contact the nurse is one sided. The options do not demonstrate that collaboration has taken place.

11. *Answer:* B

Rationale: By developing a course in which interaction would take place, the nurses would be able to gain knowledge and skills to help them become more comfortable with sexuality assessments, leading to better documentation. Eliminating the problem is avoidance and will not improve quality of care; the poster may call attention to problems, but it does not provide the nurse with a means to resolve the problem. Nurses may not be familiar with the Annon's PLISSIT sexuality assessment tool. They need some education to help them get over their discomfort with this subject.

12. *Answer:* B

Rationale: Patient navigation was initiated by Harold P. Freeman, MD, at Harlem Hospital Center in New York City for patients with breast cancer and resulted in reduced healthcare barriers, which resulted in increased screening rates among underserved populations, reduced treatment delays after diagnosis, and improved overall 5-year survival rates. Navigation is an essential component of American College of Surgeons Commission on Cancer (ACoSCoC) breast cancer treatment centers. It will be phased in by the ACoSCoC in 2015. Navigation is not addressed by the National Comprehensive Cancer Network. The Oncology Nursing Society does not have specific cancer program guidelines for optimal patient outcomes.

13. *Answer:* C

Rationale: There are four competency areas for nurse navigators as proposed by the initial component of each of the options. However, only the explanation in C is correct as written.

14. *Answer:* C

Rationale: Simplistic advocacy is the act of pleading for the cause of another. Consumer advocacy means that the nurse is required to provide the client with information and let him or her make the decision. Paternalistic advocacy means that the nurse does something for the client's own good without his or her consent. Consumer-centric advocacy means that the nurse provides information and then supports the client in her or his decision

15. *Answer:* B

Rationale: Consumer-centric advocacy is the act of a nurse providing a client with information and then supporting the client in her or his decision. Simplistic advocacy is one who pleads the cause of another. Paternalistic advocacy is doing something for or to another without that person's consent and on the premise that it serves the person's own good. Consumer advocacy supports that patients have adequate information to make their decisions.

16. *Answer:* B

Rationale: Independent actions may be restricted by nursing practice acts or state laws, thus limiting certain actions by a nurse. The availability of evidence may increase nursing awareness of advocacy but is not directly associated with risks. Nurses are indeed qualified to address controversial issues and have numerous professional resources to assist them. Although nurses may pursue ethical consultation as a component of advocating for a client, perceived lack of availability of these services is not a risk associated with client advocacy.

17. *Answer:* A

Rationale: A strong scientific base will enhance nursing's ability to function in the ever-changing healthcare system. This recommendation by the Institute of Medicine recognizes the role of adequately prepared nurses and is not an attempt to eliminate programs or control nursing education. The role of the advanced practice nurse will still be essential; nurses with bachelor's degrees may actually be more likely to recognize them as an important resource.

18. *Answer:* D

Rationale: The professional certification serves the public who may not otherwise know how to determine this information independently. Although having certified nurses on staff may upgrade the nursing services provided and improve outcomes, that is not the direct intent of certification. Also, although employers may be wise to support the pursuit of certification and recognize certified staff, they are not required to do so.